Quality of Care for
Cardiopulmonary
Conditions

A Review of the Literature
and Quality Indicators

Eve A. Kerr • Steven M. Asch
Eric G. Hamilton • Elizabeth A. McGlynn

Editors

RAND Health

Supported by the Agency for Healthcare Research and Quality

Principal funding for this report was provided by a cooperative agreement from the Agency for Healthcare Research and Quality.

ISBN: 0-8330-2921-5

Published 2000 by RAND
1700 Main Street, P.O. Box 2138, Santa Monica, CA 90407-2138
1200 South Hayes Street, Arlington, VA 22202-5050
RAND URL: http://www.rand.org/
To order RAND documents or to obtain additional information, contact Distribution Services: Telephone: (310) 451-7002;
Fax: (310) 451-6915; Internet: order@rand.org

This report is one of a series of volumes describing the QA Tools, a comprehensive, clinically based system for assessing care for children and adults. The quality indicators that comprise these Tools cover 46 clinical areas and all 4 functions of medicine—screening, diagnosis, treatment, and follow-up. The indicators also cover a variety of modes of providing care, including history, physical examination, laboratory study, medication, and other interventions and contacts.

Development of each indicator was based on a review of the literature. Each volume documents the literature on which the indicators were based, explains how the clinical areas and indicators were selected, and describes what is included in the overall system.

The QA Tools were developed with funding from public and private sponsors—the Health Care Financing Administration, the Agency for Healthcare Research and Quality, the California HealthCare Foundation, and the Robert Wood Johnson Foundation.

The other four volumes in this series are:

Quality of Care for General Medical Conditions: A Review of the Literature and Quality Indicators. Eve A. Kerr, Steven M. Asch, Eric G. Hamilton, and Elizabeth A. McGlynn, eds. MR-1280-AHRQ, 2000.

Quality of Care for Oncologic Conditions and HIV: A Review of the Literature and Quality Indicators. Steven M. Asch, Eve A. Kerr, Eric G. Hamilton, Jennifer L. Reifel, and Elizabeth A. McGlynn, eds. MR-1281-AHRQ, 2000.

Quality of Care for Children and Adolescents: A Review of Selected Clinical Conditions and Quality Indicators. Elizabeth A. McGlynn, Cheryl L. Damberg, Eve A. Kerr, and Mark A. Schuster, eds. MR-1283-AHRQ, 2000.

Quality of Care for Women: A Review of Selected Clinical Conditions and Quality Indicators. Elizabeth A. McGlynn, Eve A. Kerr, Cheryl L. Damberg, and Steven M. Asch, eds. MR-1284-AHRQ, 2000.

These volumes should be of interest to clinicians, health plans, insurers, and health services researchers. At the time of publication, the QA Tools system was undergoing testing in managed care plans,

medical groups, and selected communities. For more information about the
QA Tools system, contact RAND_Health@rand.org.

CONTENTS

ACKNOWLEDGEMENTS

Funding for this work was provided by a Cooperative Agreement (No. 5U18HS09463-02), "Adult Global Quality Assessment Tool") from the Agency for Healthcare Research and Quality. We appreciate the continued and enthusiastic support of our project officer, Elinor Walker.

We are indebted to our expert panelists who gave generously of their time, knowledge and wisdom:

Leo M. Cooney, Jr., M.D.
Chief, Section of General Internal Medicine
Humana Foundation Professor of Geriatric Medicine
Yale University School of Medicine
New Haven, Connecticut

Mark A. Hlatky, M.D., F.A.C.C.
Professor of Health Research and Policy
Stanford University School of Medicine
Palo Alto, California

Barry J. Make, M.D.
Director, Pulmonary Rehabilitation and Emphysema Programs
National Jewish Medical and Research Center
Denver, Colorado

Keith I. Marton, M.D., F.A.C.P. (Panel Chair)
Vice President, Medical Academic Affairs
St. Mary's Medical Center
San Francisco, California

Barbara Phillips, M.D., F.C.C.P.
Professor of Medicine
Division of Pulmonary and Critical Care Medicine
University of Kentucky Medical Center
Director, Sleep Apnea Center
Columbia Medical Center
Lexington, Kentucky

John Popovich, Jr., M.D.
Division Head, Pulmonary and Critical Care Medicine
Henry Ford Hospital
Clinical Associate Professor
University of Michigan
Detroit, Michigan

Rita F. Redberg, M.D., M.Sc., F.A.C.C.
Associate Professor of Medicine
UCSF Medical Center
Co-Director
UCSF National Center of Excellence in Women's Health
San Francisco, California

Douglas R. Rosing, M.D., F.A.C.C.
Clinical Professor of Medicine
George Washington University Medical School
Governor and President
American College of Cardiology, Maryland Chapter
Baltimore, MD

Sidney C. Smith, Jr., M.D., F.A.C.C., F.A.C.P.
Professor of Medicine
Chief of Cardiology
Director, Academic Center for Cardiovascular Disease
University of North Carolina at Chapel Hill
Chapel Hill, North Carolina

Our thanks also go to the following experts who reviewed and
provided consultation on specific chapters:

Anthony Steimle, MD, Kaiser Permanente Northern California (Atrial
Fibrillation and Heart Failure)

Jeffrey Saver, MD, University of California at Los Angeles
(Cerebrovascular Disease)

We are also greatly indebted to the following project staff whose
contributions made this document possible: Kenneth Clark, Landon
Donsbach, Sandy Geschwind, Kevin Heslin, Nicole Humphrey, Amy Kilbourne,
and Tammy Majeski.

INTRODUCTION

Developing and implementing a valid system of quality assessment is essential for effective functioning of the health care system. Although a number of groups have produced quality assessment tools, these tools typically suffer from a variety of limitations. Information is obtained on only a few dimensions of quality, the tools rely exclusively on administrative data, they examine quality only for users of services rather than the population, or they fail to provide a scientific basis for the quality indicators.

Under funding from public and private sponsors, including the Health Care Financing Administration (HCFA), the Agency for Healthcare Research and Quality (AHRQ), the California HealthCare Foundation, and the Robert Wood Johnson Foundation (RWJ), RAND has developed and tested a comprehensive, clinically based system for assessing quality of care for children and adults. We call this system QA Tools.

In this introduction, we discuss how the clinical areas were selected, how the indicators were chosen, and what is included in the overall system. We then describe in detail how we developed the indicators for children and adolescents.

ADVANTAGES OF THE QA TOOLS SYSTEM

QA Tools is a comprehensive, clinically based system for assessing the quality of care for children and adults. The indicators cover 46 clinical areas and all four functions of medicine including screening, diagnosis, treatment, and follow-up. The indicators also cover a variety of modes of providing care, such as history, physical examination, laboratory study, medication, and other interventions and contacts. Initial development of indicators for each clinical area was based on a review of the literature.

The QA Tools system addresses many limitations of current quality assessment tools by offering the following:

- They are clinically detailed and require data typically found only in medical records rather than just relying exclusively on data from administrative records.

- They examine quality for a population-based sample rather than for a more restricted sample of those who use care or have insurance.

- They document the scientific basis for developing and choosing the indicators.

- The QA Tools system is designed to target populations vulnerable to underutilization.

- Because of the comprehensiveness of the system, it is difficult for health care organizations to focus on a few indicators to increase their quality scores.

- QA Tools is a system that can be effective for both internal and external quality reviews. Health care organizations can use the system in order to improve the overall quality of the care provided.

- Because of the simple summary scores that will be produced, it will be an important tool for purchasers and consumers who are making choices about health care coverage and which provider to see.

Given its comprehensiveness, the QA Tools system contrasts with *leading indicators*, the most common approach to quality measurement in use today. Under the leading indicators approach, three to five specific quality measures are selected across a few domains (for example, rates of mammography screening, prevalence of the use of beta blockers among persons who have had a heart attack, and appropriateness of hysterectomy).

Leading indicators may work well for drawing general conclusions about quality when they correlate highly with other similar but unmeasured interventions and when repeated measurement and public reporting does not change the relationship of those indicators to the related interventions. However, to date no real evaluation of the utility of leading indicators in assessing health system performance has been done. We also do not know whether the selected indicators currently in use consistently represent other unmeasured practices.

By contrast, a comprehensive system can represent different dimensions of quality of care delivery by using a large number of measures applied to a population of interest and aggregated to produce index scores to draw conclusions about quality. A comprehensive system works well when evidence exists of variability within and between the diagnosis and management of different conditions and when the question being asked is framed at a high level (for instance, how well is the health system helping the population stay healthy, or how much of a problem does underuse present?).

In the 46 clinical areas they encompass, the QA Tools adequately represent scientific and expert judgment on what constitutes quality care. However, both the science and the practice of medicine continue to evolve. For the QA Tools to remain a valid tool for quality assessment over time, the scientific evidence in each area needs to be reviewed annually to determine if new evidence warrants modifying the indicators and/or clinical areas included in the system.

SELECTING CLINICAL AREAS FOR THE QA TOOLS

We reviewed Vital Statistics, the National Health Interview Survey, the National Hospital Discharge Survey, and the National Ambulatory Medical Care Survey to identify the leading causes of morbidity and mortality and the most common reasons for physician visits in the United States. We examined statistics for different age and gender groups in the population (0-1, 1-5, 6-11, 12-17, 18-50 [men and women], 50-64, 65-75, over 75).

We selected topics that reflected these different areas of importance (death, disability, utilization of services) and that covered preventive care as well as care for acute and chronic conditions. In addition, we consulted with a variety of experts to identify areas that are important to these various populations but that may be underrepresented in national data sets (for example, mental health problems). Finally, we sought to select enough clinical areas to represent a majority of the health care delivery system.

Table I.1 lists the 46 clinical areas included in the QA Tools system by population group; 20 include indicators for children and 36 for adults. The clinical areas, broadly defined, represent about 55 percent of the reasons for ambulatory care visits among children, 50 percent of the reasons for ambulatory care visits for the entire population, and 46 percent of the reasons for hospitalization among adults.

Note: Table I.1 reflects the clinical areas that were included in the system currently being tested. Several clinical areas (for example, lung cancer and sickle cell disease) for which indicators were developed were not incorporated into the current tool due to budgetary constraints.

Table I.1

Clinical Areas in QA Tools System By Covered Population Group

Clinical Areas	Children	Adults
Acne	X	
Adolescent preventive services	X	
Adult screening and prevention		X
Alcohol dependence		X
Allergic rhinitis	X	
Asthma	X	X
Atrial fibrillation		X
Attention deficit/hyperactivity disorder	X	
Benign prostatic hyperplasia		X
Breast cancer		X
Cataracts		X
Cerebrovascular disease		X
Cervical cancer		X
Cesarean delivery		X
Chronic obstructive pulmonary disease	X	X
Colorectal cancer		X
Congestive heart failure		X
Coronary artery disease		X
Depression	X	X
Developmental screening	X	
Diabetes Mellitus	X	X
Diarrheal disease	X	
Family planning and contraception	X	X
Fever of unknown origin	X	
Headache		X
Hip fracture		X
Hormone replacement therapy		X
Human immunodeficiency virus		X
Hyperlipidemia		X
Hypertension		X
Immunizations	X	X
Low back pain		X
Orthopedic conditions		X
Osteoarthritis		X
Otitis media	X	
Pain management for cancer		X
Peptic ulcer disease & dyspepsia		X
Pneumonia		X
Prenatal care and delivery	X	X
Prostate cancer		X
Tuberculosis	X	X
Upper respiratory tract infections	X	
Urinary tract infections	X	X
Uterine bleeding and hysterectomy		X
Vaginitis and sexually transmitted diseases	X	X
Well child care	X	
Total number of clinical areas	**20**	**36**

SELECTING QUALITY INDICATORS

In this section, we describe the process by which indicators were chosen for inclusion in the QA Tools system. This process involved RAND staff drafting proposed indicators based on a review of the pertinent clinical literature and expert panel review of those indicators.

Literature Review

For each clinical area chosen, we reviewed the scientific literature for evidence that effective methods of prevention, screening, diagnosis, treatment, and follow-up existed (Asch et al., 2000; Kerr et al., 2000; McGlynn et al., 2000a; McGlynn et al., 2000b). We explicitly examined the continuum of care in each clinical area. RAND staff drafted indicators that

- addressed an intervention with potential health benefits for the patient
- were supported by scientific evidence or formal professional consensus (guidelines, for example)
- can be significantly influenced by the health care delivery system
- can be assessed from available sources of information, primarily the medical record.

The literature review process varied slightly for each clinical area, but the basic strategy involved the following:

- Identify general areas in which quality indicators are likely to be developed.
- Review relevant textbooks and summary articles.
- Conduct a targeted MEDLINE search on specific topics related to the probable indicator areas.

The levels of evidence for each indicator were assigned to three categories: randomized clinical trial; nonrandomized controlled trials, cohort or case analysis, or multiple time series; and textbooks, opinions, or descriptive studies. For each proposed indicator, staff noted the highest level of evidence supporting the indicator.

Because of the breadth of topics for which we were developing indicators, some of the literature reviews relied exclusively on textbooks and review articles. Nonetheless, we believe that the reviews adequately summarize clinical opinion and key research at the time that they were conducted. The literature reviews used to develop quality indicators for children and adolescents, and for women, were conducted between January and July 1995. The reviews for general medical conditions, oncologic conditions, and cardiopulmonary conditions were conducted between November 1996 and July 1997.

For each clinical area, we wrote a summary of the scientific evidence and developed tables of the proposed indicators that included the level of evidence, specific studies in support of the indicator, and the clinical rationale for the indicator. Because the organization of care delivery is changing so rapidly, we drafted indicators that were not in most cases inextricably linked to the place where the care was provided.

Types of Indicators

Quality of care is usually determined with three types of measures:

- *Structural measures* include characteristics of clinicians (for instance, board certification or years of experience), organizations (for instance, staffing patterns or types of equipment available), and patients (for instance, type of insurance or severity of illness).

- *Process measures* include the ways in which clinicians and patients interact and the appropriateness of medical treatment for a specific patient.

- *Outcomes measures* include changes in patients' current and future health status, including health-related quality of life and satisfaction with care.

The indicators included in the QA Tools system are primarily process indicators. We deliberately chose such indicators because the system was designed to assess care for which we can hold providers responsible. However, we collect data on a number of intermediate outcomes measures (for example, glycosylated hemoglobin, blood pressure, and cholesterol) that could be used to construct intermediate clinical outcomes indicators.

In many instances, the measures included in the QA Tools system are used to determine whether interventions have been provided in response to poor performance on such measures (for instance, whether persons who fail to control their blood sugar on dietary therapy are offered oral hypoglycemic therapy).

The Expert Panel Process

We convened expert panels to evaluate the indicators and to make final selections using the RAND/UCLA Appropriateness Method, a modified Delphi method developed at RAND and UCLA (Brook 1994). In general, the method quantitatively assesses the expert judgment of a group of clinicians regarding the indicators by using a scale with values ranging from 1 to 9.

The method is iterative with two rounds of anonymous ratings of the indicators by the panel and a face-to-face group discussion between rounds. Each panelist has equal weight in determining the final result: the quality indicators that will be included in the QA Tools system.

The RAND/UCLA Appropriateness Method has been shown to have a reproducibility consistent with that of well accepted diagnostic tests such as the interpretation of coronary angiography and screening mammography (Shekelle et al., 1998a). It has also been shown to have content, construct, and predictive validity in other applications (Brook, 1994; Shekelle et al., 1998b; Kravitz et al., 1995; Selby et al., 1996).

Approximately six weeks before the panel meeting, we sent panelists the reviews of the literature, the staff-proposed quality indicators, and separate rating sheets for each clinical area. We asked the panelists to examine the literature review and rate each indicator on a nine-point scale on each of two dimensions: validity and feasibility.

A quality indicator is defined as valid if:

1. Adequate scientific evidence or professional consensus exists supporting the indicator.
2. There are identifiable health benefits to patients who receive care specified by the indicator.

3. Based on the panelists' professional experience, health professionals with significantly higher rates of adherence to an indicator would be considered higher quality providers

4. The majority of factors that determine adherence to an indicator are under the control of the health professional (or are subject to influence by the health professional—for example, smoking cessation).

Ratings of 1-3 mean that the indicator is not a valid criterion for evaluating quality. Ratings of 4-6 mean that the indicator is an uncertain or equivocal criterion for evaluating quality. Ratings of 7-9 mean that the indicator is clearly a valid criterion for evaluating quality.

A quality indicator is defined as feasible if:

1. The information necessary to determine adherence is likely to be found in a typical medical record.

2. Estimates of adherence to the indicator based on medical record data are likely to be reliable and unbiased.

3. Failure to document relevant information about the indicator is itself a marker for poor quality.

Ratings of 1-3 mean that it is not feasible to use the indicator for evaluating quality. Ratings of 4-6 mean that there will be considerable variability in the feasibility of using the indicator to evaluate quality. Ratings of 7-9 mean that it is clearly feasible to use the indicator for evaluating quality.

The first round of indicators was rated by the panelists individually in their own offices. The indicators were returned to RAND staff and the results of the first round were summarized. We encouraged panelists to comment on the literature reviews, the definitions of key terms, and the indicators. We also encouraged them to suggest additions or deletions to the indicators.

At the panel meeting, participants discussed each clinical area in turn, focusing on the evidence, or lack thereof, that supports or refutes each indicator and the panelists' prior validity rankings. Panelists had before them the summary of the panel's first round ratings and a confidential reminder of their own ratings.

The summary consisted of a printout of the rating sheet with the distribution of ratings by panelists displayed above the rating line (without revealing the identity of the panelists) and a caret (^) marking the individual panelist's own rating in the first round displayed below the line. An example of the printout received by panelists is shown in Figure I.1.

```
panelist  ; round 1;  page  1                              September 14, 1997
_____
 Chapter 1
 ASTHMA                                 Validity          Feasibility
_____

DIAGNOSIS

3. Spirometry should be measured in patients   1   1 2 3 1 1                3 4 2
with chronic asthma at least every 2 years.  1 2 3 4 5 6 7 8 9    1 2 3 4 5 6 7 8 9  ( 1- 2)
                                                         ^                    ^

TREATMENT

7. Patients requiring chronic treatment with
systemic corticosteroids during any 12 month
period should have been prescribed inhaled
corticosteroids during the same 12 month            1 6   2                  2 3 4
period.                                       1 2 3 4 5 6 7 8 9    1 2 3 4 5 6 7 8 9  ( 3- 4)
                                                         ^                    ^

10. All patients seen for an acute asthma
exacerbation should be evaluated with a
complete history including all of the
following:
                                                  2 2   3                  2 2   1 1 3
    a. time of onset                          1 2 3 4 5 6 7 8 9    1 2 3 4 5 6 7 8 9  ( 5- 6)
                                                         ^                    ^

                                                      4 1 4                      3 1 5
    b. all current medications                1 2 3 4 5 6 7 8 9    1 2 3 4 5 6 7 8 9  ( 7- 8)
                                                         ^                    ^

    c. prior hospitalizations and emergency             5 1 3                    5 1 3
       department visits for asthma           1 2 3 4 5 6 7 8 9    1 2 3 4 5 6 7 8 9  ( 9-10)
                                                         ^               -            ^

    d. prior episodes of respiratory                1 1 3 2 2              1   2   3 1 2
       insufficiency due to asthma            1 2 3 4 5 6 7 8 9    1 2 3 4 5 6 7 8 9  (11-12)
                                                         ^                            ^
_____
Scales:  1 = low validity or feasibility;  9 = high validity or feasibility
```

Figure I.1 - Sample Panelist Summary Rating Sheet

Panelists were encouraged to bring to the discussion any relevant published information that the literature reviews had omitted. In a few cases, they supplied this information which was, in turn, discussed. In several cases, the indicators were reworded or otherwise clarified to better fit clinical judgment.

After further discussion, all indicators in each clinical area were re-ranked for validity. These final round rankings were analyzed in a manner similar to past applications of the RAND/UCLA Appropriateness Method (Park et al., 1986; Brook, 1994). The median panel rating and measure of dispersion were used to categorize indicators on validity.

We regarded panel members as being in *disagreement* when at least three members of the panel judged an indicator as being in the highest tertile of validity (that is, having a rating of 7, 8, or 9) and three members rated it as being in the lowest tertile of validity (1, 2, or 3) (Brook, 1994). Indicators with a median validity rating of 7 or higher without disagreement were included in the system.

We also obtained ratings from the panelists about the feasibility of obtaining the data necessary to score the indicators from medical. This was done to make explicit that failure to document key variables required to score an indicator would be treated as though the recommended care was not provided.

Although we do not intend for quality assessment to impose significant additional documentation burdens, we wanted the panel to acknowledge that documentation itself is an element of quality particularly when patients are treated by a team of health professionals. Because of the variability in documentation patterns and the opportunity to empirically evaluate feasibility, indicators with a median feasibility rating of 4 and higher were accepted into the system. Indicators had to satisfy both the validity and feasibility criteria.

Five expert panels were convened on the topics of children's care, care for women 18-50, general medicine for adults, oncologic conditions and HIV, and cardiopulmonary conditions.

The dates on which the panels were conducted are shown in Table I.2.

Table I.2

Dates Expert Panels Convened

Children	October 1995
Women	November 1995
Cardiopulmonary	September 1997
Oncology/HIV	October 1997
General Medicine	November 1997

Tables I.3 through I.6 summarize the distribution of indicators by level of evidence, type of care (preventive, acute, chronic), function of medicine (screening, diagnosis, treatment, follow-up, continuity), and modality (for example, history, physical examination, laboratory test, medication) (Malin et al., 2000; Schuster et al., 1997).

The categories were selected by the research team and reflect terminology commonly used by health services researchers to describe different aspects of health service delivery. The categories also reflect the areas in which we intend to develop aggregate quality of care scores. However, a significant benefit of the QA Tools system is its adaptability to other frameworks.

Note: In the following tables, the figures in some columns may not total exactly 100 percent due to the rounding of fractional numbers.

Table I.3

Distribution of Indicators (%) by Level of Evidence

Level of Evidence	Children	Women	Cancer/HIV	Cardio-pulmonary	General Medicine
Randomized trials	11	22	22	18	23
Nonrandomized trials	6	16	37	4	17
Descriptive studies	72	59	26	71	57
Added by panel	12	4	15	7	4
Total	101	101	100	100	101

Table I.4
Distribution of Indicators (%) by Type of Care

Type of Care	Children	Women	Cancer/HIV	Cardio-pulmonary	General Medicine
Preventive	30	11	20	3	18
Acute	36	49	7	26	38
Chronic	34	41	74	71	44
Total	100	101	101	100	100

Table I.5
Distribution of Indicators (%) by Function of Medicine

Function of Medicine	Children	Women	Cancer/HIV	Cardio-pulmonary	General Medicine
Screening	23	18	9	3	12
Diagnosis	31	30	27	54	41
Treatment	36	43	53	36	41
Follow-up	10	12	10	8	6
Total	100	103	99	101	100

13

Table I.6

Distribution of Indicators (%) by Modality

Modality	Children	Women	Cancer/HIV	Cardio-pulmonary	General Medicine
History	19	18	4	11	23
Physical	19	10	5	21	15
Lab/Radiology	21	23	24	23	18
Medication	25	29	25	25	26
Other	17	19	42	20	17
Total	101	99	100	100	99

DEVELOPING QUALITY INDICATORS FOR CARDIOPULMONARY CONDITIONS

We now describe in more detail the process by which we developed quality indicators for cardiopulmonary conditions.

Selecting Clinical Areas

We began our selection of clinical areas by examining national data sources to identify the leading causes of mortality, morbidity, and functional limitation among adult men and women. The principal data sources for this review were Vital Statistics, the National Health Interview Survey (NHIS), the National Ambulatory Medical Care Survey (NAMCS), and the National Hospital Discharge Survey (NHDS).

From these data sources, we selected the conditions that represent the leading causes of mortality, morbidity, hospitalization, and outpatient visits. This process led to the selection of some areas that overlapped with the previously conducted women's care panel (McGlynn et al., 2000b).

To facilitate the review and rating process, we grouped the selected areas into three categories: cardiopulmonary conditions, oncologic conditions and HIV, and general medical conditions. Table I.7 lists the clinical areas covered by each of these categories.

"Supportive Care for Oncologic Conditions" was not among the originally selected clinical areas, but was added during the panel process as a result of strong recommendations from several oncology panelists.

Table I.7

Clinical Areas Covered by each Expert Panel

Cardiopulmonary (N=12)	Oncology and HIV (N=11)	General Medicine (N=22)
Asthma*	Breast Cancer Screening	Acne*
Atrial Fibrillation	Breast Cancer Diagnosis	Alcohol Dependence*
Cerebrovascular Disease	and Treatment*	Allergic Rhinitis*
Chronic Obstructive	Cervical Cancer	Benign Prostatic
Pulmonary Disease	Screening*	Hyperplasia
Cigarette Counseling*	Colorectal Cancer	Cataracts
Congestive Heart	Screening	Cholelithiasis
Failure	Colorectal Cancer	Dementia
Coronary Artery Disease	Diagnosis and Treatment	Depression*
Diagnosis and Screening	HIV Disease	Diabetes Mellitus*
Coronary Artery Disease	Lung Cancer	Dyspepsia and Peptic
Prevention and	Prostate Cancer	Ulcer Disease
Treatment	Screening	Hormone Replacement
Hyperlipidemia	Prostate Cancer	Therapy
Hypertension*	Diagnosis and Treatment	Headache*
Pneumonia	Skin Cancer Screening	Hip Fracture
Upper Respiratory	Cancer Pain and	Hysterectomy
Infections*	Palliation	Inguinal Hernia
		Low Back Pain (Acute)*
		Orthopedic Conditions
		Osteoarthritis
		Preventive Care*
		Urinary Tract
		Infections*
		Vaginitis and Sexually
		Transmitted Diseases*
		Vertigo and Dizziness

  * Previously addressed by the panel on quality of care for women (McGlynn et al., 2000b).

Conducting Literature Reviews

The literature reviews were conducted as described earlier in this Introduction by a team of 14 physician investigators, many with clinical expertise in the conditions selected for this project. Each investigator then drafted a review of the literature for his or her topic area, focusing on important areas for quality measurement (as opposed to a clinical review of the literature, which would focus on clinical management) and drafted potential indicators.

Every indicator table was reviewed by Drs. Asch or Kerr for content, consistency, and the likely availability of information necessary to score adherence to the indicator from the medical record. On a few occasions, when questions remained even after detailed literature review, we requested that a clinical leader in the field read and comment on the draft review and indicators.

In addition, the physician investigators updated the 16 clinical areas carried over from the previous women's care panel. This included reading the reviews and indicators, updating the supporting literature from 1995 to 1997, and modifying the pre-existing indicators as was appropriate.

In most cases few changes were made, but indicators were deleted if the evidence changed or if our implementation experience proved that it was not feasible to collect the data necessary to score adherence to an indicator. Indicators were added if strong evidence since 1995 supported the need for a new criterion. In the clinical areas previously addressed by the women's care panel, the expert panel for cardiopulmonary conditions rated only those indicators that had been added or significantly revised (indicated by bold type in the indicator tables in the chapters that follow).

This quality assessment system is intended to encompass a substantial portion of the inpatient and ambulatory care received by the population. In order to estimate the percentage of ambulatory care visits covered by this system, we aggregated applicable ICD-9 codes into the clinical areas for which we are developing quality indicators. We then calculated the number of adult visits for each condition in the 1993 National Ambulatory Medical Care Survey (NAMCS). We used the same method to estimate the percentage of inpatient admissions accounted for by each clinical area in the 1992 National Hospital Discharge Survey.

Aggregating ICD-9 codes into the clinical areas covered by this system was an imprecise task, requiring a rather broad definition of what is "included" in each clinical area. The clinical conditions covered by this quality measurement system encompass 50 percent of all ambulatory care visits and 46 percent of non-federal inpatient hospital admissions.

Developing Indicators

In each clinical area investigators developed indicators defining the explicit criteria by which quality of care [per your edits. ND] would be evaluated. These indicators focus on technical processes of care for the various conditions and are organized by function: screening, diagnosis, treatment and follow-up. Although we have developed indicators across the continuum of management for each condition, we have not attempted to cover every important area or every possible clinical circumstance. The indicators were designed to apply to the average patient with the specified condition who is seeing the average physician.

Our approach makes a strong distinction between indicators of quality care and practice guidelines (see Table I.8). Whereas guidelines are intended to be comprehensive in scope, indicators are meant to apply to specific clinical circumstances in which there is believed to be a strong link between a measurable health care process and patient outcomes.

Indicators are not intended to measure all possible care for a condition. Furthermore, guidelines are intended to be applied prospectively at the individual patient level, whereas indicators are applied retrospectively and scored at an aggregate level. Finally, indicators must be written precisely in order to be *operationalized* (that is, to form useful measures of quality based on medical records or administrative data).

Table I.8

Clinical Guidelines versus Quality Indicators

Guidelines	Indicators
Comprehensive: Cover virtually all aspects of care for a condition.	**Targeted**: Apply to specific clinical circumstances in which there is evidence of a process-outcome link.
Prescriptive: Intended to influence provider behavior prospectively at the individual patient level.	**Observational:** Measure past provider behavior at an aggregate level.
Flexible: Intentionally allow room for clinical judgment and interpretation.	**Operational:** Precise language that can be applied systematically to medical records or administrative data.

The indicator tables at the end of each chapter of this book
- note the population to whom the indicators apply
- list the indicators themselves
- provide a "grade" for the strength of the evidence that supports each indicator
- list the specific literature used to support each indicator
- provide a statement of the health benefits of complying with each indicator
- include comments to further explain the purpose or reasoning behind each indicator.

Selecting Panel Participants

We requested nominations for potential expert panel participants in the from the relevant specialty societies: the American College of Physicians, American Academy of Family Physicians, American Geriatrics Society, American College of Cardiology, American College of Chest Physicians, American Thoracic Society, and the Society of General

Internal Medicine. We received a total of 206 nominations for the panels on general medicine, oncology and HIV, and cardiopulmonary conditions.

Each nominee was sent a letter summarizing the purpose of the project and indicating which group recommended them. Interested candidates were asked to return a curriculum vitae and calendar with available dates for a two-day panel meeting. We received positive responses from 156 potential panelists. The quality of the recommended panelists was excellent.

We sought to ensure that each panel was diverse with respect to type of practice (academic, private practice, managed care organizational practice), geographic location, gender, and specialty. The cardiopulmonary panel included four cardiologists, three pulmonologists, a geriatrician and a general internist. Dr. Keith Marton, a general internist, was selected by RAND staff to chair this panel. (See the Acknowledgements at the front of this book for the list of panelists.)

Selecting and Analyzing the Final Set of Indicators

The panel process was conducted as described earlier in this Introduction.

A total of 319 quality indicators were reviewed by the cardiopulmonary expert panel. All 47 of the indicators retained from the women's care panel were accepted by the cardiopulmonary panel on the basis of the women's panel's ratings. Three indicators were deleted before the final panel ratings in response to comments by panelists before or during the panel meeting. Of the remaining 269 indicators that received final ratings from this panel, 50 were added by the panel itself. This occurred either when panelists agreed that a new indicator should be written to cover an important topic, or, more frequently, as a result of splitting a staff-proposed indicator.

One reason for the large number of indicators added by the cardiopulmonary panel was an active discussion during the meeting regarding the appropriate populations to which some indicators should be applied. Rather than attempting to resolve issues that remain controversial in the medical community at large, the panel chose to move

19

forward by splitting several indicators by the age or gender of the target population, thus allowing the panelists to register their opinions on these issues through their ratings.

The panel accepted 209 (78%) of the 269 indicators it rated. Sixty indicators (22%) were dropped due to low ratings: 56 for low validity scores and 4 for substantial disagreement on validity.

Table I.9 summarizes the disposition of all 319 proposed cardiopulmonary quality indicators by the strength of their supporting evidence. The final set consists of 256 indicators (209 rated by this panel and 47 approved based on ratings by the women's care panel), or 80 percent of those proposed. Table I.9 reveals that indicators that are not based on clinical trials (that is, Level III indicators) were much more likely to be rejected by the panel. Moreover, indicators proposed by the panelists themselves fared poorly. This pattern has been observed consistently across several RAND quality of care panels.

Table I.9

Disposition of Proposed Cardiopulmonary Quality Indicators by Strength of Evidence

Strength of Evidence	Total Proposed	Indicator Disposition			
		Accepted	Retained from Women's Panel	Drop before rating	Drop due to low rating
I. Randomized controlled trials	47 (100%)	40 (85%)	5 (11%)	0 (0%)	2 (4%)
II. Non-randomized trials	10 (100%)	3 (30%)	7 (70%)	0 (0%)	0 (0%)
III. Opinions, descriptive studies, or textbooks	212 (100%)	147 (69%)	35 (17%)	3 (1%)	27 (13%)
IV. Added by Clinical Panel	50 (100%)	19 (38%)	0 (0%)	0 (0%)	31 (62%)
Total	319 (100%)	209 (66%)	47 (15%)	3 (1%)	60 (19%)

The summary ratings sheets for cardiopulmonary conditions are shown in Appendix A.

Figure I.2 provides an example of a final summary rating sheet. The chapter number and clinical condition are shown in the top left margin. The rating bar is numbered from 1 to 9, indicating the range of possible responses. The number shown above each of the responses in the rating bar indicates how many panelists provided that particular rating for the indicator. Below the score distribution, in parentheses, the median and the mean absolute deviation from the median are listed. Each dimension is assigned an A for "Agreement", D for "Disagreement", or I for "Indeterminate" based on the score distribution.

Note: We recommend caution when reviewing the ratings for each indicator. The overall median does not tell us anything about the extent to which the indicators occur in clinical practice. To determine that, actual clinical data to assess the indicators must be collected and analyzed.

COMMUNITY-ACQUIRED PNEUMONIA	Validity	Feasibility
DIAGNOSIS, CONT.		

7. Hospitalized persons with pneumonia should have the following documented on the first and second days of hospitalization:

    a. temperature
```
                1 3 5                1 1 7
1 2 3 4 5 6 7 8 9   1 2 3 4 5 6 7 8 9   ( 29- 30)
   (9.0, 0.6, A)       (9.0, 0.3, A)
                2 3 4                2 1 6
```
    b. lung examination
```
1 2 3 4 5 6 7 8 9   1 2 3 4 5 6 7 8 9   ( 31- 32)
   (8.0, 0.7, A)       (9.0, 0.6, A)
```

TREATMENT

8. Non-hospitalized persons <= 65 years of age diagnosed with pneumonia without a known bacteriologic etiology and without coexisting illnesses should be offered an oral empiric macrolide, unless allergic.
```
              1 3 2 3              3 4 2
1 2 3 4 5 6 7 8 9   1 2 3 4 5 6 7 8 9   ( 33- 34)
   (8.0, 0.9, A)       (8.0, 0.6, A)
```

9. Non-hospitalized persons > 65 years of age diagnosed with pneumonia without a known bacteriologic etiology or with coexisting illnesses should be offered one of the following oral empiric antibiotic regimens:
  - a second generation cephalosporin
  - trimethoprim-sulfamethoxazole
  - a beta-lactam/beta-lactamase inhibitor combination
```
              1 4   4              2 4 3
1 2 3 4 5 6 7 8 9   1 2 3 4 5 6 7 8 9   ( 35- 36)
   (7.0, 1.0, A)       (8.0, 0.6, A)
```

10. Hospitalized persons with non-severe pneumonia without a known bacteriologic etiology should be offered one of the following empiric antibiotic regimens:

  - a second or third generation cephalosporin
  - a beta-lactam/beta-lactamase inhibitor combination.
```
              1 4 1 3              2 3 4
1 2 3 4 5 6 7 8 9   1 2 3 4 5 6 7 8 9   ( 37- 38)
   (7.0, 0.9, A)       (8.0, 0.7, A)
```

11. Hospitalized persons with severe pneumonia without a known bacteriologic etiology should be offered one of the following antibiotic regimens:

  - a macrolide and a third generation cephalosporin with anti-Pseudomonas activity
  - a macrolide and another anitpseudomonal agent such as imipenem/ciliastin, ciprofloxacin
```
              1 3 2 3              1 4 4
1 2 3 4 5 6 7 8 9   1 2 3 4 5 6 7 8 9   ( 39- 40)
   (8.0, 0.9, A)       (8.0, 0.6, A)
```

12. Persons with CAP should be offered antibiotics for 10-14 days, with the exception of azithromycin, which may be given for 5 days.
```
1 1 4 2     1    1 1   1   3 2 1
1 2 3 4 5 6 7 8 9   1 2 3 4 5 6 7 8 9   ( 41- 42)
   (3.0, 1.1, I)       (7.0, 1.9, D)
```

FOLLOW-UP

13. Persons treated for pneumonia should have follow-up contact with a provider within 6 weeks after discharge or diagnosis.
```
              1 6   2              1 3 2 3
1 2 3 4 5 6 7 8 9   1 2 3 4 5 6 7 8 9   ( 43- 44)
   (7.0, 0.6, A)       (8.0, 0.9, A)
```

Scales: 1 = low validity or feasibility; 9 = high validity or feasibility

Figure I.2 - Sample Rating Results Sheet

The tables in Appendix B show the changes made to each indicator during the panel process, the reasons for those changes, and the final disposition of each indicator. Wherever possible, we have tried to briefly summarize the discussion that led the panel to either modify or drop indicators. These explanations are based on extensive notes taken by RAND staff during the panel process, but should not be considered representative of the views of all of the panelists, nor of any individual.

Because this quality assessment system is designed to produce aggregate scores for various dimensions of health care, it is useful to examine the distribution of the final indicators across some of these dimensions. Table I.10 summarizes the distribution of quality indicators by type of care (preventive, acute, and chronic), the function of the medical care provided (screening, diagnosis, treatment, and follow-up), and the modality by which care is delivered (history, physical examination, laboratory or radiologic study, medication, other interventions,[1] and other contacts[2]).

Indicators were assigned to only one type of care, but could have up to two functions and three modalities. Indicators with more than one function or modality were allocated fractionally across categories. For example, one indicator states, "For patients who present with a complaint of sore throat, a history/physical exam should document presence or absence of: a) fever; b) tonsillar exudate; c) anterior cervical adenopathy." This indicator was allocated 50 percent to the history modality and 50 percent to the physical modality.

---

[1] Other interventions include counseling, education, procedures, and surgery.

[2] Other contacts include general follow-up visit or phone call, referral to subspecialist, or hospitalization.

Table I.10

**Distribution of Final Cardiopulmonary Quality Indicators by
Type of Care, Function, and Modality**

	Number of Indicators	Percent of Indicators
Type		
Preventive	7	3%
Acute	66	26%
Chronic	183	71%
Function		
Screening	7	3%
Diagnosis	138	54%
Treatment	91	36%
Follow-up	20	8%
Modality		
History	28	11%
Physical	53	21%
Laboratory or Radiologic Study	59	23%
Medication	64	25%
Other Intervention	39	15%
Other Contact	13	5%
Total	**256**	**100%**

CONCLUSION

This report provides the foundation for a broad set of quality indicators covering cardiopulmonary health care. The final indicators presented here cover a variety of clinical conditions, span a range of clinical functions and modalities, and are rated by the level of evidence in the supporting literature. When combined with the indicators approved by the women's care, child and adolescent care, oncology/HIV, and general medicine expert panels, the complete quality assessment system will be more comprehensive than any system currently in use.

The comprehensive nature of this system is demonstrated by the broad scope of the indicators. Of the 319 indicators reviewed by the cardiopulmonary expert panel, 256 (80%) were retained. These indicators cover a mix of preventive, acute, and chronic care. They address all four functions of medicine, including screening, diagnosis, treatment and follow-up. Moreover, the indicators cover a variety of modes of care provision, such as history, physical examination, laboratory study, and medication.

There are many advantages to a global quality assessment system. Not only does it cover a broad range of health conditions experienced by the target population, but it is also designed to detect underutilization of needed services. In addition, because of its broad scope, it will be difficult for health care organizations to improve their quality scores by focusing their improvement efforts on only a few indicators or clinical areas.

Finally, this system can be effective for both internal and external quality reviews. There is sufficient clinical detail in the system that health plans will be able to use the resulting information to improve care, while the simple summary scores that it generates will be an important tool for health care purchasers and consumers.

ORGANIZATION OF THIS DOCUMENT

The rest of this volume is organized as follows:

- Each chapter summarizes
  - Results of the literature review for one condition.
  - Provides a table of the staff's recommended indicators based on that review.
  - Indicates the level of scientific evidence supporting each indicator along with the specific relevant citations.
- Appendix A provides the summary rating sheets for each condition.
- Appendix B shows the changes made to each indicator during the panel process, the reasons for those changes, and the final disposition of each indicator.

REFERENCES

Asch, S. M., E. A. Kerr, E. G. Hamilton, J. L. Reifel, E. A. McGlynn (eds.), *Quality of Care for Oncologic Conditions and HIV: A Review of the Literature and Quality Indicators,* Santa Monica, CA: RAND, MR-1281-AHRQ, 2000.

Brook, R. H., "The RAND/UCLA Appropriateness Method," *Clinical Practice Guideline Development: methodology perspectives,* AHCPR Pub. No. 95-0009, Rockville, MD: Public Health Service, 1994.

Kerr E. A., S. M. Asch, E. G. Hamilton, E. A. McGlynn (eds.), *Quality of Care for General Medical Conditions: A Review of the Literature and Quality Indicators,* Santa Monica, CA: RAND, MR-1280-AHRQ, 2000b.

Kravitz R. L., M. Laouri, J. P. Kahan, P. Guzy, et al., "Validity of Criteria Used for Detecting Underuse of Coronary Revascularization," *JAMA* 274(8):632-638, 1995.

Malin, J. L., S. M. Asch, E. A. Kerr, E. A. McGlynn. "Evaluating the Quality of Cancer Care: Development of Cancer Quality Indicators for a Global Quality Assessment Tool," *Cancer 2000,* 88:701-7, 2000.

McGlynn E. A., C. Damberg, E. A. Kerr, M. Schuster (eds.), *Quality of Care for Children and Adolescents: A Review of Selected Clinical Conditions and Quality Indicators,* Santa Monica, CA: RAND, MR-1283-HCFA, 2000a.

McGlynn E. A., E. A. Kerr, C. Damberg, S. M. Asch (eds.), *Quality of Care for Women: A Review of Selected Clinical Conditions and Quality Indicators,* Santa Monica, CA: RAND, MR-1284-HCFA, 2000b.

Park R. A., Fink A., Brook R. H., Chassin M. R., et al., "Physician Ratings of Appropriate Indications for Six Medical and Surgical Procedures," *AJPH* 76(7):766-772, 1986.

Schuster M. A., S. M. Asch, E. A. McGlynn, et al., "Development of a Quality of Care Measurement System for Children and Adolescents: Methodological Considerations and Comparisons With a System for

Adult Women," *Archives of Pediatrics and Adolescent Medicine,* 151:1085-1092, 1997.

Selby J. V., B. H. Fireman, R. J. Lundstrom, et al., "Variation among Hospitals in Coronary-Angiography Practices and Outcomes after Myocardial Infarction in a Large Health Maintenance Organization," *N Engl J Med,* 335:1888-96, 1996.

Shekelle P. G., J. P. Kahan, S. J. Bernstein, et al., "The Reproducibility of a Method to Identify the Overuse and Underuse of Medical Procedures," *N Engl J Med,* 338:1888-1895, 1998b.

Shekelle P. G., M. R. Chassin, R. E. Park, "Assessing the Predictive Validity of the RAND/UCLA Appropriateness Method Criteria for Performing Carotid Endarterectomy," *Int. J Technol Assess Health Care,* 14(4):707-727, 1998a.

1. ASTHMA[1]

Eve A. Kerr, MD, MPH and Kenneth A. Clark, MD, MPH

The general approach to developing quality indicators for asthma diagnosis and treatment was based on *Guidelines for the Diagnosis and Management of Asthma* (NAEPP, 1997). These guidelines, issued by the National Heart, Lung, and Blood Institute (NHLBI), are based on expert consensus and scientific literature review.[2] They are updates of the original guidelines published in 1991. The guidelines are being submitted for publication as of the time of this writing. The expert panel was convened by the Coordinating Committee of the National Asthma Education and Prevention Program (NAEPP). We also reviewed the standards issued by the American Thoracic Society for the diagnosis and care of patients with chronic obstructive pulmonary disease and asthma.[3] Further, we conducted a MEDLINE literature search to identify randomized controlled trials related to asthma and its treatment or the prevention and control of asthma exacerbations published in English between January, 1991 and April, 1997. We reviewed select articles dealing with areas where management controversy exists.

IMPORTANCE

NHLBI defines asthma as "a chronic inflammatory disorder of the airways in which many cells and cellular elements play a role, in particular, mast cells, eosinophils, T lymphocytes, macrophages, neutrophils, and epithelial cells. In susceptible individuals, this inflammation causes recurrent episodes of wheezing, breathlessness, chest tightness, and cough, particularly at night and in the early morning. These episodes are usually associated with widespread but variable airflow obstruction that is often reversible either

---

[1] This chapter is a revision of one written for an earlier project on quality of care for women and children (Q1). The expert panel for the current project was asked to review all of the indicators, but only rated new or revised indicators.
[2] Material reviewed is current to February 24, 1997.
[3] American Thoracic Society adopted the standards in November, 1986.

spontaneously or with treatment. The inflammation also causes an associated increase in the existing bronchial hyperresponsiveness to a variety of stimuli" (NAEPP, 1997). Asthma affects between 14 and 15 million Americans, and total estimated asthma-related health care expenditures for 1990 exceeded $6 billion in the United States (NAEPP, 1997; Weiss et al., 1992).

SCREENING

The reviewed literature does not support screening for asthma in asymptomatic patients.

DIAGNOSIS

The diagnosis of asthma is based on the patient's medical history, physical examination, and laboratory test results. Symptoms include cough, wheezing, shortness of breath, chest tightness, and sputum production. Precipitating and/or aggravating factors may include viral respiratory infections, exposure to environmental or occupational allergens, irritants, cold air, and drugs (e.g., aspirin), exercise, and endocrine factors. Severity of disease ranges widely, with some patients having rare symptoms and others having severe limitation of daily activity with frequent exacerbations. Consequently, the use of health care services and the impact of asthma on an individual's quality of life also vary widely.

Patients with a diagnosis of asthma should have a detailed medical history that addresses identification of possible precipitating factors such as viral respiratory infections, environmental exposures, inhalant allergens (NAEPP, 1997) (Indicator 1).

Spirometry, to document severity of airflow obstruction and establish acute bronchodilator responsiveness, should be performed for all patients in whom the diagnosis of asthma is being considered (NAEPP, 1997). The NHLBI guidelines recommend spirometry at the time of initial assessment (Indicator 2), and at least every one to two years to assess the maintenance of airway function (Indicator 3)(NAEPP, 1997). When considering alternative diagnoses, additional laboratory testing, such as chest x-rays and complete pulmonary function studies, may be considered in some patients. Skin testing and in vitro testing, to determine the presence of specific IgE antibodies to common allergens, is recommended for patients with persistent asthma who require daily therapy (NAEPP, 1997).

Measurement of peak expiratory flow (PEF) with a peak flow meter is generally a sufficient assessment of pulmonary function, particularly in cases of mild intermittent, mild persistent, and moderate persistent asthma. PEF provides a simple, quantitative, and reproducible measure of the existence and the severity of airflow obstruction. PEF meters are designed as tools for monitoring, not for diagnosis (NAEPP, 1997).

Since different brands of peak flow meters can give significantly different values and because lung function varies across racial and ethnic populations, there is no universal normative standard for PEF (NAEPP, 1997).

Peak flow monitoring can be used for short-term monitoring, management of exacerbations, and daily long-term monitoring. Two recent studies have shown that asthma self-management programs using peak flow monitoring as a component achieved improvements in health outcomes (Ignacio-Garcia and Gonzalez-Santos, 1995 and Lahdensuo et al., 1996). To date, however, studies that have isolated comparisons between PEF and symptom monitoring have not been sufficient to assess the relative contributions of each to asthma management (NAEPP, 1997).

TREATMENT

According to the NHLBI, asthma therapy has several components: patient education, control of factors contributing to severity, and pharmacological therapy, as well as the use of objective measures to assess the severity of disease and monitor the course of therapy (NAEPP, 1997).

Patient Education

Patient education is an essential component of successful asthma management. It should begin at the time of diagnosis and be integrated into every step of medical care (NAEPP, 1997). Asthma education programs have led to improved patient outcomes, including reduced hospitalizations and emergency room visits (Lawrence, 1995), fewer asthma symptoms and physician visits, and improvement in asthma

31

management skills (Kotses et al., 1995). However, the performance and adequacy of education is not easily assessed through medical record review. Therefore, the review and the indicators that follow will not focus on the patient-education component of care.

Pharmacological Therapy

Corticosteroids

Corticosteroids are the most potent and the most effective anti-inflammatory medication currently available. Inhaled forms are used for long-term control, while systemic corticosteroids are often used to obtain prompt control of the disease when beginning long-term therapy (NAEPP, 1997). Inhaled corticosteroids, at currently approved doses, are safe and effective for the treatment of asthma and are being utilized more frequently as primary therapy.

In any patient requiring chronic treatment with oral corticosteroids (i.e., exceeding one month in duration), a trial of inhaled corticosteroids should be attempted in an effort to reduce or eliminate oral steroids (Indicator 7). High doses of inhaled steroids should be used if conventional doses fail to permit oral steroid tapering. Pulmonary functions (PEF or FEV_1) should be monitored during tapering. Prolonged daily use of oral corticosteroids is reserved for patients with severe asthma despite use of high-dose inhaled corticosteroids. In patients on long-term oral corticosteroids, pulmonary function tests should be used to objectively assess efficacy.

Cromolyn Sodium and Nedocromil

Cromolyn sodium and nedocromil are mild-to-moderate nonsteroidal anti-inflammatory medications with a strong safety profile. Both compounds have been shown to reduce asthma symptoms, improve morning peak flow, and reduce the need for quick-relief $beta_2$-agonists. The clinical response to cromolyn and nedocromil is less predictable than the response to inhaled corticosteroids (NAEPP, 1997).

$Beta_2$-agonists

Inhaled short-acting $beta_2$-agonists are the medication of choice for the prevention of exercise-induced bronchospasm and for the immediate treatment of acute asthma exacerbations (Indicator 4)(NAEPP,

1997). There appears to be some consensus in the medical community that regular (i.e., four times daily) use of beta$_2$-agonists should be discouraged in favor of anti-inflammatory treatment (Indicator 5)(Executive Committee of the American Academy of Allergy and Immunology, 1993). One case-control study found an increased risk of death and near death from asthma associated with regular use of inhaled beta$_2$-agonist bronchodilators (Spitzer et al., 1992).

Inhaled long-acting beta$_2$-agonists are used as an adjunct to anti-inflammatory therapy for providing long-term control of symptoms, especially nocturnal symptoms, and to prevent exercise-induced bronchospasm (NAEPP, 1997). Long-acting beta$_2$-agonists are not to be used for exacerbations. The frequency of beta-agonist use can be a useful monitor of disease activity (NAEPP, 1997). Patient education regarding correct use is critical.

Methylxanthines

Theophylline, the methylxanthine principally used in treating asthma, provides mild-to-moderate bronchodilation. Monitoring serum theophylline concentrations is essential to ensure that therapeutic, but not toxic, doses are achieved (NAEPP, 1997). Recent evidence suggests that low serum concentrations of theophylline are mildly anti-inflammatory (Kidney, 1995). Sustained-release theophylline is mainly used as adjuvant therapy, and is particularly useful for controlling symptoms of nocturnal asthma. When there are issues concerning cost or adherence to regimens using inhaled medication, sustained-release theophylline can be considered as an alternative long-term preventive therapy, but is not preferred. Patients on chronic theophylline should have a serum theophylline determination at least once each year to decrease the risk of theophylline toxicity (NAEPP, 1997) (Indicator 8).

Leukotriene Modifiers

Leukotriene modifiers can be considered an alternative therapy to low doses of inhaled steroids or cromolyn or nedocromil for patients 12 years of age of older with mild persistent asthma. However, additional clinical experience and study are needed to establish their roles in asthma therapy (NAEPP, 1997).

Anticholinergics

Ipratropiium bromide may be an alternative bronchodilator for some patients who do not tolerate inhaled beta$_2$-agonists. It may also provide some additive benefit to inhaled beta$_2$-agonists during severe exacerbations (NAEPP, 1997).

Control of Factors Affecting Severity

Allergens and irritants may play a significant role in the symptoms of asthma for some persons. Because of the importance of allergens and their control in asthma morbidity and management, the NHLBI Expert Panel recommends that patients with asthma at any level of severity be questioned about exposures to inhalant allergens (e.g., animal allergens, house-dust mites, outdoor allergens). For persons with persistent asthma who require daily therapy, the Expert Panel also recommends skin testing or in vitro testing to determine the presence of specific IgE antibodies to indoor allergens (NAEPP, 1997).

Once it is determined (through history and/or ancillary testing) that allergy plays a role in the person's asthma, allergen avoidance should be the first recommendation (NAEPP, 1997). However, when avoidance is not possible and appropriate medication fails to control symptoms of allergic asthma, immunotherapy should be considered (NAEPP, 1997). A meta-analysis of 20 randomized, placebo-controlled studies has substantiated the effectiveness of immunotherapy in asthma (Abramson, 1995). Because immunotherapy is absolutely indicated in only a small subset of asthma patients, we have not developed an indicator on this topic.

Other factors that influence asthma severity should also be considered. Intranasal corticosteroids are recommended for the treatment of chronic rhinitis in patients with persistent asthma. Adult patients with asthma should be questioned about bronchoconstriction that is precipitated by aspirin or other nonsteroidal anti-inflammatory drugs. Nonselective beta-blockers (e.g., atenol and propranolol) can cause asthma symptoms and should be avoided by patients with asthma (Indicator 6).

Treatment of Asthma by Severity

The NHLBI guidelines state that therapeutic agents to prevent or reverse airway hyperresponsiveness are considered first-line therapy. Specific asthma therapy must be selected to fit the needs of individual patients. Treatment recommendations are based on severity of disease. However, it must be recognized that grading severity is not always straightforward. Criteria for determining the severity of asthma have been suggested by the NAEPP Expert Panel. They are summarized below and are based on 1997 NHLBI guidelines. The severity classification has been changed from the chronic mild, chronic moderate, and chronic severe groupings in the 1991 NHLBI guidelines to a four step system.

Mild Intermittent Asthma

According to NHLBI, mild intermittent asthma is characterized by:

- intermittent, brief (less than 1 hour) wheezing, coughing, or dyspnea up to two times weekly;
- asymptomatic status and normal PEF between exacerbations;
- brief exacerbations (from a few hours to a few days) with variable intensity; and
- infrequent nocturnal symptoms (no more than two times a month).

For these patients, asthma symptoms often occur following exercise, exposure to irritants or allergens, or respiratory infections. For patients with mild intermittent asthma, the use of short-acting inhaled beta$_2$-agonists on an as-needed basis usually suffices. However, if significant symptoms recur or beta$_2$-agonists are required for quick relief more than two times a week (except for exacerbations caused by viral infections or exercise-induced bronchospasm), the patient should be moved to the next step of care. Patients who experience exercise-induced bronchospasm benefit from taking inhaled beta$_2$-agonists, cromolyn, or nedocromil shortly before exercise (NAEPP, 1997).

Mild Persistent Asthma

According to NHLBI, mild persistent asthma is characterized by:

- symptoms greater than two times a week but less than one time a day;
- exacerbations that may affect activity; and

- nocturnal symptoms more than two times a month.

The NHLBI Expert Panel recommends that patients with persistent asthma at any level of severity should receive daily long term control medication. For persons with mild persistent asthma this is inhaled corticosteroids at a low dose, cromolyn, or nedocromil. Sustained-release theophylline is an alternative, but not a preferred, long-term control therapy. Leukotriene modifiers can also be considered, but their place in therapy is not fully established. Short-acting inhaled beta$_2$-agonists should be used as needed to relieve symptoms (NAEPP, 1997).

Moderate Persistent Asthma

According to NHLBI, moderate persistent asthma is characterized by:
- daily symptoms;
- daily use of inhaled short-acting beta$_2$-agonists;
- exacerbations that affect activity;
- exacerbations greater than or equal to two times a week that may last days; and
- nocturnal symptoms more than once a week.

There are at least three options for patients with moderate persistent asthma. The first option is increasing inhaled corticosteroids to a medium dose. Most patients will benefit from this strategy, though infrequent adverse effects may arise. The second option is adding a long-acting bronchodilator to a low-to-medium dose of inhaled corticosteroids. The bronchodilator may be either a long-acting inhaled beta$_2$-agonist (e.g., salmeterol) or sustained-release theophylline. Long-acting beta$_2$-agonist tablets, although not preferred, may be considered. The third option is to establish control with medium-dose inhaled corticosteroids, then lower the dose and add nedocromil. The panel reviewed literature on this third option and found some benefit in three studies and no benefit in another study. Therefore, this treatment option is not preferred. If symptoms are not initially controlled with these therapy options, then daily long-term control medications should be increased to a high dose of inhaled corticosteroids and a long-acting bronchodilator should be added (NAEPP, 1997).

Severe Persistent Asthma

According to NHLBI, severe persistent asthma is characterized by:

- continual symptoms;
- limited physical activity; and
- frequent exacerbations;
- frequent nocturnal symptoms.

Patients who are not controlled on maximal doses of long-acting bronchodilators and high doses of inhaled anti-inflammatory agents will also need oral systemic corticosteroids on a routine, long-term basis. The lowest possible dose must be sought and should be administered under the supervision of an asthma specialist (NAEPP, 1997).

Other Management Measures

The U.S. Preventive Services Task Force (USPSTF) recommends pneumococcal vaccination and regular influenza vaccination for those with chronic cardiac or pulmonary disease (USPSTF, 1996). The updated NHLBI guidelines recommend annual influenza vaccinations for patients with persistent asthma, but their earlier support for pneumococcal vaccine has been dropped due to insufficient evidence of benefit (Indicator 9)(NAEPP, 1997).

Care of an Acute Asthma Exacerbation

Patients at high risk of death from exacerbations should be counseled to seek immediate medical care rather than initiate home therapy. Patients at high risk include those with a history of:

- past sudden severe exacerbation;
- prior intubation;
- two or more hospitalizations for asthma in past year;
- three or more emergency care visits for asthma in the past year;
- prior admission for asthma to an intensive care unit;
- hospitalization or emergency care visit within the past month;
- current use of systemic corticosteroids or recent withdrawal from systemic corticosteroids;

- comorbidity from cardiovascular or chronic obstructive pulmonary diseases;
- serious psychiatric or psychosocial problems (NAEPP, 1997).

The NAEPP recommends that all patients seen in the emergency department or other urgent care setting should be evaluated with a complete history in order to identify factors related to high risk of mortality. This history should include:

- time of onset and cause of current exacerbation;
- severity of symptoms;
- all current medications;
- prior hospitalizations and emergency department visits for asthma;
- prior episodes of respiratory insufficiency due to asthma (Indicator 10); and,
- other potentially complicating illnesses such as cardiac or pulmonary disease or diseases worsened by systemic corticosteroid therapy (NAEPP, 1997).

Further, the NAEPP recommends that all patients presenting to the emergency department with an asthma exacerbation should be evaluated with at least one measurement of airflow obstruction:

- peak expiratory flow rate measured with a peak flow meter; or
- one-second forced expired volume (FEV1) determined by spirometry (NAEPP, 1997) (Indicator 11).

These measures are important for determining appropriate treatment. NAEPP recommendations also state that all patients with an exacerbation should have an initial physical examination of the chest to assess airflow (NAEPP, 1997) (Indicator 13). At the time of the exacerbation, patients on theophylline should have serum theophylline level measured (Indicator 12). All patients should receive initial treatment with inhaled $beta_2$-agonists (Indicator 14). Patients treated with $beta_2$-agonists who have an FEV_1 less than 70 percent of baseline should have an FEV_1 or PEF repeated prior to discharge (NAEPP, 1997) (Indicator 15). Patients should be re-evaluated, including PEF or FEV_1, after the initial dose of bronchodilator and after three doses of inhaled bronchodilator (60 to 90 minutes after initiating treatment). Patients who have persistent symptoms, diffuse wheezes audible on chest auscultation, and a PEF or FEV_1 < 40 percent of predicted or baseline should be admitted to the hospital because of higher risks of complications and mortality (Indicator 17) (McFadden and Hejal, 1995). Patients with a good response to inhaled $beta_2$-agonist treatment should be observed for 30 to 60 minutes after the last treatment to ensure stability prior to discharge (NAEPP, 1997).

Listed below are the NAEPP follow-up care recommendations for a patient who has been stabilized after an acute exacerbation:

- Treatment should be given for at least three days (NAEPP, 1997).
- Treatment regimen should include systemic corticosteroids for all patients with an FEV_1 or PEF less than 70 percent of baseline (or predicted) at discharge, and for all patients at increased risk for potential life-threatening deterioration (Indicator 16).
- A follow-up medical appointment should occur within three to five days of discharge (NAEPP, 1997).

Care of Patients Hospitalized for Asthma

Patients whose airflow obstruction does not respond to intensive bronchodilator treatment require close attention in the hospital. They should be closely monitored and should have oxygen saturation measured (Indicator 18). Supplemental oxygen should be given to most patients to maintain the oxygen saturation greater than 90 percent. Hospitalized patients should be followed during the acute phase of the exacerbation with lung function measurement (PEF or FEV_1) before and after bronchodilator therapy. Thereafter, PEF or FEV_1 should be measured at least once a day until discharge (NAEPP, 1997).

All patients with asthma who are admitted to the hospital should receive systemic corticosteroids (preferably via intravenous route) (Indicator 19) and $beta_2$-agonists (Indicator 20). The administration of intravenous methylxanthines to hospitalized adults is controversial (Huang, 1993), and is not generally recommended by the NHLBI guidelines (NAEPP, 1997). Oxygen should be given to all patients with an oxygen saturation less than 90 percent (Indicator 21); or with an FEV_1 or PEF less than 50 percent of predicted when arterial oxygen monitoring is not available. Patients with a pCO_2 greater than 40 should receive at least one additional blood gas measurement to evaluate response to treatment (Indicator 22). Chest physical therapy has not been found to be helpful for most patients, and is not recommended in the literature. Use of mucolytics (e.g., acetylcysteine, potassium iodide) should be avoided because they may worsen cough or airflow obstruction. Sedation (i.e., with anxiolytics and hypnotic drugs) should be avoided because of its respiratory depressant effect (Indicator 23). Since bacterial and mycoplasmal respiratory infections are thought to contribute only infrequently to severe exacerbations of asthma, use of antibiotics should be reserved for those patients with purulent sputum and/or fever (NAEPP, 1997).

FOLLOW-UP

Before discharge from the hospital, the patient's medication should be adjusted to an oral and/or inhaled regimen. This should occur when the patient is minimally symptomatic and has little wheezing on chest exam. The NHLBI recommends close medical follow-up during the tapering period, but does not specify a follow-up interval. Since the taper of most patients will be finished within 14 days, a follow-up visit within that time seems reasonable (Indicator 24) but is not supported by any clinical trial evidence. Discharge medications should include a short-acting inhaled beta$_2$-agonist and enough oral corticosteroid to complete a course of therapy or to continue until a follow-up visit. If inhaled corticosteroids are to be given, they should be started before the course of oral corticosteroids is completed (NAEPP, 1997).

REFERENCES

Abramson MJ, P. R. 1995. Is allergen immunotherapy effective in asthma? *American Journal of Respiratory Critical Care Medicine* 151: 969-974.

Barach Eric M. February 1994. Asthma in ambulatory care: use of objective diagnostic criteria. *Journal of Family Practice* 38 (2): 161-5.

Barker, LR. 1991. In: *Principles of Ambulatory Medicine*, Third ed. Baltimore, MD: Williams and Wilkins.

Casey K. June 1995. Acute severe asthma. How to recognize and respond to a life-threatening attack. *Postgraduate Medicine* 97 (6): 71-78.

Executive Committee of the American Academy of Allergy and Immunology. 1993. Inhaled beta-2-adrenergic agonists in asthma. *Journal of Allergy and Clinical Immunology* 91: 1234-7.

Huang D, et al. 1993. Does aminophylline benefit adults admitted to the hospital for an acute exacerbation of asthma? *Annuals of Internal Medicine* 119: 1155-1160.

Ignacio-Garcia J. 1995. Asthma self management education program by home monitoring of peak expiratory flow. *American Journal of Respiratory Critical Care Medicine* 151: 353-359.

Kidney J, et al. 1995. Immunomodulation by theophylline in asthma. *American Journal of Respiratory Critical Care Medicine* 151: 1907-1914.

Kotses H, et al. February 1995. A self-management program for adult asthma. Part I: Development and evaluation. *Journal of Allergy and Clinical Immunology* 95 (2): 529-40.

Lahdensuo A, et al. 1996. Randomised comparison of guided self management and traditional treatment of asthma over one year. *British Medical Journal* 312: 748-52.

Lawrence G. January 1995. Asthma self-management programs can reduce the need for hospital-based asthma care. *Respiratory Care* 40 (1): 39-43.

McFadden Jr ER. 13 May. Asthma. *The Lancet* 345: 1215-1220.

Nathan, RA. 1992. Beta-2 agonist therapy: Oral versus inhaled delivery. *Journal of Asthma* 29 (1): 49-54.

National Asthma Education and Prevention Program. February 1997. Expert Panel Report II: Guidelines for the diagnosis and management of asthma.

Rees J, et al. May 1995. Chronic Asthma-General Management. *British Medical Journal* 310 (27): 1400-1401.

Sherman C. December 1995. Late-onset asthma: Making the diagnosis, choosing drug therapy. *Geriatrics* 50 (12): 24-33.

Spitzer WO, et al. 20 February. The use of B-agonists and the risk of death and near death from asthma. *The New England Journal of Medicine* 326 (8): 501-506.

Weiss KB, et al. 26 March 1992. An economic evaluation of asthma in the United States. *New England Journal of Medicine* 326 (13): 862-6.

RECOMMENDED QUALITY INDICATORS FOR ASTHMA

These indicators apply to men and women age 18 and older who have chronic asthma, and exclude patients with only exercise-induced bronchospasm. Only the indicators in bold type were rated by this panel; the remaining indicators were endorsed by a prior panel.

Indicator	Quality of Evidence	Literature	Benefits	Comments
Diagnosis				
1. Patients with the diagnosis of moderate-to-severe asthma should have had some historical evaluation of asthma precipitants[1] within six months (before or after) of diagnosis.	III	NAEPP, 1997	Decrease baseline shortness of breath. Improve exercise tolerance. Decrease steroid toxicity.[2] Decrease number of exacerbations.[3]	This may result in improved control of asthma and less need for medications such as steroids, which have undesirable toxicities.[2]
2. Patients with the diagnosis of moderate-to-severe asthma should have baseline spirometry or peak flow performed within six months of diagnosis.	III	NAEPP, 1997	Decrease baseline shortness of breath.	By documenting the diagnosis with spirometry, one can initiate the appropriate therapy, minimize inappropriate use of medications, and assess future worsening or improvement.
3. Spirometry should be measured in patients with chronic asthma at least every 2 years.	III	NAEPP, 1997	Decrease shortness of breath. Improve exercise tolerance.	Sequential measurement spirometry is useful for therapeutic decisions. Knowing the person's baseline is useful for treatment of exacerbations.
Treatment (Therapy)				
4. Patients with the diagnosis of moderate-to-severe asthma should have been prescribed a beta2-agonist inhaler for symptomatic relief of exacerbations to use as needed.	III	NAEPP, 1997	Decrease shortness of breath. Prevent need for emergency room treatment.	Beta2-agonists are first-line therapy for asthma exacerbations. Asthmatics should have ready access to this therapy.

43

	Indicator	Quality of Evidence	Literature	Benefits	Comments
5.	Patients who report using a beta2-agonist inhaler more than 3 times per day on a daily basis (not only during an exacerbation) should be prescribed a longer acting bronchodilator (theophylline) and/or an anti-inflammatory agent (inhaled corticosteroids, cromolyn).	III	Executive Committee of the American Academy of Allergy and Immunology, 1993	Decrease baseline shortness of breath. Improve exercise tolerance.	This is somewhat controversial since some clinicians are still advocating chronic treatment with beta$_2$-agonists. However, chronic treatment with beta$_2$-agonists appears to increase bronchial reactivity and may contribute to asthma mortality.
6.	Patients with moderate-to-severe asthma should not receive beta-blocker medications (e.g., atenolol, propranolol).	III	NAEPP, 1997	Prevent worsening of shortness of breath.	Beta-blockade promotes airway reactivity.
7.	Patients requiring chronic treatment[4] with systemic corticosteroids during any 12 month period should have been prescribed inhaled corticosteroids during that same 12 month period.	III	NAEPP, 1997	Decrease steroid toxicities.[2]	There is a great deal of focus in the guidelines on the use of inhaled steroids and on reducing dependence on systemic corticosteroids.
8.	Patients on chronic theophylline (dose > 600 mg/day for at least 6 months) should have at least one serum theophylline level determination per year.	III	NAEPP, 1997	Decrease shortness of breath. Improve exercise tolerance. Prevent theophylline toxicity.	Clearance of theophylline can vary even within the same individual. Patients may therefore become sub-therapeutic or toxic on doses that were previously therapeutic. Toxicities include tremulousness and agitation, nausea, vomiting, and cardiac arrhythmias.
9.	Patients with the diagnosis of moderate-to-severe asthma should have a documented flu vaccination in the fall/winter of the previous year (September - January).	III	NAEPP, 1997; CDC, 1993	Prevent pneumonia secondary to influenza infection. Prevent asthma exacerbation.[3]	Influenza can precipitate exacerbations and lead to secondary pneumonia in patients with asthma.

Indicator	Quality of Evidence	Literature	Benefits	Comments
Diagnosis and Treatment of Exacerbations				
10. All patients seen for an acute asthma exacerbation should be evaluated with a complete history including all of the following: a. time of onset, b. all current medications, c. prior hospitalizations and emergency department visits for asthma, d. prior episodes of respiratory insufficiency due to asthma.	III	NAEPP, 1997	Prevent complications and medication toxicities. Reduce chance for future exacerbations. Prevent mortality.	Objective measurements are useful for treatment decisions. They help initiate appropriate level of therapeutic intervention and help direct treatment strategies.
11. Patients presenting to the physician's office with an asthma exacerbation or historical worsening of asthma symptoms should be evaluated with PEF or forced expiratory volume at 1 second (FEV_1).	III	NAEPP, 1997	Decrease shortness of breath.	Objective measurements are useful for treatment decisions. They help initiate appropriate level of therapeutic intervention, whether that be with beta2-agonists, steroids, or hospitalization.
12. At the time of an exacerbation, patients on theophylline should have theophylline level measured.	III	NAEPP, 1997	Decrease shortness of breath.	Theophylline clearance may vary to a great degree. Subtherapeutic levels in persons on chronic treatment may add to an exacerbation.
13. A physical exam of the chest should be performed on patients presenting with an asthma exacerbation in the physician's office or emergency room.	III	NAEPP, 1997; McFadden and Hejal, 1995	Prevent mortality due to asthma.	A silent chest may predict more severe asthma. A physical exam helps guide therapy by evaluating severity.
14. Patients presenting to the physician's office or ER with an FEV_1 or PEF < 70% of baseline should be treated with beta2-agonists before discharge.	III	NAEPP, 1997	Decrease shortness of breath.	The percentage cut-off for this and the next three indicators are achieved through expert opinion; 70% is generally felt to be a cut-off for moderately severe exacerbations. It is generally agreed, however, that beta2-agonists are first-line drugs in an exacerbation. Lack of improvement indicates the need for additional therapy. If baseline is not available, predicted will be used.

45

	Indicator	Quality of Evidence	Literature	Benefits	Comments
15.	Patients who receive treatment with beta$_2$-agonists in the physician's office or ER for FEV$_1$ < 70% of baseline should have an FEV$_1$ or PEF repeated prior to discharge.	III	NAEPP, 1997	Decrease shortness of breath.	Repeat measures assess response (or lack thereof) to therapy.
16.	Patients with an FEV$_1$ or PEF < 70% of baseline after treatment for asthma exacerbation in the physician's office should be placed on an oral corticosteroid taper.	III	NAEPP, 1997; McFadden and Hejal, 1995	Decrease shortness of breath.	Steroids have been shown to improve recovery, but little objective data exists to back up the appropriate cut-off. If patients do not improve significantly with beta$_2$-agonists alone, then the severity of the exacerbation warrants steroid treatment.
17.	Patients who have a PEF or FEV$_1$ < 40% of baseline after treatment with beta$_2$-agonists should not be discharged from the physician's office.	III	NAEPP, 1997; McFadden and Hejal, 1995	Prevent mortality from asthma.	The cut-off, though arbitrary, reflects severe asthma exacerbation. These patients require close supervision to prevent mortality.
Inpatient Treatment					
18.	Patients admitted to the hospital for asthma exacerbation should have oxygen saturation measured.	III	NAEPP, 1997	Prevent mortality. Prevent cardiac ischemia. Decrease shortness of breath.	Oxygen saturation identifies patients who are hypoxemic and for whom oxygen therapy should be initiated.
19.	Hospitalized patients should receive systemic steroids (either PO or IV).	III	NAEPP, 1997	Prevent mortality. Decrease shortness of breath.	Steroids improve recovery from severe asthma exacerbation. There is a debate regarding the preference of IV versus PO steroids.
20.	Hospitalized patients should receive treatment with beta$_2$-agonists.	III	NAEPP, 1997	Prevent mortality. Decrease shortness of breath.	These are first-line agents for treatment of broncho-constriction.
21.	Hospitalized patients with oxygen saturation < 90% should receive supplemental oxygen, unless pCO$_2$ > 40 is previously documented.	III	NAEPP, 1997	Prevent mortality. Prevent cardiac ischemia. Decrease shortness of breath.	90% is a conservative cut-off.

46

Indicator	Quality of Evidence	Literature	Benefits	Comments
22. Hospitalized patients with pCO$_2$ > 40 should receive at least one additional blood gas measurement to evaluate response to treatment, unless pCO$_2$ > 40 is previously documented.	III	NAEPP, 1997	Decrease shortness of breath. Prevent mortality.	CO$_2$ retention indicates poor gas exchange and fatigue, and these patients should be monitored closely for treatment response.
23. Hospitalized patients should not receive sedative drugs (e.g., anxiolytics), except if on a ventilator, physiologically dependent on sedatives, or in alcohol withdrawal.	III	NAEPP, 1997	Prevent worsening of shortness of breath.	Sedation may worsen exacerbation.
Follow Up				
24. Patients with a hospitalization for asthma exacerbation should receive outpatient follow-up contact within 14 days.	III	NAEPP, 1997	Prevent exacerbation recurrence.	NHLBI recommends follow-up but does not state a time interval. Two weeks seems reasonable since a taper off steroids is usually for approximately 2 weeks. Four weeks would be the outside range.

Definitions and Examples

[1] Asthma precipitants include pollens, molds, viral infections, exercise, animals with fur, birds, and house-dust mites (mattresses, pillows, carpets, and upholstered furniture).

[2] Toxicities of glucocorticoid therapy include fluid/electrolyte disturbances, peptic ulcer disease, ulcerative esophagitis, diabetes mellitus, glaucoma, psychosis, myopathy, osteoporosis, pancreatitis, impaired wound healing, adrenal atrophy, cataracts, and increased susceptibility to infections. (Barker et al., 1991).

[3] An asthma exacerbation is characterized by acute obstruction to airflow. Exacerbations may be initiated through exposure to allergens and irritants, influenza, pneumonia, as well as other unidentified factors. Patients become acutely short of breath, tachycardic, and if severe, use accessory muscles of respiration. Exacerbation could lead to death if improperly treated. Treatment for an exacerbation should begin at home with beta$_2$-agonists. Physicians need to evaluate the severity of the exacerbation in order to initiate appropriate treatment.

[4] Chronic treatment with systemic corticosteroids is defined as at least two prescriptions for systemic corticosteroids in a one year period or any continuous treatment with systemic corticosteroids for 30 days or more.

Quality of Evidence Codes
I   RCT
II-1   Nonrandomized controlled trials
II-2   Cohort or case analysis
II-3   Multiple time series
III   Opinions or descriptive studies

2. ATRIAL FIBRILLATION

Arleen Brown, MD

The quality indicators for atrial fibrillation were developed from recent reviews (Pritchett, 1992; Kudenchuk, 1996); results from the Framingham Study (Wolf, 1978; Kannel, 1982; Brand, 1985; Wolf 1991); and a consensus statement from the American Heart Association (Prystowsky, 1996). Additional sources were used for the anticoagulation quality indicators: guidelines from the Fourth American College of Chest Physicians (ACCP) Consensus Conference on Antithrombotic Therapy (Laupacis, 1995) and an analysis of pooled data from five randomized controlled trials of antithrombotic therapy in atrial fibrillation (Atrial Fibrillation Investigators, 1994). Where these core references cited studies to support individual indicators, we have referenced the original sources. We also performed narrow MEDLINE searches of the medical literature from 1985 to 1997 to supplement these references for particular indicators.

IMPORTANCE

Atrial fibrillation (AF) is the most common sustained arrhythmia encountered in clinical practice, with a prevalence of approximately five percent in persons over the age of 65 in the United States (Halperin, 1988; Furberg, 1994; Prystowsky, 1996). Hospital stays are longer than for any other arrhythmia, and in 1990, atrial fibrillation was the primary diagnosis in approximately 180,000 hospital admissions (Bialy, 1992).

The incidence of atrial fibrillation increases markedly with age. Data from the Framingham Study suggest that the prevalence of atrial fibrillation is 0.5 percent in the 50 to 59 year old age group and rises to 8.8 percent among 80-89 year olds (Kannel, 1982; Wolf, 1991). In addition to increasing age, atrial fibrillation is also associated with the presence of structural heart disease (such as rheumatic heart disease, heart failure, and coronary heart disease) and non-cardiac disorders. Valvular atrial fibrillation arises in the presence of valvular heart disease, most commonly rheumatic mitral stenosis. Nonvalvular atrial fibrillation occurs in the absence of mitral stenosis or valvular prostheses. With the decline of rheumatic valvular heart disease in this country, atrial fibrillation is most commonly found in patients with hypertensive and ischemic heart disease and heart failure.

Atrial fibrillation is associated with a significant increase in morbidity and mortality. There are a myriad of symptoms that may accompany atrial fibrillation, many of which can be disabling. In addition, the dysrhythmia is associated with a marked increase in risk of stroke, systemic emboli, and death. The rate of stroke in untreated patients with atrial fibrillation is approximately five times that of persons without atrial fibrillation. The attributable risk of stroke from atrial fibrillation is 1.5 percent for 50 to 59 year olds, rising to 30 percent for those aged 80 to 89 (Wolf, 1987). Risk factors for thromboembolism in persons with atrial fibrillation are discussed below.

SCREENING

There is no role for screening asymptomatic patients for atrial fibrillation.

DIAGNOSIS

Although many persons with atrial fibrillation may be asymptomatic, with the rhythm disturbance noted incidentally (Brand, 1985), others present with clear symptoms. Symptoms include fatigue, palpitations, dyspnea, chest discomfort, presyncope, and dizziness, but are often non-specific and may be difficult to attribute to atrial fibrillation. This is particularly true in persons with comorbid cardiac or pulmonary disease. While the symptoms of atrial fibrillation occur more frequently at heart rates over 150 beats per minute, some patients, particularly the elderly, may be symptomatic at normal heart rates because of a loss of organized atrial contractile activity.

Isolated atrial fibrillation tends to be transient and reversible and occurs in the presence of another event or illness, such as hyperthyroidism, acute alcohol intoxication, cholinergic intoxication, pulmonary conditions that produce hypoxemia (such as pulmonary embolus), and non-cardiac surgery. Atrial fibrillation is found in 9 to 22 percent of patients with thyrotoxicosis (Woeber, 1992). One study found that 13 percent of patients in atrial fibrillation with no obvious cardiovascular cause had thyrotoxicosis (Forfar, 1979). It is estimated that 35 percent of atrial fibrillation is due to alcoholism and binge drinking, especially in younger patients (Kostinen, 1990; Lowenstein, 1992). Stimulant drug use may also play an important role in atrial fibrillation in this age group.

Paroxysmal atrial fibrillation occurs intermittently and is unrelated to an acute event or illness. It may proceed to chronic atrial fibrillation, in which atrial fibrillation is the predominant rhythm. Primary (or "lone") atrial fibrillation, which denotes atrial fibrillation that arises in the absence of other preexisting conditions and with normal left ventricular function by echocardiogram, is a diagnosis of exclusion (Prystowsky, 1996). The majority of this chapter will focus on chronic or paroxysmal nonvalvular atrial fibrillation.

There is controversy about the prognosis of lone atrial fibrillation. Data from Framingham revealed that the relative risk of stroke was 4.1 compared with control subjects (Brand, 1985); while data from Olmsted County, Minnesota (Kopecky, 1987) showed no increased risk of stroke. However, the two studies defined lone atrial fibrillation differently and the study populations were significantly different. In Framingham, lone atrial fibrillation was defined as atrial fibrillation occurring in adults in the absence of an acute precipitating factor, coronary heart disease, congestive heart failure, rheumatic heart disease, or hypertensive heart disease. In contrast, the Olmsted County participants were all under 60 years old, included children, and excluded patients with hypertension, diabetes mellitus, chronic obstructive pulmonary disease, and other patients who were "ill." The Framingham patients were thus older and more likely to be chronically ill than those in the Minnesota study.

Because many conditions can precipitate atrial fibrillation, patients with new onset atrial fibrillation should be carefully evaluated for reversible causes. They should be closely questioned about stimulant drug use and alcohol use (Indicator 1). In addition, a laboratory evaluation for hyperthyroidism should be performed, including

51

a thyroid stimulating hormone (TSH) level (Forfar, 1979; Woeber,1992; Prystowsky,1996) (Indicator 2). A chest radiograph should be taken to evaluate the patient for cardiomegaly, left atrial enlargement, pulmonary edema, and other pulmonary processes that may predispose to atrial fibrillation (Indicator 3). Although echocardiograms have been recommended to evaluate the presence of structural disease when there is no evidence of underlying systemic or metabolic disease (Prystowsky, 1996), there are no studies on when echocardiogram is indicated in the management of atrial fibrillation.

TREATMENT

Physicians must consider three therapeutic goals for patients with new onset atrial fibrillation: 1) control of ventricular rate, 2) restoration and maintenance of sinus rhythm, and 3) prevention of thromboembolism. While rate control is the initial goal of management, the risks and benefits of therapy to restore sinus rhythm and prevent thromboembolism are largely determined individually. Therapy to maintain normal sinus rhythm remains particularly controversial. There is an ongoing NIH trial, Atrial Fibrillation Follow-up Investigation of Rhythm Management (AFFIRM), that will evaluate the relative benefits and risks of rate control alone versus attempting to maintain sinus rhythm (Prystowsky, 1996). The prevention of thromboembolism will be discussed in the "Follow-up" section.

Control of Ventricular Rate

Emergent electrical cardioversion is indicated in patients with new onset atrial fibrillation and a rapid ventricular rate complicated by concomitant hypotension, pulmonary edema, or evidence of ongoing myocardial ischemia or infarction. Electrical cardioversion is the treatment of choice for new atrial fibrillation when emergent rate and rhythm control are required.

In hemodynamically stable patients with chest pain or mild heart failure secondary to a rapid ventricular response, intravenous medications are indicated. Intravenous calcium antagonists (such as diltiazem or verapamil) or beta blockers (such as esmolol, propranolol, or metoprolol) often result in rapid rate control. Intravenous digoxin slows the heart rate at rest, but has a delayed onset of action, with onset at 60 minutes and full effect requiring up to six hours.

Restoration and Maintenance of Sinus Rhythm

There are limited data on how and whether sinus rhythm should be restored and maintained in treating new onset atrial fibrillation. Restoration of sinus rhythm may improve symptoms and hemodynamics, and may be associated with increased cerebral blood flow (Prystowsky, 1996). In patients with atrial fibrillation who have hypertrophic cardiomyopathy and other forms of severe diastolic dysfunction, restoring the atrial contribution to ventricular filling may alleviate the symptoms of heart failure and syncope, and reduce mortality (Kudenchuk, 1996). It is also assumed that maintaining sinus rhythm lessens the risk of stroke. However, the data for the efficacy of maintaining sinus rhythm on stroke prevention are limited.

Cardioversion may be achieved through electrical or chemical means. It is extremely difficult to compare methods and drugs for cardioversion based on the published literature. Recent-onset or paroxysmal atrial fibrillation often reverts spontaneously, and most patients with atrial fibrillation can be transiently cardioverted to normal sinus rhythm (Lown, 1967). However, after cardioversion, there are high rates of reversion back to atrial fibrillation, with less than 25 percent of patients maintaining sinus rhythm at one year (Suttorp, 1993). Electrical cardioversion has success rates of 70 to 85 percent, in selected populations, with declining rates as patient age and the duration of atrial fibrillation increases (Arnold, 1992; Van Gelder, 1991).

There are minimal data from randomized clinical trials comparing the efficacy of any one drug over the others for restoration and maintenance of sinus rhythm in new onset atrial fibrillation. Therefore, selection of an antiarrhythmic agent should be individualized and will depend in part on renal and hepatic function, concomitant illnesses and drugs, and cardiovascular function (Prystowsky, 1996). In addition, as discussed above, the efficacy of maintaining normal sinus

53

rhythm is unproven. For these reasons, our indicators will not focus on maintenance of sinus rhythm.

FOLLOW-UP

Chronic atrial fibrillation is defined as atrial fibrillation of greater than 48 hours known duration.

Rate Control

For long term rate control, there are several potential treatment options. Patients with depressed atrioventricular node function may have adequate ventricular rate control and have no need for further therapy. However, even among patients whose heart rate is controlled at rest, changes in autonomic tone may result in excessive rates during exercise and may contribute to a tachycardia-mediated cardiomyopathy.

While several studies have compared heart rates of patients on digoxin, beta blockers, and calcium antagonists, there are no data from randomized clinical trials comparing the efficacy of any one of these drugs over the others for controlling symptoms or maintaining quality of life (Prystowsky, 1996). Therefore, our indicators will not focus on methods for rate control in chronic atrial fibrillation.

Prevention of Thromboembolism

Thromboembolism is a common and potentially devastating complication of chronic atrial fibrillation. Seventy-five percent of the thromboembolic events associated with atrial fibrillation involve the brain (Kudenchuk, 1995). Stroke in the majority of patients with atrial fibrillation is believed to be due to embolization of stasis-induced thrombi formed in the left atrium, especially the left atrial appendage. However, large percentages of patients with atrial fibrillation also have hypertension and carotid artery stenosis, both of which are additional risk factors for stroke. As a result, 25 percent of strokes in this population are believed to be due to intrinsic cerebrovascular disease, other cardiac sources of embolism, and aortic arch atheroma. It is also noteworthy that there does not appear to be a difference in the stroke rates of atrial fibrillation patients with and without carotid stenosis. Thus, the literature does not support routine carotid ultrasound for patients with atrial fibrillation (Prystowsky, 1996).

Studies show that two groups of patients should definitely receive anticoagulant therapy: patients with valvular atrial fibrillation and those undergoing elective cardioversion. Patients with atrial fibrillation secondary to mitral valve disease (particularly mitral valve stenosis) have a 17-fold higher risk of a thromboembolic complications than age-, sex-, and blood pressure-matched controls, with 30 to 75 percent of this group sustaining an embolic event in the absence of anticoagulation (Wolf, 1978; Sherman, 1986; Siegel, 1987). Patients with chronic atrial fibrillation undergoing elective cardioversion without anticoagulation have a seven times higher risk of thromboembolism than those on anticoagulant therapy (Bjerkelund, 1969).

Recommendations for the majority of patients with chronic or paroxysmal atrial fibrillation, who do not fit into either of the above categories, are less clear cut. These patients can be stratified into those at low risk and those at high risk for thromboembolism. Pooled data from five randomized controlled trials suggest that the risk factors for stroke in patients with atrial fibrillation include prior stroke or transient ischemic attack (TIA), diabetes, a history of hypertension, age over 65, congestive heart failure, and coronary heart disease (Atrial Fibrillation Investigators, 1994; Stroke Prevention in Atrial Fibrillation Investigators, 1992a). In these patients, the annual risk of stroke is five percent or more. Age is a particularly important risk factor, and in patients over the age of 75, the risk of stroke without oral anticoagulation appears to outweigh the risk of intracranial hemorrhage on warfarin. In contrast, patients with atrial fibrillation under 65 years of age, who do not have risk factors for stroke, have an annual stroke risk of one percent or less. An intermediate group of patients, those between the ages of 65 and 75, have an annual risk of stroke of two to four percent. Additional echocardiographic predictors of stroke include left atrial enlargement and impaired left ventricular function (Stroke Prevention in Atrial Fibrillation Investigators, 1992b). The clinical factors and transthoracic echocardiogram can be combined to identify patients in atrial fibrillation with high risk of thromboembolism.

Transesophageal echocardiogram provides better visualization of the left atrial appendage and may identify thrombi or areas of stasis in the left atrial or left atrial appendage. However, there are insufficient clinical data to recommend routine transesophageal echocardiography for risk stratification for patients with atrial fibrillation (Prystowsky, 1996), and our indicators do not specify any mandatory use for transesophageal echocardiogram.

Use of Anticoagulation

Several recent randomized controlled trials have evaluated the efficacy of oral anticoagulation and antiplatelet agents for stroke prevention in atrial fibrillation. An intention-to-treat analysis of five randomized controlled trials[1] that evaluated warfarin compared to placebo showed a mean reduction in ischemic stroke of approximately 70 percent on therapy, using international normalized ratios (INRs) ranging from 1.8 to 4.2 (Atrial Fibrillation Investigators, 1994). There was an even greater reduction in the on-therapy analysis, and warfarin decreased the rate of death by 33 percent.

Warfarin can be difficult to take, requires frequent monitoring, and may require substantial dietary modification. However, the most significant risk of warfarin therapy is the risk of bleeding. Risk factors for bleeding on oral anticoagulants for atrial fibrillation vary from study to study, depending on the patient population (Fihn, 1993; Levine, 1995; Fihn, 1996; The Stroke Prevention in Atrial Fibrillation Investigators, 1996). Known risk factors for bleeding in patients on anticoagulant therapy include the intensity of the anticoagulation, the duration of therapy, and the use of other drugs that affect hemostasis (Levine, 1995; Fihn, 1996). There is some disagreement over the

---

[1] Atrial Fibrillation, Aspirin, And Anticoagulant Therapy Study (AFASAK), Boston Area Anticoagulation Trial for Atrial Fibrillation (BAATAF), Canadian Atrial Fibrillation Anticoagulation (CAFA), Stroke Prevention in Atrial Fibrillation (SPAF), Stroke Prevention in Nonrheumatic Atrial Fibrillation (SPINAF).

association between hemorrhage on warfarin and several other factors, among them increasing patient age, hypertension, prior gastrointestinal hemorrhage, renal disease, and a history of cerebrovascular disease (Levine, 1995; Fihn, 1993). In the five randomized controlled trials of warfarin and aspirin, a bleed was labeled major if it required a transfusion or hospitalization or if it involved a critical anatomic region, such as an intracranial or paraspinal hemorrhage (Laupacis, 1995). The combined risk of major bleeding for the patients in these five studies (mean age 65 years) was 1.0 percent in the control patients and 1.3 percent in the warfarin-treated patients. Among patients over 75, there was only one intracranial hemorrhage. However, other data suggest that older patients and those who are less closely monitored are more likely to have major bleeding. One study found that patients over 75 had a much higher risk of major hemorrhage during anticoagulation, using INRs of 2.0 to 4.5 (mean 2.7), than those younger than 75 (SPAF II, 1994).

The effectiveness of stroke prevention in atrial fibrillation is less clear for aspirin than for warfarin. Three clinical trials have evaluated aspirin versus placebo for stroke prevention. Using doses of aspirin ranging from 75 to 325 mg per day, there was an overall risk reduction of 25 percent (range 14 to 44 percent) (Petersen, 1989; SPAF, 1991; EAFT, 1993). However, direct comparisons have found aspirin to be significantly less effective than warfarin for preventing atrial fibrillation-related stroke (Petersen, 1989; SPAF, 1991; EAFT, 1993).

The following recommendations have been made by the American College of Chest Physicians (ACCP) Consensus Conference on Antithrombotic Therapy (Laupacis, 1995):

- All patients over 65 years old with atrial fibrillation and those patients under 65 years old with one or more risk factors for stroke (such as previous TIA or stroke; a history of hypertension, even if controlled; heart failure; diabetes; coronary heart disease; or thyrotoxicosis) should be strongly considered for oral anticoagulant therapy with a target INR of 2.0 to 3.0.

- Patients over 65 years old with atrial fibrillation and those patients under 65 years old with one or more risk factors for stroke who have contraindications to anticoagulation or who decline warfarin should receive aspirin at a dose of 325 mg per day.

- For patients in atrial fibrillation between 65 and 75 years old who do not have any risk factors for stroke, the decision between oral anticoagulants and aspirin should be based on patient and physician assessment of the potential benefits relative to the risk and inconvenience of therapy.

- Patients under 65 years of age with no risk factors for stroke can receive aspirin alone or no antithrombotic therapy.

Our proposed indicators on anticoagulation for atrial fibrillation stem from these recommendations (Indicators 4, 5, and 6).

Anticoagulation for Cardioversion

Both electrical and chemical cardioversion of atrial fibrillation can be complicated by systemic emboli. The risk of stroke in this situation is three to five percent. The likelihood of thromboembolism increases in older persons and in persons with a history of prior embolic events, coronary heart disease, heart failure, hypertension, and long duration atrial fibrillation (Bjerkelund, 1969; Prystowsky, 1996). No randomized controlled trials have evaluated the effectiveness of anticoagulation prior to cardioversion, however, as stated above, the rates of thromboembolism without anticoagulation range from 30 to 75 percent (Wolf, 1978; Sherman, 1986; Siegel, 1987).

Patients with atrial fibrillation of unknown duration or for more than 48 hours should receive at least three weeks of anticoagulation with warfarin prior to either electrical or pharmacological cardioversion and at least four weeks after cardioversion. Alternatively, immediate cardioversion preceded by intravenous heparin and followed by four weeks of warfarin may be used in those without thrombi on transesophageal echocardiography. Those with atrial thrombi should get warfarin if they are candidates for anticoagulation. If not, they should receive aspirin. The Assessment of Cardioversion Using

Transesophageal Echocardiography (ACUTE) Pilot Study suggested that transesophageal echocardiography (guided cardioversion with short term anticoagulation) was a safe means of providing cardioversion earlier than would be possible with conventional therapy (Klein, 1997). Although it is routinely suggested that persons with atrial fibrillation of recent onset (less than 48 hours) can be cardioverted without anticoagulation, emboli have been seen in patients cardioverted from atrial fibrillation of only a few days duration (Arnold, 1992). However, a recent study suggests that in patients who are clinically estimated to have had atrial fibrillation for less than 48 hours, there is a low likelihood of thromboembolism related to cardioversion (Weigner, 1997) (Indicators 7 and 8).

Monitoring anticoagulation

Patterns of monitoring warfarin are highly variable, and it is not known how frequently the INR must be monitored to attain stable control. Patients with atrial fibrillation newly started on warfarin should have an INR checked within one week (Errichetti, 1984). Most patients are followed at intervals ranging from two to five weeks. Patients with a stable INR can be followed at intervals of up to eight to ten weeks (Fihn, 1994). However, frequent monitoring may not always be necessary; in one study, 89 percent of patients required no change in warfarin dose on more than 50 percent of visits (Errichetti, 1984). Therefore, our indicators on monitoring anticoagulation focus on initiation of warfarin or changing warfarin in dose (Indicators 9 and 10).

REFERENCES

Arnold AZ, et al. 1992. Role of prophylactic anticoagulation for direct current cardioversion in patients with atrial fibrillation or flutter. *Journal of the American College of Cardiology* 19: 851-855.

Atrial Fibrillation Investigators. 1994. Risk factors for stroke and efficacy of antithrombotic therapy in atrial fibrillation: analysis of pooled data from five randomized controlled trials. *Archives of Internal Medicine* 154: 1449-1457.

Bialy D, et al. 1992. Hospitalization for arrhythmas in the United States: importance of atrial fibrillation. *Journal of the American College of Cardiology* 19: 41A.

Bjerkelund C. 1969. The efficacy of anticoagulant therapy in preventing arrhythmias due to DC electrical conversion of atrial fibrillation. *American Journal of Cardiology* 23: 208-216.

Brand FN, A. R., et al. 1985. Characteristics and prognosis of lone atrial fibrillation — 30-year follow-up in the Framingham study. *Journal of the American Medical Association* 254: 3449-3453.

Connolly SJ, et al. 1991. Canadian atrial fibrillation anticoagulation (CAFA) study. *Journal of the American College of Cardiology* 18: 349-355.

EAFT Study Group. 1993. European Atrial Fibrillation secondary prevention of vascular events in patients with nonrheumatic atrial fibrillation and a recent transient ischemic attack or minor ischemic stroke. *Lancet* 342: 1255-1262.

Errichetti AM, et al. 1984. Management of oral anticoagulant therapy. *Archives of Internal Medicine* 144: 1966-1968.

Ezekowitz MD, et al. 1992. Warfarin in the prevention of stroke associated with atrial fibrillation. *New England Journal of Medicine* 327: 1406-1412.

Fihn SD, et al. 1994. A computerized intervention to improve timing of outpatient follow-up: a multicenter randomized trial in patients treated with warfarin. National Consortium of Anticoagualtion Clinics. *Journal of General Internal Medicine* 9: 131-139.

Fihn SD, et al. 1996. The risk for and severity of bleeding complications in elderly patients treated with warfarin. *Annals of Internal Medicine* 124: 970-979.

Forfar JC and Toft AD. 1979. Occult thyrotoxicosis: a correctable cause of "idiopathic" atrial fibrillation. *American Journal of Cardiology* 44: 9-12.

Furberg CD, et al. 1994. Prevalence of atrial fibrillation in elderly subjects (the Cardiovascular Health Study). *American Journal of Cardiology* 74: 236-241.

Halperin JL, et al. 1988. Atrial fibrillation and stroke -- new ideas, persisting dilemmas. *Stroke* 19: 937-941.

Kannel WB, et al. 1982. Epidemiologic features of chronic atrial fibrillation: the Framingham study. *New England Journal of Medicine* 306: 1018-1022.

Klein AL, et al. 1997. Cardioversion guided by transesophageal echocardiography: the ACUTE pilot study. *Annals of Internal Medicine* 126: 200-209.

Kopecky SL, et al. 1987. The natural history of lone atrial fibrillation — A population-based study over three decades. *New England Journal of Medicine* 317: 669-674.

Koskinen P. 1990. The role of alcohol in recurrences of atrial fibrillation. *American Journal of Cardiology* 66: 954-958.

Kudenchuk PJ. 1996. Atrial fibrillation -- pearls and perils of management. *Western Journal of Medicine* 164: 425-434.

Laupacis A, et al. 1995. Antithrombotic therapy in atrial fibrillation. *Chest* 108: 352S-359S.

Levine MN, et al. 1995. Hemorrhagic complications of anticoagulant treatment. *Chest* 108: 276S-290S.

Lowenstein S, et al. 1992. The role of alcohol in new-onset atrial fibrillation. *Archives of Internal Medicine* 116: 388-390.

Lown B. 1967. Electrical reversion of cardiac arrhythmias. *British Heart Journal* 29: 469-489.

Petersen P, et al. 1989. Placebo-controlled, randomised trial of warfarin and aspirin for prevention of thromboembolic complications in chronic atrial fibrillation — the Copenhagen AFASAK study. *Lancet* 1: 175-178.

Pritchett ELC. 1992. Management of atrial fibrillation. *New England Journal of Medicine* 326: 1264-1271.

Prystowsky EN, et al. 1996. Management of patients with atrial fibrillation: a statement for healthcare professionals from the subcommittee on electrocardiography and electrophysiology, American Heart Association. *Circulation* 93: 1262-1277.

Sherman DG, 1986. The secondary prevention of stroke with atrial fibrillation. *Archives of Neurology* 43: 68-70.

Siegel R, et al. 1987. Effects of anticoagulation recurrent systemic emboli in mitral stenosis. *American Journal of Cardiology* 60: 1191-1192.

Stroke Prevention in Atrial Fibrillation Investigators 1991. Stroke prevention in atrial fibrillation study — final results. *Circulation* 84: 527-539.

Stroke Prevention in Atrial Fibrillation Investigators. 1992. Predictors of thromboembolism in atrial fibrillation: I. Clinical features of patients at risk. *Annals of Internal Medicine* 116: 1-5.

Stroke Prevention in Atrial Fibrillation Investigators. 1992. Predictors of thromboembolism in atrial fibrillation: II. Echocardiographic features of patients at risk. *Annals of Internal Medicine* 116: 6-12.

Stroke Prevention in Atrial Fibrillation Investigators. 1993. Risk factors for complications of chronic anticoagulation. *Annals of Internal Medicine* 118: 511-520.

Stroke Prevention in Atrial Fibrillation Investigators. 1994. Warfarin versus aspirin for prevention of thromboembolism in atrial fibrillation: Stroke prevention in atrial fibrillation II study. *Lancet* 343: 687-691.

Stroke Prevention in Atrial Fibrillation Investigators. 1996. Bleeding during antithrombotic therapy in patients with atrial fibrillation. *Archives of Internal Medicine* 156: 401-16.

Suttorp MJ, et al. 1993. Recurrence of paroxysmal atrial fibrillation or flutter after successful cardioversion in patients with normal left ventricular function. *American Journal of Cardiology* 71: 710-713.

The Boston Area Anticoagulation Trial for Atrial Fibrillation Investigators. 1990. The effect of low-dose warfarin on the risk of stroke in patients with nonrheumatic atrial fibrillation. *New England Journal of Medicine* 323: 1505-1511.

Van Gelder IC, et al. 1991. Prediction of uneventful cardioversion and maintenance of sinus rhythm from direct-current electrical cardioversion of atrial fibrillation and flutter. *American Journal of Cardiology* 68: 41-46.

Weigner MJ, et al. 1997. Risk for clinical thromboembolism associated with conversion to sinus rhythm in patients with atrial fibrillation lasting less than 48 hours. *Annals of Internal Medicine* 126: 615-620.

Woeber K. 1992. Thyrotoxicosis and the heart. *New England Journal of Medicine* 327: 94-98.

Wolf PA, et al. 1978. Epidemiologic assessment of chronic atrial fibrillation and risk of stroke: The Framingham study. *Neurology* 28: 973-977.

RECOMMENDED QUALITY INDICATORS FOR ATRIAL FIBRILLATION

These indicators apply to men and women age 18 and older who have atrial fibrillation.

Indicator	Quality of Evidence	Literature	Benefits	Comments
Diagnosis				

1. Patients presenting with new-onset atrial fibrillation[1] or atrial fibrillation of unknown duration should have documentation of the following in the medical record at the time of presentation:
  a. alcohol use; and
  b. stimulant drug use.
	III	Kostinen, 1990; Lowenstein, 1992; Prystowsky, 1996	Guide management; decrease symptoms.	No controlled trials directly evaluate the elements of quality in the history and physical for persons in atrial fibrillation. Identification of causes of isolated atrial fibrillation may eliminate the need for further evaluation. There is no evidence in support of the suggested time period.

2. Patients presenting with new-onset atrial fibrillation or atrial fibrillation of unknown duration should have a thyroid stimulating hormone (TSH) level checked within the first week of presentation.	III	Forfar, 1979; Woeber, 1992; Prystowsky, 1996	Guide management; decrease symptoms.	Atrial fibrillation is found in 9-22% of patients with thyrotoxicosis, a potentially transient and reversible cause of atrial fibrillation. There is no evidence in support of the suggested time period.
3. Patients presenting with new-onset atrial fibrillation or atrial fibrillation of unknown duration should have a chest radiograph performed in the first 24 hours after presentation.	III	Prystowsky, 1996	Guide management; decrease symptoms.	Chest x-ray assists further evaluation and treatment. No clinical trials directly assess the role of the chest radiograph in the evaluation of new onset atrial fibrillation. There is no evidence in support of the suggested time period.

64

Indicator	Quality of Evidence	Literature	Benefits	Comments
Treatment				

4. Patients with atrial fibrillation of greater than 48 hours duration who do not have contraindications to warfarin[3] should receive warfarin if they are:
  a. under 65 with one or more other risk factors for stroke;[2] or,
  b. 65 years of age or older.
	I, II-1, II-2, III	Petersen, 1989; BATAAF, 1990; Connolly, 1991; SPAF, 1991; Wolf, 1991; Ezekowitz, 1992; SPAF, 1992a; SPAF, 1992b; EAFT, 1993; Atrial Fibrillation Investigators, 1994; SPAF II, 1994; Laupacis, 1995; SPAF, 1996	Prevent stroke.	In a pooled, intention-to-treat analysis of five randomized controlled trials, control patients had an annual stroke rate of 4.5% while patients on warfarin had a 1.4% annual stroke rate. The risk of stroke must be balanced against the risk of major bleeding.

5. Patients with chronic atrial fibrillation[4] who have contraindications to warfarin or have declined warfarin therapy should receive aspirin if they are:
  a. under 65 with one or more other risk factors for stroke;[2] or,
  b. age 65 years or older.
	I, II-1, III	Petersen, 1989; Atrial Fibrillation Investigators, 1994; SPAF II, 1994; Laupacis, 1995	Prevent stroke.	The combined results of two primary prevention studies (AFASAK and SPAF II) show a 36% risk reduction on aspirin compared to placebo, but aspirin is less efficacious than warfarin.

6. Patients with atrial fibrillation who do not have contraindications to warfarin should be started on warfarin within one month of presenting with either of the following:
  a. new onset ischemic or embolic stroke; or
  b. new onset transient ischemic attack.
	I	SPAF, 1992b; EAFT, 1993; Atrial Fibrillation Investigators, 1994;	Prevent stroke.	In a pooled, intention-to-treat analysis of five randomized controlled trials, control patients had an annual stroke rate of 4.5% while patients on warfarin had a 1.4% annual stroke rate.

7. Patients with atrial fibrillation of greater than 48 hours duration who are undergoing elective electrical or chemical cardioversion should receive anticoagulation for at least 3 weeks prior to cardioversion.	II-2, III	Bjerkelund, 1969; Laupacis, 1995	Prevent stroke.	No randomized trials of anticoagulation prior to cardioversion; however, one cohort study (Bjerkelund) and several descriptive studies (see Laupacis) suggest that anticoagulants are indicated prior to elective cardioversion. Thrombus takes about 2 weeks to organize and become firmly adherent to the atrial wall.

65

	Indicator	Quality of Evidence	Literature	Benefits	Comments
8.	All patients with atrial fibrillation should receive anticoagulation for at least 4 weeks after cardioversion unless there are contraindications to anticoagulation.[3]	III	Bjerkelund, 1969; Laupacis, 1995	Prevent stroke.	In the postcardioversion period, forceful atrial and atrial appendage contractions may not resume until 2-3 weeks after sinus rhythm has returned. Anticoagulation prevents the formation of fresh thrombus in the left atrial appendage after cardioversion if the resumption of atrial contraction is delayed and/or if atrial fibrillation recurs after successful cardioversion.
Follow-up					
9.	Patients with atrial fibrillation started on warfarin should have an INR checked within 1 week of the first dose.	III	Errichetti, 1984; Fihn, 1994	Prevent stroke; prevent hemorrhage.	There is no evidence in support of the suggested time period. Timing of follow-up of INRs is rather arbitrary. Studies suggest that frequent monitoring is not always necessary, and that many visits and INR measurements were not associated with a change in warfarin dosage.
10.	Patients on warfarin should have an INR checked a minimum of every three months.	III	Errichetti, 1984; Fihn, 1994	Prevent stroke; prevent hemorrhage.	There is no evidence from RCTs in support of the suggested time period, but there is some expert consensus.

Definitions and Examples
_____

[1] New onset atrial fibrillation is defined as the first presentation of atrial fibrillation of known duration less than 48 hours.

[2] High risk for stroke includes one or more of the following risk factors (Atrial Fibrillation Investigators, 1994):

  a. Prior stroke
  b. Diabetes mellitus
  c. Hypertension - any of the following:

- At least three measurements on different days with a mean SBP>140 mm Hg and/or a
- mean DBP>90 mm Hg documented in the medical record
- A diagnosis of hypertension mentioned in the chart
- Documentation of chronic antihypertensive therapy

  d. Age >65 years old
  e. Heart failure — any charted diagnosis of heart failure
  f. Clinical coronary heart disease (angina or myocardial infarction mentioned in the chart)
  g Mitral stenosis
  h. Prosthetic heart valves
  i. Echo criteria:
  j. Left atrial enlargement (>4.5 cm)
  k. Impaired left ventricular function (ejection fraction <50% or LV dyskinesis, hypokinesis, or akinesis)

[3] Potential contraindications to warfarin: These may be either specifically documented in the medical record or may use clinician assessment of the contraindication:

   a. Previous hemorrhagic stroke at any time or non-hemorrhagic stroke within 1 month

   b. Known intracranial neoplasm, mass, or other intracerebral pathology (e.g. aneurysm, abscess)

   c. Bleeding within the past 4 weeks (including gastrointestinal bleeding, melena, epistaxis, any bleeding requiring transfusion; excluding menses and occult hemoglobin in stools)

   d. Suspected aortic dissection

   e. Bleeding diathesis (e.g. dysfunctional platelets, von Willebrand's disease, thrombocytopenia, clotting factor deficiency, hemophilia)

   f. Pregnancy

   g. Allergy/hypersensitivity to warfarin

   h. Notation of frequent falls in the medical record

   i   Concern about the patient's mental status and ability to adhere to the regimen and follow-up

   j. Any mention of contraindications to anticoagulation in the medical record

[4] Chronic atrial fibrillation: Atrial fibrillation of greater than 48 hour duration or of unknown duration.

Quality of Evidence Codes

I	Randomized Controlled Trial (RCT)
II-1	Nonrandomized controlled trials
II-2	Cohort or case analysis
II-3	Multiple time series
III	Opinions or descriptive studies

3. CEREBROVASCULAR DISEASE

Beatrice A. Golomb, MD, PhD

The development of quality indicators for stroke prevention and treatment began with a MEDLINE search of English language review articles from 1992 to 1996. More targeted searches on carotid endarterectomy, hypertension, antiplatelet therapy, anticoagulation, and thrombolysis were then performed to supplement the original group of articles. In addition, selected clinical studies referenced in review articles were retrieved when relevant to the development of specific preventive or therapeutic indicators.

IMPORTANCE

Stroke is a leading cause of death and disability in developed countries (Feinberg, 1996). The incidence of stroke is estimated at one to ten per 1000 persons aged 60 years and older (Brodedrick, Phillips et al., 1989; Phillips and Whisnant, 1992). New or recurrent stroke affects approximately 550,000 persons in the U.S. each year, for an average of approximately one stroke each minute (Post-Stroke Rehabilitation Guideline Panel, 1995; Brickner, 1996). Stroke is the third leading cause of mortality in the U.S. (Brickner, 1996), accounting for approximately 150,000 deaths each year (Taylor et al., 1996). Stroke accounts for ten to 12 percent of all deaths in industrialized countries (Bonita, 1992). Mortality among those who have had a stroke is approximately 17 to 34 percent at one month, and 25 to 40 percent at one year (Post-Stroke Rehabilitation Guideline Panel, 1995). Eighty-eight percent of deaths attributed to stroke occur in people over the age of 65 (Bonita, 1992). Stroke is also the leading cause of serious disability in the U.S. with over three million people living with disability from stroke (Post-stroke Rehabilitation Guideline Panel. 1995). Of those who survive to one year after the incidence of stroke, one-third will no longer be able to live independently (Humphrey, 1995). The economic burden of stroke was estimated to be $30 billion in 1993, with $17 billion in direct medical costs and $13 billion in costs associated with lost earnings (Taylor et al., 1996).

"Stroke" is a generic term for a clinical syndrome that includes focal cerebral infarction (ischemic stroke), focal hemorrhage in the brain, and subarachnoid hemorrhage. "Infarction" refers to necrosis defined at microscopic examination and inferred from neuroimaging (Phillips, 1992). Transient ischemic attacks (TIAs) are arbitrarily distinguished from strokes, and refer to ischemic deficits (acute, focal neurologic symptoms resulting from vascular disease) that persist for less than 24 hours (Humphrey, 1995; Gress 1994). The majority of TIAs last from five to 15 minutes (Kelley et al., 1992). Some events designated as TIAs by this clinical definition will have infarction demonstrated by computed tomography (CT) or magnetic resonance imaging (MRI) studies (Gress, 1994). The incidence of TIAs is 0.5 per 1000 people (Humphrey, 1995). The risk of stroke after TIA is highest in the first year, and approximately 30 percent in five years (Humphrey, 1995). In patients with carotid stenosis of unspecified degree, the risk of stroke is approximately ten to 12 percent in the first year after TIA (Humphrey, 1995).

SCREENING

Screening for reversible risk factors for cerebrovascular disease (CVD), specifically hypertension and cigarette smoking, is widely advocated because it may lead to treatment that reduces the rates of stroke and death. Hypertension and smoking are risk factors not only for cerebrovascular but for cardiovascular and other diseases, which increases the utility of screening for these factors. Additional discussion of the benefits of intervention for these risk factors is discussed below in the section on Primary and Secondary Prevention.

The physical exam (auscultation) for carotid bruits is neither sensitive nor specific for carotid stenosis. In one evaluation, specificity was 70 percent and sensitivity was 57 percent for 70 to 99 percent of stenosis cases (Humphrey, 1995; Brown et al., 1994). Because data do not clearly support intervention (i.e., carotid endarterectomy) to reverse even tight stenosis in asymptomatic patients, the utility of screening asymptomatic patients for CVD through auscultation of carotid bruits is currently limited (UPSTF, 1996).

Primary and Secondary Prevention

Hypertension

The most well-identified predictor of stroke, hypertension is a factor in nearly 70 percent of strokes (Bronner, 1995). Meta-analysis has shown a 10 to 12-fold increase in the risk of stroke for people in the high category of diastolic blood pressure (mean: 105 mm Hg) compared with the lowest category (mean: 76 mm Hg) (Bronner, 1995). Moreover, reduction in diastolic blood pressure has been shown to reduce the risk of cardiovascular events, particularly stroke, in persons aged 60 to 79 years (Phillips, 1992). Screening and treatment for hypertension are covered in another Chapter 5.

Smoking

Cigarette smoking is a major independent risk factor for both ischemic and hemorrhagic stroke. Smokers have a significant (50%) increased risk of stroke compared with nonsmokers, and the risk appears to increase in a dose-response manner (Bronner et al., 1995). The risk of stroke for former smokers is lower than that for current smokers, with reductions of 30 to 40 percent in the first two to five years after smoking cessation (Bronner et al., 1995). Screening for smoking, and smoking cessation, are covered in another chapter.

Anticoagulation for Atrial Fibrillation

Atrial fibrillation affects about one percent of the general population, six percent of people over age 65, and ten percent of those over age 75. Nonvalvular atrial fibrillation is estimated to cause 75,000 strokes each year in the U.S., with an annual stroke risk of approximately three to eight percent (Gorelick, 1995). Warfarin reduces the risk of arterial thromboembolism by an average of 70 percent (Feinberg, 1996; MAST-I Group 1995; Gorelick, 1995). There is consensus that anticoagulation in selected patients should be used to reduce risk of stroke with atrial fibrillation (Indicator 3 and 4) (Dalen, 1994). Use of anticoagulation for atrial fibrillation is covered in another chapter.

Other Measures

Although glucose intolerance is associated with increased risk of stroke, the preventive role of strict glycemic control remains uncertain (Bronner, 1995). The population attributable risk of stroke associated with obesity is 15 to 25 percent (Bronner, 1995). Some of this effect is probably modified by hypertension, dyslipidemia, and glucose intolerance, although an independent association has also been observed (Bronner, 1995). However, the effect of obesity control on stroke is uncertain. Evidence of the relationship between serum cholesterol level and risk of stroke is mixed. If trials with clofibrate are excluded, no appreciable association has been found between cholesterol-lowering treatment and risk of fatal or nonfatal stroke, although some studies have shown a trend toward benefit (Scandinavian Simvastatin Survival Study Group, 1994; Shepherd et al., 1995). Trials have shown clofibrate to be associated with an increased risk of fatal stroke and a decreased risk of nonfatal stroke (Bronner, 1995).

Observational studies have shown physical activity to be inversely related to risk of ischemic and hemorrhagic stroke in men and women (Bronner, 1995); however, this relationship could be mediated in part by a reduced ability to exercise in those with preexisting atherosclerotic disease. Use of aspirin in primary prevention in middle-aged individuals failed to demonstrate a significant positive or negative effect on the incidence of all types of stroke in two large trials. Moreover, in the Physician's Health Study, a significant increase in hemorrhagic stroke and a trend to increase in all types of stroke was noted. In the British Doctor's Trial, a significant increase in disabling stroke was seen. A meta-analysis of observational studies found no apparent association between risk of stroke and post-menopausal estrogen replacement therapy (Bronner, 1995). The role of antioxidants in stroke remains to be clarified. Because each of these associations are either weak or inconclusive, we will not address them in the quality indicators.

DIAGNOSIS

Neurological Examination

Stroke and TIA are largely clinical diagnoses, often primarily based on history. Current review articles delineating the diagnostic process for stroke and TIA do not focus on -- indeed, often fail to mention -- the neurological examination (Poole, 1994; Pryse-Phillips 1994). Evidence from one study on the utility of clinical examination found that history and physical exam together allowed accurate diagnosis in 77 percent of cases (Chimowitz et al., 1990); however, the majority of this may be derived from history alone, and 77 percent may be too low a sensitivity to preclude the need for routine use of neuroimaging. Formal scored neurologic exams such as the National Institutes of Health Stroke Scale or the Canadian Neurological Scale have been found to: 1) correlate with infarct size (Brott et al., 1989); 2) predict prognosis; and 3) demonstrate utility in guiding treatment -- for example, by identifying patients at higher risk of hemorrhagic transformation if treated with heparin or tissue plasminogen activator (TPA) (Toni et al., 1996). Findings from a neurological examination may appear consistent with a nonstroke etiology and may direct evaluation toward other diagnoses. Furthermore, an initial neurological examination will permit ongoing assessment of subsequent recovery or deterioration. Nonetheless, there are no data to verify that the physical examination changes therapeutic management if neuroimaging is routinely performed. Moreover, the difficulty of rating the neurological physical examination retrospectively on chart review is formidable enough to warrant excluding it from the quality indicators.

CT Scan or MRI

After a presumed stroke, CT or MRI studies are commonly recommended to differentiate hemorrhagic from ischemic stroke, because management for the two types of stroke may differ (Humphrey, 1995; Brown et al., 1994). Debate remains on whether CT is indicated in all instances of presumed stroke or TIA. The American Heart Association (AHA), like many others (Wardlaw, 1994), advocates the use of CT or MRI in all patients acutely, as seen in its Guidelines for Management of Patients with Acute

Ischemic Stroke (AHA, 1994). Opponents of this position cite the costs of CT and the data indicating that CT does not affect the rate of misdiagnosis (Allison, 1994). For this reason, we do not propose an indicator for routine use of CT in patients presenting with stroke, although routine use of neuroimaging is probably appropriate. However, thrombolytic, anticoagulant, and antiplatelet therapy are clearly inappropriate in hemorrhagic stroke, and an estimated 24 percent of hemorrhagic strokes may have been misdiagnosed as infarcts in the pre-CT era (Phillips, 1992; Drury et al., 1984). Because of this, we have included an indicator requiring that CT or MRI be performed before initiation of each of these treatments (Indicators 1 and 2).

TREATMENT

Treatment of Acute Stroke

There is no proven medical treatment for acute stroke. Dextran has not been shown to be beneficial, and trials of calcium antagonists, steroids, and glycerol are inconclusive (Humphrey, 1995). Heparin has been used for many years in the treatment of stroke, but the data supporting its use are inadequate (Wityk et al., 1994). Although many elect to treat mild stroke cases acutely with anticoagulation (Humphrey, 1995), there is currently no clear indication for heparin in acute stroke (Wityk et al., 1994; AHA, 1994). Therefore, we have not developed an indicator for the use of heparin. Thrombolytic therapy (which is discussed below) and neuroprotective agents may prove useful in selected patients, but investigation is ongoing to clarify the patient population for whom benefit most clearly exceeds risk. Data on aspirin have, until this year, been equivocal. However, results of the International Stroke Trial and the Chinese Aspirin Stroke Trial being reported this year will, it appears, give conclusive evidence in support of aspirin treatment (Dr. Jeff Saver, personal communication). Nonetheless, it would not be appropriate at present to include use of aspirin as a quality indicator.

Thrombolysis

Early studies failed to uniformly demonstrate benefit to stroke outcomes with thrombolytic therapy (Levine, 1992). Although instances

74

of sustained and significant neurological improvement have been demonstrated with thrombolysis (Hund, 1995), identification of the patient subgroup most likely to benefit is difficult (e.g., those with moderate-to-severe neurologic deficit and without extended infarct signs on initial CT scan) (Hacke et al., 1995). Recent results have not entirely settled the matter. Four trials of early thrombolysis after stroke were identified in MEDLINE for the period 1995 to 1996. One trial found a nonsignificant trend toward worse outcomes (i.e., both death and disability) in those assigned to thrombolysis (Donnan, 1996). A second trial found an increase in mortality in the group assigned to thrombolysis at ten days (p < .002) and at six months (p < .06) (Europe Study Group, 1996). Another trial found a "marginal" nonsignificant reduction in both death and severe disability with thrombolysis (MAST-I, 1995). The fourth trial found that some functional measures and neurologic outcome were improved with thrombolysis in selected patients; however, the authors cautioned that identification of the appropriate subgroup was difficult and that "therefore, since treating ineligible patients is associated with an unacceptable increase of hemorrhagic complications and death, intravenous thrombolysis cannot currently be recommended for use in an unselected population of acute ischemic stroke patients" (Hacke, 1995). Data suggest that there is benefit in moderate-dose TPA given early. Indeed, national guidelines on TPA use have been published by the AHA (1994) and the American Academy of Neurology (1996). Continued efforts may clarify more effectively which patients are suitable candidates for thrombolytic treatment, and the use of TPA as thrombolytic therapy may be appropriate for a quality indicator in the future.

Treatment of Hypertension in Acute Stroke

High blood pressure after acute stroke is common and often resolves spontaneously. Reduction in blood pressure may worsen outcome (Reid, 1993). Because of concerns that ischemic brain damage may be worsened with efforts to control blood pressure after stroke (Powers, 1993), the AHA recommends that hypertension in the setting of acute ischemic stroke be treated rarely and cautiously (Emergency Cardiac Care Committee and

Subcommittees 1992; O'Connell, 1996). Treatment may be acceptable in the following circumstances:

1) systolic blood pressure exceeding 220 mm Hg, or diastolic blood pressure exceeding 130 mm Hg;

2) presumed hypertensive encephalopathy;

3) myocardial ischemia;

4) congestive heart failure;

5) worsening renal function;

6) aortic dissection;

7) proven cerebral hemorrhage (Humphrey, 1995; Wityk, 1994).

Some maintain that pre-stroke antihypertensive treatment should be continued in the post-stroke period (O'Connell, 1996), but there is agreement that no treatment should be added merely for management of acute elevations of blood pressure, barring exceptional circumstances. Because of the difficulties of retrospectively ascertaining by chart review an exceptional circumstance such as "presumed hypertensive encephalopathy," and because of the ongoing debate on the advisability of continuing prior antihypertensive treatment during the acute stroke period, no indicator on the use of antihypertensive treatment in acute stroke has been formulated.

Treatment of Known Cerebrovascular Disease: Secondary Prevention

The risk of stroke in patients with a carotid stenosis who have had a TIA is approximately ten percent per year (Humphrey, 1995). The risk of stroke in patients with a previous hemispheric stroke is five to 20 percent per year, with an average five-year recurrence rate of 50 percent. (Moore, 1993). Therefore, there is a need for interventions that reduce the high rates of stroke in those with prior symptomatic CVD.

Carotid Doppler/Duplex Ultrasound to Detect Carotid Stenosis

The North American Symptomatic Carotid Endarterectomy Trial (NASCET, 1991) and the European Carotid Surgery Trial (ECST, 1991) found that patients with a TIA or nondisabling stroke involving carotid symptoms, and with 70 to 99 percent internal carotid stenosis on the appropriate side, had 75 percent fewer strokes after carotid endarterecomy than with antiplatelet medication alone over a two to three year follow-up period. The risk of post-TIA stroke was reduced to two to three percent per year (Humphrey, 1995; North American Symptomatic Carotid Endarterectomy Trial Collaborators, 1991; European Carotid Surgery Trialists' Collaborative Group 1991) with an absolute risk reduction in ipsilateral stroke of 17 percent in NASCET (North American Symptomatic Carotid Endarterectomy Trial Collaborators, 1991). For this reason, it is recommended that patients who have suffered a TIA or stroke with recovery and who have a tight symptomatic stenosis should be offered surgery, with an explanation of the risks and benefits (Humphrey, 1995; Ad Hoc Committee, 1995). The reported benefits depended on a perioperative (30 day) complication rate of stroke or death of no more than six percent, and a perioperative rate of major stroke or death of less than two percent (Barnett, 1995). Surgical risk of carotid endarterectomy varies from one to 25 percent (Humphrey, 1995) and is institution- and surgeon-specific. Benefit is greatest if surgery is performed soon after TIA or stroke with recovery, because the risk of a recurrent event is highest in the first six months after an initial event. Therefore, it has been recommended that patients be assessed within a few days of symptoms and prepared for surgery, if appropriate, within two weeks after TIA and six to eight weeks after strokes with recovery (Indicator 6) (Humphrey, 1995).

In a European trial of carotid surgery, the surgical risk was found to outweigh the benefit if there was symptomatic carotid stenosis of 29 percent or less (European Carotid Surgery Trialists' Collaborative Group, 1991). The AHA has issued guidelines that identify carotid endarterectomy as inappropriate in patients with the following conditions:

1) moderate stroke with stenosis of less than 50 percent, not on aspirin;

2) single TIA with stenosis of less than 50 percent, not on aspirin;

3) high-risk patient with multiple TIAs and stenosis of less than 50 percent, not on aspirin;

4) high-risk patient with mild or moderate stroke and stenosis of less than 50 percent, not on aspirin;

5) global ischemic symptoms with stenosis of less than 50 percent; or,

6) acute dissection, asymptomatic on heparin (Ad Hoc Committee AHA, 1995).

The relative harm or benefit associated with carotid endarterectomy in patients with intermediate degrees of stenosis remains to be clarified.

Experts agree that the results of Doppler/duplex ultrasound are highly operator-dependent. Nonetheless, patients with carotid-distribution TIAs, small stroke, or stroke with recovery merit evaluation with Doppler/duplex ultrasound to detect severe carotid stenosis, so that candidacy for carotid endarterectomy can be determined (Indicator 5) (Humphrey, 1995; Wityk, 1994). There is no consensus that routine arteriography is needed before carotid endarterectomy (Dawson, 1993). Because morbidity and mortality from carotid endarterectomy is operator-dependent, the surgeon's skill must be taken into account in the final decision to perform carotid endarterectomy; however, referral for endarterectomy is clearly appropriate. Because of the potential difficulties of operationalizing "small stroke" and "stroke with recovery," we have confined our quality indicator to referral for carotid endarterectomy in persons diagnosed with TIA.

Antiplatelet Agents

Patients with TIA or stroke with recovery merit antiplatelet treatment, usually with aspirin. Patients with monocular or hemispheric TIAs have a stroke risk of ten to 30 percent within one year of symptom onset, which continues at six percent per year thereafter, and an overall stroke risk of 35 to 50 percent within five years of symptom onset (Moore, 1993). In multiple studies (The Canadian Cooperative Study Group, 1978; Bousser et al., 1983; UK-TIA Study Group, 1991; ESPS, 1987; ATC, 1994) and one meta-analysis (Sze et al., 1988), aspirin has been shown to reduce the combined risk of stroke and death in patients with TIA by 15 to 42 percent. Data are inconclusive on the optimal dose of aspirin. Ticlopidine may be more effective than aspirin but may cause skin rash, diarrhea, and reversible neutropenia or, occasionally, irreversible bone marrow failure (Humphrey, 1995). Therefore, it is usually reserved for patients who are allergic to aspirin or who have had cerebrovascular events while taking aspirin. Some studies have shown little or no effect of aspirin on stroke risk in women (The Canadian Cooperative Study Group, 1978; Sherman, 1992; UK-TIA Study Group, 1988), which is akin to the finding by some of no benefit from aspirin for secondary prevention of myocardial infarction in women (Breddin et al., 1980). However, other trials, such as the French "AICLA" studies, have found aspirin to provide a magnitude of stroke risk reduction in women comparable with that seen in men (Bousser et al., 1983).

Anticoagulation

In patients with TIA, nonhemorrhagic small stroke, or stroke with recovery, warfarin is indicated for persons with definite cardiac emboli or atrial fibrillation (Humphrey, 1995). In these persons, warfarin has been found to reduce the risk of subsequent stroke by 60 to 70 percent compared with placebo (Antiplatelet Trialists' Collaboration, 1994). The risk of serious bleeding was three percent per year, with 1.2 percent intracranial bleeds. This compares with a non-significant, 17 percent reduction in stroke with 300 mg/day of aspirin. Anticoagulation for atrial fibrillation is addressed in another chapter. Difficulty in identifying the presence or absence of a definite cardiac source from chart abstraction precludes development of a quality indicator for anticoagulation for embolic disease. Moreover, while some recommend immediate anticoagulation for mild defects, with an 11 day delay in initiation for more severe defects (Humphrey, 1995), timing will not be included in the quality indicators because of the potential difficulties in quantifying severity of stroke from medical record abstraction.

FOLLOW-UP

Antihypertensive Treatment

Data on the treatment of hypertension after stroke are mixed. Some evidence suggests that there is benefit in blood pressure reduction. Other studies have found a J-shaped relationship between post-stroke diastolic blood pressure and stroke recurrence, with an optimal diastolic pressure of 80 to 85 mm Hg. One study found no reduction in recurrence with antihypertensive treatment (O'Connell, 1996). Current evidence does not demonstrate that benefits of blood pressure reduction after stroke clearly exceed risks. For this reason, no indicator has been generated regarding blood pressure reduction as a secondary prevention measure.

Rehabilitation

It is widely agreed that efforts to restore function through post-stroke rehabilitation are important, and guidelines such as those by the Agency for Health Care Policy and Research have been issued (DHHS, 1995). Most gains occur within the first six months, although minimal additional improvement may occur for an additional six months. Patients are viewed as unsuitable for rehabilitation if their functional loss is minimal, or if their "rehabilitation potential" is low due to loss of cognitive skills or other severe deficits in which meaningful recovery is unlikely. Unfortunately, assessment of the potential for rehabilitation is an inexact science (Post-stroke Rehabilitation Guideline Panel, 1995; Brummel-Smith, 1995) and would be difficult to ascertain from medical record review. Therefore, no indicators have been developed on the use of post-stroke rehabilitation.

Smoking Cessation

Smoking promotes atherosclerosis and is a leading risk factor for CVD (DHHS, 1989). General counseling of smokers is covered in another chapter. Although no studies exist to demonstrate the benefit of smoking cessation in known CVD, smoking has been shown to be related to the likelihood of first stroke in a dose-dependent manner (Bronner et al., 1995). Additionally, there is general consensus that patients at risk for stroke should not smoke. Our indicators specify the need for smoking cessation counseling in patients who have presented with TIA (Futrell and Millikan, 1996) (Indicators 7 and 8). Although it is appropriate to provide smoking cessation counseling to patients who have had a small stroke and who remain functional, the difficulty of estimating the stroke size and of understanding patients post-stroke functional status from a retrospective review of the medical record

80

makes it complicated to write a counseling indicator for all post-stroke patients.

REFERENCES

Ad Hoc Committee American Heart Association. 1995. Guidelines for carotid endarterectomy. *Stroke* 26: 188-201.

Allison S. 1994. Is routine computed tomography in strokes unnecessary? Costs outweight benefits. *British Medical Journal* 309: 1498-1500.

Antiplatelet Trialists' Collaboration. 1994. Collaborative overview of randomised trials of antiplatelet therapy--I: Prevention of death, myocardial infarction, and stroke by prolonged antiplatelet therpay in various categories of patients. *British Medical Journal* 308: 81-106.

Barnett H, and Meldrum H. 1995. Update on carotid endarterectomy. *Current Opinion in Cardiology* 10: 511-516.

Bonita R. 1992. Epidemiology of stroke. *The Lancet* 339: 342-344.

Bousser M, Eschwege E, Haguenau M, et al. 1983. "AICLA" controlled trial of aspirin and dipyridamole in the secondary prevention of atherothrombotic cerebral ischemia. *Stroke* 14: 5-14.

Breddin K, Loew D, Lechner K, et al. 1980. The German-Austrian Aspirin trial: a comparison of acetylsalicylic acid, placebo and phenprocoumon in secondary prevention of myocardial infarction. *Circulation* 62 (suppl V): V63-71.

Brickner M. 1996. Cardioembolic stroke. *American Journal of Medicine* 100: 465-74.

Brodedrick J, Phillips S, et al. *Stroke* 1611-1626.

Bronner L, Kanter D, and Manson J. 1995. Primary prevention of stroke. *The New England Journal of Medicine* 333: 1392-1400.

Brott T, Adams H, et al. 1989. Developing measurements of acute cerebral infarction: a clinical examination scale. *Stroke* 20: 864-870.

Brown R, Evans B, and Wiebers D et al. 1994. Transient ischemic attack and minor ischemic stroke: An algorithm for evaluation and treatment. *Mayo Clinic Proceedings* 1027-39.

Brummel-Smith K. 15 February. Management of the poststroke patient. *Hospital Practice* 42-52.

Chimowitz, M, E Logigian, et al. 1990. The accuracy of bedside neurological diagnosis. *Annals of Neurology* 28: 78-85.

Dalen J. 1994. Atrial fibrillation: reducing stroke risk with low-dose anticoagulation. *Geriatrics* 49: 24-32.

Dawson D, Zierler E, Strandness E, Clowes A, and Kohler T. The role of duplex scanning and arteriography before carotid endarterectomy: A prospective study. *Journal of Vascular Surgery* 193 (18): 673-83.

Donnan G, Davis S, Chambers B, et al. 1996. Streptokinase for acute ischemic stroke with relationship to time of administration: Australian Streptokinase (ASK) Trial Study Group. *Journal of the American Medical Association* 276: 961-6.

Drury I, Whisnant J, and Garraway W. 1984. Primary intracerebral hemorrhage: impact of CT on incidence. *Neurology* 34: 653-657.

Emergency Cardiac Care Committee and Subcommittees AHA. 1992. Guidelines for cardiopulmonary resuscitation and emergency cardiac care. Part IV. Special resuscitation situations: stroke. *Journal of the American Medical Association* 268: 2242-4.

Europe Study Group. 1996. Thrombolytic therapy with streptokinase in acute ischemic stroke.The Multicenter Acute Stroke Trial--Europe Study Group. *New England Journal of Medicine* 335: 145-5.

European Carotid Surgery Trialists' Collaborative Group. 1991. MRC European Carotid Surgery Trial: interim results for symptomatic patients with severe (70-99%) or with mild (0-29%) carotid stenosis. *The Lancet* 337: 1235-1243.

European Stroke Prevention Study Group. 1987. ESPS: principal end points. *The Lancet* 2: 1351-54.

Feinberg W. 1996. Primary and secondary stroke prevention. *Current Opinion in Neurology* 9: 46-52.

Gorelick P. 1995. Stroke prevention. *Archives of Neurology* 52: 347-355.

Gress D. 1994. Stroke: Revolution in therapy. *Western Journal of Medicine* 161: 288-291.

Hacke W, Kaste M, Fieschi C, et al. 1995. Intravenous thrombolysis with recombinant tissue plasminogen activator for acute hemispheric stroke. The European Cooperative Acute Stroke Study (ECASS). *Journal of the American Medical Association* 274: 1017-25.

Humphrey P. 1995. Management of transient ischaemic attacks and stroke. *Postgraduate Medical Journal* 71: 577-84.

Hund E, Grau A, and Hacke W. 1995. Neurocritical care for acute ischemic stroke. *Neurol Clin* 13: 511-527.

Kelley R, and Berger J. 1992. TIA and minor stroke. *Postgraduate Medicine* 91: 197-202.

Levine S, and Brott T. 1992. Thrombolytic therapy in cerebrovascular disorders. *Progress in Cardiovascular Diseases* 34: 235-262.

Meissner I, and Meyer F. 1994. Carotid stenosis and carotid endarterectomy. *Cerebrovascular and Brain Metabolism Review* 6: 163-179.

Moore W. 1993. Carotid endarterectomy for prevention of stroke. *Western Journal of Medicine* 159: 37-43.

Multicentre Acute Stroke Trial--Italy (MAST-I) Group. 1995. Randomised controlled trial of streptokinase, aspirin, and combination of both in treatment of acute ischaemic stroke. *Lancet* 346: 1509-14.

North American Symptomatic Carotid Endarterectomy Trial Collaborators. 1991. Beneficial effect of carotid endarterectomy in symptomatic patients with high-grade stensosis. *New England Journal of Medicine* 325: 445-453.

O'Connell J, and Gray C. 1996. Treatment of post-stroke hypertension: A practical guide. *Drugs and Aging* 8: 408-415.

Phillips S, and Whisnant J. 1992. Hypertension and the brain. *Archives of Internal Medicine* 152: 938-945.

Poole R, and Chimowitz M. 1994. Ischemic stroke and TIA: Clinical clues to common causes. *Geriatrics* 49: 37-42.

Post-stroke Rehabilitation Guideline Panel. 1995. Post-stroke rehabilitation: Assessment, referral and patient management. *American Family Physician* 52: 461-470.

Powers W. 1993. Acute hypertension after stroke. *Neurology* 43: 461-7.

Pryse-Phillips W, and Yegappan M. 1994. Management of acute stroke. *Postgraduate Medicine* 96: 75-85.

Quality Standards Subcommittee of the American Academy of Neurology. 1996. Practice advisory -- throbolytic therapy for acute ischemic stroke. *Neurology* 47: 835-839.

Reid J. 1993. Hypertension and stroke: opportunities for prevention and prospects for protection. *Journal of Hypertension* 11: S2-S6.

Scandinavian Simvastatin Survival Study Group. 1994. Randomised trial of cholesterol lowering in 4444 patients with coronary heart disease: The Scandinavian Simvastatin Survival Study (4S). *Lancet* 344: 1383-9.

Schneider L, Libman R, and Kanner R. 1996. Utility of repeat brain imaging in stroke. *American Journal of Neuroradiology* 17: 1259-1263.

Shepherd J, Cobbe S, et al. 1995. Prevention of coronary heart disease with pravastatin in men with hypercholesterolemia. *New England Journal of Medicine* 333 (20): 1301-7.

Sherman DG, Dyken ML, Fisher M, Gent M, Harrison M, and Hart RG. 1992. Antithrombotic therapy for cerebrovascular disorders. *Chest* 102: 529S-537S.

Special Writing Group of the Stroke Council: American Heart Association (1994) "Guidelines for the management of patients with acute ischemic stroke" Stroke 25: 1901-1914.

Special Writing Group of the Stroke Council: American Heart Association (1994) "Guidelines for thrombolytic therapy for acute stroke" Stroke 27: 1711-1718.

Sze P, Reitman D, Pincus M, Sacks H, and Chalmers T. 1988. Antiplatelet agents in the secondary prevention of stroke: Meta-analysis of the randomized controlled trials. *Stroke* 19: 436-442.

Taylor T, Davids P, Torner J, Holmes J, Meyer J, and Jacobson M. 1996. Lifetime cost of stroke in the United States. *Stroke* 27: 1459-1466.

The Canadian Cooperative Study Group. 1978. A randomized trial of aspirin and sulfinpyrazone in threatened stroke. *New England Journal of Medicine* 9: 309-18.

Toni, D, M Fiorelli, et al. 1996. Hemorrhagic transformation of brain infarct; predictability in the first 5 hours from stroke onset and influence on clinical outcome. *Neurology* 46: 341-345.

UK-TIA Study Group. 1991. The United Kingdom transient ischaemic attack (UK-TIA) aspirin trial: final results. *J Neurol Neurosurg Psychiatry* 54: 1044-54.

UK-TIA Study Group. 1988. United Kingdom transient ischaemic attack (UK-TIA) aspirin trial: interim results. *British Medical Journal* 296: 315-20.

US Department of Health and Human Services. Clinical practice guideline #16: Post-stroke rehabilitation. *AHCPR*

US Preventative Services Task Force. 1996. *Guide to Clinical Preventative Services, 2nd ed.* Baltimore: Williams & Wilkins.

Wardlaw J. 1994. Is routine computed tomography in strokes unnecessary. *British Medical Journal* 309: 1498-500.

RECOMMENDED QUALITY INDICATORS FOR CEREBROVASCULAR DISEASE

These indicators apply to men and women age 18 and older.

Indicator	Quality of Evidence	Literature	Benefits	Comments
Diagnosis				
1. Patients who receive thrombolytic therapy[4] for treatment of acute stroke should receive a head CT or MRI after presenting with stroke and before initiation of thrombolytic treatment.	III	Phillips, 1992	Reduce complications of treatment.	CT or MRI is needed to reliably distinguish hemorrhagic from thrombotic stroke. Thrombolysis is contraindicated in the presence of hemorrhagic stroke.
2. Patients who receive anticoagulant or antiplatelet therapy[2] for treatment of acute stroke within 7 days of presentation should receive a head CT or MRI prior to the initiation of anticoagulant or antiplatelet treatment.	III	Phillips, 1992	Reduce complications of treatment.	CT or MRI is needed to reliably distinguish hemorrhagic from thrombotic stroke. Anticoagulation is contraindicated in the presence of hemorrhagic stroke.
Treatment				
3. Patients newly diagnosed with a stroke or TIA who are not already on antiplatelet[2] or antithrombotic[3] treatment should be started on antiplatelet therapy or antithrombotic therapy within 1 month of the diagnosis unless a contraindication is documented.[6,7]	I	Sze, 1988; Antiplatelet Trialists' Collaboration, 1994	Reduce risk of second stroke. Reduce risk of death from stroke.	Aspirin has been shown to reduce risk of second stroke. Ticlid is used in some patients who are sensitive to aspirin or have had a cerebrovascular event while taking aspirin. If patients are placed on antithrombotic treatment (e.g., for atrial fibrillation), additional antiplatelet treatment is not needed.
4. Patients with a documented history of stroke or TIA should be on daily antiplatelet[2] or antithrombotic[3] treatment, unless a contraindication to antithrombotic treatment is documented.[7]	I	Sze, 1988; Antiplatelet Trialists' Collaboration, 1994	Reduce risk of second stroke. Reduce risk of death from stroke.	Aspirin reduces risk of second stroke. Anticoagulants (e.g., coumadin) reduce stroke incidence in patients with atrial fibrillation and other conditions. Antiplatelet agents are not needed in patients receiving anticoagulation.

Indicator	Quality of Evidence	Literature	Benefits	Comments
5. Patients presenting for care with carotid artery symptoms[1] who are diagnosed with TIA or stroke should have a carotid artery imaging study within 6 months before or 1 month after the event, unless the medical record documents, in the same time period, that the patient is not a candidate for carotid surgery.	I	NACET, 1991; ECST, 1991; Humphrey, 1995	Reduce recurrent stroke.	Carotid endarterectomy benefits patients with symptoms of a carotid with 70-99% stenosis, if the surgeon's perioperative complication rate is < 6%. The more promptly endarterectomy is carried out, the greater the benefit.
6. Patients presenting for care with carotid artery symptoms,[1] who are diagnosed with carotid imaging evidence of >=70% stenosis on the side corresponding to the symptoms, should receive endarterectomy or referral for endarterectomy within 2 weeks of the diagnostic study.	I	NACET, 1991; ECST, 1991; Humphrey, 1995	Reduce recurrent stroke.	Carotid endarterectomy benefits patients with symptoms of a carotid with 70-99% stenosis, if the surgeon's perioperative complication rate is < 6%. The more promptly endarterectomy is carried out, the greater the benefit.

Follow-Up

Indicator	Quality of Evidence	Literature	Benefits	Comments
7. Patients who smoke and present with TIA but are not hospitalized should be counseled to stop smoking at the time they present with TIA.	III	Futrell & Millikan, 1996	Reduce mortality. Reduce stroke recurrence.	Smoking cessation reduces overall and cardiovascular mortality. To our knowledge, no data explicitly shows that smoking cessation reduces risk of second cerebrovascular event. However, there is no evidence that TIA and stroke patients are resistant to the mortality benefits of smoking cessation. Some stroke patients may not have adequate mental faculties to receive information regarding smoking cessation; thus, the indicator is confined to those with TIA.
8. Patients who smoke and are admitted to the hospital with a TIA should be counseled to stop smoking before hospital discharge.	III	Futrell & Millikan, 1996	Reduce mortality. Reduce stroke recurrence.	As above.

Definitions and Examples

[1] Carotid artery symptoms: From Humphrey (1995), common symptoms of carotid TIA and stroke include hemiparesis (complete or partial); hemisensory loss (complete or partial); dysphasia; and loss of vision in one eye (amaurosis fugax). Apraxia and visuospatial problems may also occur, and severe deficits may be accompanied by homonymous hemianopia and gaze palsy.

[2] Antiplatelet therapy: Aspirin or ticlopidine (ticlid).

[3] Antithrombotic therapy: coumadin or, less commonly, heparin.

[4] Thrombolytic therapy: Tissue plasminogen activator, streptokinase, urokinase.

[5] Carotid Artery Imagining Study: carotid duplex or angiography.

[6] Contraindications to aspirin/ antiplatelet agents:
   a. Hypersensitivity/ allergy to salicylates (rare).
   b. Bleeding within the past 4 weeks. This includes gastrointestinal bleeding, melena, epistaxis, any bleeding requiring transfusion; excluding occult hemoglobin in stools, or menses.

[7] Potential contraindications to heparin:
   a. Previous hemorrhagic stroke at any time or non-hemorrhagic stroke within 1 month.
   b. Known intracranial neoplasm, mass, or other intracerebral pathology (e.g. aneurysm, abscess).
   c. Bleeding within the past 4 weeks. This includes gastrointestinal bleeding, melena, epistaxis, any bleeding requiring transfusion; this does not include occult hemoglobin in stools, or menses.
   d. Suspected aortic dissection.
   e. Current use of anticoagulants in therapeutic doses.
   f. Bleeding diathesis (e.g., dysfunctional platelets, von Willebrand's disease, thrombocytopenia, clotting factor deficiency, hemophilia).
   g. Received streptokinase, APSAC, or urokinase during the current admission.

[8] Potential contraindications to thrombolytics:
   a. Previous hemorrhagic stroke at any time or non-hemorrhagic stroke within 1 month.
   b. Known intracranial neoplasm, mass, or other intracerebral pathology (e.g., aneurysm, abscess).
   c. Bleeding within the past 4 weeks. This includes gastrointestinal bleeding, melena, epistaxis, any bleeding requiring transfusion; this does not include occult hemoglobin in stools, or menses.
   d. Suspected aortic dissection.
   e. Current use of anticoagulants in therapeutic doses (e.g. coumadin with INR).
   f. Bleeding diathesis (e.g., dysfunctional platelets, von Willebrand's disease, thrombocytopenia, clotting factor deficiency, hemophilia).
   g. Blood pressure > 180/110.
   h. Trauma within 4 weeks (head trauma, concussion, bone fracture).
   i. CPR within 4 weeks.
   j. Surgery within 4 weeks (excluding cataract surgery).
   k. Pregnancy.

Quality of Evidence Codes

I	RCT
II-1	Nonrandomized controlled trials
II-2	Cohort or case analysis
II-3	Multiple time series
III	Opinions or descriptive studies

4. CHRONIC OBSTRUCTIVE PULMONARY DISEASE

Beatrice Golomb, MD, PhD

The approach to developing quality indicators for the diagnosis and treatment of chronic obstructive pulmonary disease (COPD) was based primarily on an evaluation of English language review articles. In addition, targeted MEDLINE literature searches identified randomized controlled trials published between 1992 and 1996 on the prevention and treatment of COPD and its exacerbations. Selected articles were reviewed in areas where randomized trials have demonstrated benefit to therapy, and in areas where management controversy exists.

IMPORTANCE

COPD is estimated to affect at least 15 million Americans (Fromm, 1994), causing 75,000 deaths and 900,000 hospitalizations each year (Rosen, 1992). COPD is second only to arthritis as the leading cause of long-term disability and functional impairment (Heath, 1993), and it is the third most frequent diagnosis (after congestive heart failure and stroke) for patients receiving home care (ATS, 1995). The mortality rate ten years after diagnosis is greater than 50 percent (Ferguson, 1993). COPD is the fifth leading cause of death in the US (Ferguson, 1993) causing eight percent of all deaths (Heath, 1993). The death rate for COPD has risen by 22 percent in the last decade (Ferguson, 1993).

Definitions

COPD is characterized by the presence of airflow obstruction due to chronic bronchitis or emphysema. The airflow obstruction is generally progressive, may be accompanied by airway hyperreactivity, and may be partially reversible (ATS, 1995). Chronic bronchitis is defined clinically as a chronic productive cough for three months in each of two successive years in a patient in whom other causes of chronic cough have been excluded (ATS, 1995). Emphysema is defined anatomically as abnormal permanent enlargement of the airspaces distal to the terminal bronchioles, with accompanying destruction of their walls and no obvious fibrosis. Destruction is defined as lack of uniformity in the pattern of respiratory airspace enlargement; the orderly appearance of the acinus and its components is disturbed and may be lost (ATS, 1995). Some diagnosticians include small airways disease in the definition of COPD (Angstman, 1992), noting that airways obstruction as gauged by forced expiratory volume at one second (FEV_1) results from airway narrowing or collapse and/or loss of elastic recoil of the lungs. They also note that the small noncartilaginous conducting airways that show pathologic changes of inflammation, fibrosis, mucus production, and narrowing are the major site of airflow obstruction in COPD. Nonetheless, early small airways disease is not reliably detected by currently available tests (Angstman, 1992), and most investigators refer exclusively to emphysema and bronchitis in discussions of COPD (ATS, 1995).

Prevention of COPD

Smoking is the principal risk factor for development of COPD (Angstman, 1992), and it accounts for 80 to 90 percent of COPD deaths (Rosen, 1992). Other identified risk factors include air pollution (sulfur dioxide and other respiratory irritants) (Heath, 1993); certain occupational exposures (Angstman, 1992) such as airborne silica (Heath, 1993); alpha1-antitrypsin deficiency (Angstman, 1992); and history of childhood respiratory trouble (Angstman, 1992). Age and reduced lung function also seem to have an effect on development of COPD (Angstman, 1992). Of these risk factors, cigarette smoking is the most amenable to change, and smoking prevention and cessation are primary targets for preventive efforts.

Smoking Cessation

COPD is closely linked to smoking. There is a strong relationship between airway obstruction (reduced FEV_1) and a high number of pack-years of smoking (Angstman, 1992). The relative risk of chronic bronchitis for smokers versus nonsmokers is 8.8 for men and 5.9 for women (Heath, 1993). In a British study of respiratory symptoms, 80 percent of male subjects who reported symptoms of chronic bronchitis were tobacco smokers (Heath, 1993). For these reasons, COPD prevention is focused on smoking prevention and cessation. Indicators for smoking cessation are included in Chapter 5.

SCREENING

There are no current recommendations in the reviewed literature for screening asymptomatic individuals for COPD.

DIAGNOSIS

History

Principal symptoms of COPD include dyspnea, chronic mucus production, decreased exercise and work tolerance, and cough (Nesse, 1992). COPD should be considered in patients with a history of smoking who present with these symptoms. Therefore, in a patient presenting with dyspnea, mucus production, or cough, a history of smoking should be elicited (Angstman, 1992) and documented in the record at the time of the presenting respiratory complaint (Indicator 1). History may provide evidence of other diseases, such as bronchiectasis, idiopathic pulmonary fibrosis, pulmonary sarcoidosis, pneumoconiosis, coccidiomycosis, and pulmonary tuberculosis (Angstman, 1992). Therefore, some information on other possible sources of exposure and occupational history should be elicited.

Physical Exam

Certain elements in the physical exam may help to confirm a diagnosis of COPD. A lung exam may provide evidence of wheezing or airflow limitation, or evidence suggestive of other pulmonary conditions. Therefore, in patients presenting with dyspnea, cough, or wheezing in whom the diagnosis of COPD is made or considered, a lung examination should be documented on first presentation with a respiratory complaint (Indicator 2).

Spirometry

Spirometry is important for detecting the presence of an obstructive defect and for establishing lack of reversibility, which distinguishes COPD from asthma. This distinction has important implications for treatment (Indicator 3). An obstructive ventilatory

93

impairment is seen on spirometry in COPD, indicated by a low FEV_1 to FVC (forced vital capacity) ratio. Typically the FEV_1 is reduced, and the FVC is normal or increased; however, in end-stage COPD it may be found that the FVC is decreased, leading to false normalization of the FEV_1:FVC ratio (Angstman, 1992). Thus the FEV_1 to FVC ratio is most useful in evaluation of mild disease. With disease progression FEV_1 worsens (Angstman, 1992), and an FEV_1 reading that is lower than predicted and declines more rapidly than expected over time (i.e., by more than 25 ml/yr) is an additional spirometric indicator of COPD (Jacobs, 1994). In COPD, impairment persists despite medical therapy, distinguishing COPD from asthma (Angstman, 1992). Although airway obstruction may reverse partially with bronchodilators, it does not do so completely (Angstman, 1992).

Indicators of Oxygenation: Complete Blood Count, Hemoglobin, Arterial Blood Gas

Oxygen treatment has been shown to improve morbidity and mortality in hypoxemic patients with COPD (Nocturnal Oxygen Therapy Trial Group 1980; The Medical Research Council Working Party, 1981; Anthonisen, 1983). For example, nocturnal treatment with oxygen for sleep desaturation in COPD patients with daytime normoxemia (PaO_2 > 60 mm Hg) slowed or reversed the progression of pulmonary hypertension (Fletcher et al., 1992). Long-term oxygen treatment in a group of COPD patients with hypoxemia (PaO_2 < 55 mm Hg) led to significantly increased survival compared with a control group (Corrado et al., 1994). Therefore, experts agree that detection of hypoxemia in patients with COPD is important.

An arterial blood gas (ABG) has been recommended for detection of hypoxemia in the following instances: 1) if there is evidence of cor pulmonale, cyanosis, erythrocytosis, or if FEV_1 is less than one liter (Angstman, 1992); or, 2) if there are ongoing symptoms of COPD. ABG results may suggest the need for long-term therapy and allow for better evaluation of the severity of respiratory deterioration during an acute exacerbation (Hagedorn, 1992) (Indicators 4 and 5).

Chest Radiograph

A chest x-ray should be considered part of the diagnostic evaluation for COPD. Although not itself diagnostic for COPD, a chest x-ray may exclude other causes of chronic airway obstruction (Angstman, 1992). Performing a chest x-ray may guide COPD therapy, as it can detect other lung conditions that, as with COPD, present as cough or dyspnea. Such conditions, not all of which produce obstructive defects, include sarcoidosis, coccidiomycosis, pulmonary tuberculosis, pneumoconiosis, pulmonary fibrosis, or lung nodules indicative of primary or metastatic cancer. Because smoking places patients at increased risk for lung cancer, which may present with dyspnea or cough, detection of an obstructive defect on spirometry does not guarantee that new symptoms result solely from COPD. The possibility of alternative or coexisting pathology has led to recommendations that a standard baseline posterior-anterior chest radiograph be obtained in the diagnostic evaluation of COPD (Listello, 1992). However, we have found no evidence to gauge the frequency with which this test identifies other pathology.

TREATMENT

Smoking Cessation

Smoking cessation is the primary therapy for chronic bronchitis in smokers (Griffith, 1993). It has also been called the most challenging intervention for both the patient and physician (Listello, 1992). Various forms of therapy are available, including group sessions, behavioral modification, hypnosis, and pharmacotherapy (Listello, 1992). Abstinence from smoking reduces the symptoms that define chronic bronchitis (cough, sputum production, wheezing, and dyspnea). Improvement with smoking cessation varies by age, smoking history, bronchial hyperreactivity, and degree of fixed airflow obstruction. Smoking cessation decreases the rate of decline in pulmonary function typically seen with sustained smoking (Griffith, 1993). Although the FEV_1 does not revert to normal on smoking cessation, the rate of decline falls back from 50-60 cc/yr to the normal rate of 20 cc/yr. The health benefits of smoking cessation include improved life expectancy;

decreased risk of cancer (lung, larynx, oral cavity, esophagus, pancreas, bladder); reduced risk of myocardial infarction; improved outcome after myocardial infarction; reduced risk of cerebrovascular and peripheral vascular disease; reduced respiratory symptoms (cough, sputum, wheezing, dyspnea); decreased mortality from respiratory infections; decreased rate of pulmonary decline; improved healing of duodenal ulcers; and, where pertinent, improved fetal birth weight (Griffith, 1993). Therefore, counseling or referral for smoking cessation should be documented on the chart for all smokers within three months of diagnosis or initiation of therapy for COPD (Indicator 6).

Inhaled Bronchodilators: Anticholinergics

High levels of safety and efficacy have made inhaled ipratropium a standard first-line drug for the treatment of patients with COPD. Bronchodilation begins about 15 minutes after use, and the duration of action is three to five hours (Nesse, 1992). Although some maintain that the drug's slow onset of action not only mandates regular use but clearly indicates inappropriate use for episodic bronchospasm (Nesse 1992), others state that onset is comparable to that seen with beta-agonists, with a longer duration of action (Griffith, 1993). The margin of safety for ipratropium is extremely large, and tachyphylaxis has not been reported. In addition, the bronchodilating effects of ipratropium in patients with chronic bronchitis are comparable or superior to those of beta-adrenergic agents in patients with chronic bronchitis (Griffith, 1993). Ipratropium has the additional theoretical advantage of producing an anticholinergic-mediated reduction of secretions (Heath, 1993), making this the bronchodilator of choice for initial treatment of chronic bronchitis (Griffith, 1993) and emphysema (Indicator 7). The most common side effects are cough and throat irritation (Griffith, 1993). As with other inhaled agents, individual patient response may dictate a higher dose, up to four puffs four times a day (Nesse, 1992).

Inhaled Bronchodilators: Beta-2 Selective Agonists

Efficacy of selective beta-agonists as bronchodilators has been unequivocally demonstrated in chronic bronchitis (Griffith, 1993). Inhaled therapy is the preferred method of administration (Griffith,

1993). No evidence clearly favors any one inhaled agonist over another (Nesse, 1992). Relatively recently it was recommended that these agents be given as two puffs four times a day, or up to six puffs or more at a time (Nesse, 1992). However, a British study found that continuous inhaled beta-agonist therapy was no more effective than "as-needed" treatment (Heath, 1993). In addition, side effects are more troublesome than those of ipratropium, and include tremor, tachycardia and increased cardiac output, though these are less problematic with inhaled than with oral therapy (Nesse, 1992; Griffith, 1993). In the asthmatic population, regular use may cause tachyphylaxis and may even increase mortality (Griffith, 1993). Although combination therapy continues to be advocated for maximal effect in acute exacerbations (Heath, 1993), the combination of ipratropium and a beta-agonist has not been found to achieve greater bronchodilation than a maximal dose of either agent alone. For this reason, routine use of ipratropium is recommended first (Griffith, 1993). Selective beta-agonists are still regarded as useful in several circumstances: 1) as needed for exacerbations of bronchospasm; 2) as an alternative first-line bronchodilator for patients who do not tolerate or do not respond to ipratropium; and 3) routinely in combination with ipratropium (both in relatively low doses) for patients who do not tolerate maximal doses of either agent (Griffith, 1993).

Instructions on Bronchodilator Usage

A metered dose inhaler (MDI) is as effective as a nebulizer for most patients (Griffith, 1993), if it is used correctly or with a spacer device. A spacer device (e.g., a simple extension tube or a proprietary device such as InspirEase) improves delivery by optimizing inhaled particle size, allowing large particles to settle out. This prevents the need for coordination of breathing and inhaler use, which is an important consideration in the elderly (Griffith, 1993). Some recommend using a spacer device for virtually all patients (Nesse, 1992). In the absence of a spacer, the factor that most limits efficacy of inhaled bronchodilators is inadequate dosage resulting from inefficient use; proper delivery requires an alert cooperative patient who has been

adequately educated in the technique, with follow-up (Nesse, 1992).
Sixty-two percent of adult outpatients with COPD use the metered dose
inhaler incorrectly (Hofford, 1992). Following a single instruction in
correct use, 77 to 80 percent demonstrate the correct technique for
using the inhaler (Hofford, 1992). Additional verbal instruction,
followed by a time during which the patient practices proper use of the
inhaler, further improves patient performance (Hofford, 1992) (Indicator
8).

Theophylline

Treatment with theophylline is controversial for the following
reasons: 1) a low toxic-to-therapeutic index, 2) wide variation in
rates of absorption and metabolism, resulting in significantly different
serum levels even in the same person over time, and 3) a large number of
pharmaceutical and other factors (such as age, smoking or smoking
cessation, diet, coexisting medical conditions) that influence the serum
level (Nesse, 1992). The risk of life-threatening complications with
theophylline therapy has been estimated at 0.5 percent per year (Nesse
1992). Severe side effects such as cardiac arrhythmias and seizures can
occur even with "therapeutic" serum levels. One study found that
theophylline added little benefit to otherwise maximal therapy, with
several adverse side effects (Griffith, 1993). Although theophylline
produces only moderate bronchodilation, efficacy in relief of dyspnea
and improvement in arterial oxygen pressure, ventilation, and functional
level have been significant even without discernible alteration in
pulmonary function tests. This may be due to factors such as
improvement in diaphragmatic muscle activity, reduced vascular and
pulmonary bronchiolar resistance, and protection against episodic
bronchospasm (Nesse, 1992).

A serum theophylline level of ten to 13 mg/mL provides at least 90
percent of the bronchodilatory benefit of higher serum levels and
reduces the likelihood of toxic side effects (Nesse, 1992). Typically,
serum levels of theophylline are checked two to five days after a
significant change in dose, and should be measured whenever symptoms
suggest toxicity (Nesse, 1992). Patients should be educated to

recognize and report to their physicians any early signs of toxicity such as nausea and tachycardia (Nesse, 1992) (Indicators 9 and 10).

Oral Corticosteroids

Corticosteroid use remains controversial for COPD. Although airway inflammation is also part of the pathophysiology of COPD, the inflammation is characterized by neutrophil excess and not by the lymphocyte traffic and eosinophilic infiltration characteristic of asthma. As a consequence, the airway inflammation of COPD and the clinical course of COPD do not appear to be amenable to corticosteroid treatment in the majority of patients (Chapman, 1996). Only about ten percent of patients with COPD will benefit from either systemic or inhaled steroid therapy according to one recent meta-analysis (Chapman, 1996). Those patients most likely to benefit from steroid therapy show significant (i.e., greater than 15 percent) improvement in flow rates after bronchodilation (Jacobs, 1994). A meta-analysis has concluded that steroids are useful in patients with severe but stable COPD who remain symptomatic with maximum bronchodilation. Therefore, oral corticosteroid therapy should be reserved for patients in whom primary bronchodilator therapy fails to provide adequate control of symptoms and in whom steroids are beneficial.

Inhaled Corticosteroids

In many or most patients who respond to systemic corticosteroids, substitution of inhaled for oral steroids is not adequate (Jacobs, 1994; Griffith, 1993). However, results of studies have shown that some patients with chronic bronchitis do respond favorably to inhaled steroids (Griffith, 1993). Such patients can only be identified by therapeutic trial. Advent of more powerful inhaled steroids may improve the likelihood of response in steroid responsive patients, though this remains to be documented. In light of favorable studies, some have recommended inhalation therapy with beclomethasone dipropionate, four to six puffs four times a day, while attempting to taper or discontinue oral prednisone; however, others have questioned whether adequate evidence supports this (Nesse, 1992).

Antibiotics

Recommendations for antibiotic use in chronic bronchitis are mixed. The role of prophylactic antibiotic therapy on both a seasonal and continuous basis has been studied repeatedly, without a clear consensus as to its effectiveness (Heath, 1993). Some note that a subgroup of chronic bronchitis patients with frequent exacerbations have shown fewer exacerbations while taking prophylactic antibiotic therapy (Griffith, 1993).

Vaccination

Hemophilus influenza: Vaccination against *H. influenzae* is believed to reduce the number of episodes of bronchitic exacerbation (Griffith, 1993). Nonetheless, data regarding this benefit are sparse.

Influenza: No data from controlled trials demonstrate a decrease in disease from use of influenza virus vaccine in patients who have chronic bronchitis exclusively (Griffith, 1993). However, one nursing home study found that those residents who received influenza vaccine had a significant reduction in lower respiratory tract disease, hospitalization, and mortality compared with those who had not been vaccinated (Griffith, 1993). Another rationale for vaccine use is potential reduction in postviral bacterial colonization of the tracheobronchial tree (Griffith, 1993). Although efficacy has not been conclusively demonstrated, it is believed that the risk-benefit ratio for influenza vaccine favors its use in chronic bronchitis (Griffith, 1993).

Pneumovax: Pneumococcal pneumonia probably occurs in patients with chronic airflow obstruction more often than in the general population, but does not appear to predispose patients to excessive pneumococcal bacteremia or increased mortality (Griffith, 1993). There are no data suggesting that the vaccine is beneficial for prevention of pneumonia or bronchitic exacerbations in this population. It has not been subjected to large-scale trials to demonstrate reduced morbidity or mortality in a COPD population, and small trials have been inconclusive (Jacobs, 1994). However, most specialists advocate its use (Chapman, 1996), believing the risk-benefit ratio to be favorable (Heath, 1993; Chapman, 1996).

Quality indicators for vaccinations are included in Volume III of this series (see "Chapter 19: Preventive Care").

Exercise Rehabilitation

Exercise rehabilitation addresses diverse factors that may contribute to dyspnea such as abnormal pulmonary mechanics, respiratory muscle fatigue, poor nutritional status, misperception of dyspnea, and even smoking cessation. Specific exercise techniques include general exercise conditioning, targeted respiratory muscle training, breathing retraining, and techniques in energy conservation (Griffith, 1993). These interventions also allow symptom monitoring by a respiratory therapist who can provide support and education for the symptomatic patient (Heath, 1993). Some maintain that exercise rehabilitation may be beneficial for patients with chronic airflow obstruction who, in spite of aggressive medical management, continue to have significant dyspnea (Griffith, 1993). However, rehabilitation techniques do not affect pulmonary function per se (Griffith, 1993) and, although they can improve exercise tolerance (Griffith, 1993), they have not been proved to alter disease progression (Heath, 1993).

Supplemental Oxygen

Supplemental oxygen has been shown to improve survival and quality of life in hypoxemic patients with chronic obstructive lung disease (Nocturnal Oxygen Therapy Trial Group, 1980; The Medical Research Council Working Party, 1981; Anthonisen, 1983; Griffith, 1993; O'Donohue, 1996). Long-term oxygen therapy may increase lifespan by six to seven years in patients who have COPD with hypoxemia and cor pulmonale. Survival and subjective improvement increase when patients use oxygen for 19 to 24 hours per day (Listello et al., 1992). Overnight oxygen improves mortality compared with no oxygen in chronically hypoxic COPD patients (Chapman, 1996), and continuous oxygen improves survival compared with overnight oxygen (Chapman, 1996). Benefits include improved survival; improved neuropsychiatric function; amelioration of polycythemia, pulmonary hypertension, and cor pulmonale; and enhanced exercise performance (Jacobs 1994; O'Donohue, 1996).

In 1993, there were approximately 616,000 people in the U.S. receiving home oxygen at a cost of $1.4 billion (O'Donohue, 1996). The indications for continuous long-term oxygen therapy for patients with hypoxemia at rest developed by the Health Care Financing Administration (HCFA) are generally accepted by third party payers throughout the U.S. These include $PaO_2 \leq 55$ mm Hg, $SaO_2 \leq 88$ percent, or PaO_2 56 to 59 mm Hg or $SaO_2 \leq 89$ percent in cases with edema caused by heart failure, with evidence of cor pulmonale, or with elevated hematocrit (> 56 percent).

Indications for use of intermittent oxygen, during sleep or at rest, are somewhat less widely accepted. Indications for oxygen with exercise by HCFA's standards are $PaO_2 \leq 55$ mm Hg, or $SaO_2 \leq 88$ percent documented during exercise. Indications for nocturnal oxygen only, according to HCFA, are $PaO_2 \leq 55$ mm Hg or $SaO_2 \leq 88$ percent during sleep; a decrease in PaO_2 of greater than 10 mm Hg; or a decrease in SaO_2 greater than five percent with signs or symptoms of hypoxemia (defined as impaired cognition, restlessness, or insomnia) (O'Donohue, 1996). These recommendations agree closely with most published recommendations (Heath, 1993; Ferguson, 1993; Listello 1992; Chapman, 1996). Measurement should be made at times of clinical stability. If patients require oxygen therapy on discharge from the hospital, oxygen saturation should be retested one to three months after recovery from the acute illness (Chapman, 1996; O'Donohue, 1996).

HCFA requires retesting 61 to 90 days after discharge with oxygen only if the initial $PaO_2 \geq 56$ mm Hg, or if $SaO_2 \geq 89$ percent (O'Donohue, 1996). Oxygen should be given at a rate sufficient to produce oxygen saturation consistently greater than 90 percent (Indicators 11, 19, and 20).

Bullectomy

Bullectomy has been suggested for improving airflow and gas exchange and reducing dyspnea in selected patients with bullae larger than one-third of the hemithorax and associated with lung compression. Laser bullectomy techniques have been described. Risks and benefits have not been clearly established (Ferguson, 1993).

102

Treatment of Acute Exacerbations of COPD

The American Thoracic Society's Standards for the Diagnosis and Care of Patients with Chronic Obstructive Pulmonary Disease recommend that emergency evaluation of acute exacerbation of COPD include elements of history, physical exam, and laboratory evaluation (ATS, 1995). Attention should be paid to factors with documented prognostic value, particularly those that identify patients at high risk of relapse after outpatient medical management. In one study, these factors were found to include medical visits for dyspnea within the previous week; number of doses of bronchodilator therapy given in the evaluation setting; use of home oxygen; previous relapse rate; administration of aminophylline; and use of corticosteroids and antibiotics at the time of discharge from the medical setting (ATS, 1995).

According to recommendations of the American Thoracic Society and others, a history should include information on:

- *Outpatient medications* (ATS, 1995) - to assess use of home O_2 (which influences risk), use of theophylline (which signifies need for theophylline testing), and use of beta-blockers (which may exacerbate bronchospasm);

- *Recent medical visits and hospitalizations for COPD exacerbations* - to assess risk;

- *The presence of other symptoms* (such as fever or new cough that might signify presence of pneumonia or other infection) - to direct the evaluation and management of risk for continued respiratory compromise and, therefore, need for hospitalization; and,

- *Comorbid medical conditions* (ATS, 1995) - which also guide the risk stratification of the patient.

A physical examination should include:

- *Documentation of vital signs* (ATS, 1995) - to indicate hemodynamic stability, evaluate tachypnea (and correlate respiratory rate with pCO_2 from ABG), and to assess for presence of fever suggestive of coexisting infection;

- *A lung and chest exam* (ATS 1995) - to document the presence of airflow restriction or wheezing, which may guide severity assessment. Crackles or egophony suggestive of consolidation will guide risk stratification, while the absence of lung sounds bilaterally may signify poor prognosis. The absence of lung sounds unilaterally may indicate the need for evaluation of pneumothorax.

- *Documentation of the presence or absence of paradoxical abdominal muscle use or accessory muscle use* (ATS, 1995) - which will indicate severity of breathing difficulty and influence severity assessment (Indicator 12).

According to American Thoracic Society 1995 standards, laboratory evaluation and other tests should include:

- *ABG* - to evaluate oxygenation status and ventilatory status;
- *EKG* - to assess for cor pulmonale and to rule out concomitant ischemia or arrhythmia that could exacerbate shortness of breath (Indicator 13);
- *Theophylline level* - if outpatient theophylline is prescribed (Indicator 14); and,
- *Chest x-ray* - to be documented within the past year, including a lateral view within the past year.

Acute treatment in the medical setting should begin with bronchodilator therapy, including beta-2 agonists and/or ipratropium by inhalation using a MDI with or without spacer or jet nebulizer (Indicator 15). The role of antibiotics remains under debate, although antibiotics are usually given. In one study, clinical deterioration was ten percent in patients treated with antibiotics, compared with 19 percent in patients who received placebo; and clear improvement occurred in 68 percent of patients treated with antibiotics versus 55 percent in the placebo group (Anthonisen et al., 1987). The advantage of antibiotic therapy was most pronounced in patients with increased dyspnea, increased sputum volume, and purulent sputum, and did not occur in subjects with only one of the three. Nonetheless, determination of who requires antibiotics and how antibiotics should be selected remain subjects of debate (Verghese, 1994).

Corticosteroids and theophylline are commonly given in acute exacerbations of COPD. However, the utility of steroids in the acute setting remains a topic of debate, with some studies showing improvement and others not (Rosen, 1992). With respect to aminophylline, one meta-analysis of 13 controlled aminophylline studies found no evidence to support its use in the acute setting (Littenberg, 1988). However, a subsequent double-blind placebo-controlled randomized trial found that aminophylline, in doses producing levels just below the level commonly accepted as therapeutic, reduced the hospital admission rate among patients with asthma or COPD exacerbations by a factor of three (Wrenn et al., 1991). Oxygen should be administered if hypoxemia is present (oxygen saturation < 88 percent on ABG or pulse oximetry, and/or PO_2 < 55 mm Hg on ABG) (Indicator 16).

A patient should be hospitalized if the acute exacerbation is characterized by increased dyspnea, cough, or sputum production plus any of several factors that indicate a more severe course or more marked clinical compromise. These factors indicate heightened risk of respiratory failure or inability of the patient to care for him- or herself at home. Although these factors have not been subjected to formal testing for prognostic utility, most physicians would acknowledge these factors as clinical indicators of severity or risk. Among the recommended factors indicating heightened risk and meriting hospitalization (ATS, 1995) those that can be operationalized as quality measures include: documentation of a serious co-morbid condition (documented ischemia; documented pneumonia); altered cognition; worsening hypoxemia (saturation below baseline and below 88 percent; or PaO_2 below baseline and below 55 mm Hg); or new or worsening hypercarbia (pCO_2 at least 5 mm Hg above baseline, and above 60 mm Hg)(Indicator 17).

A patient with acute COPD exacerbation and increasing respiratory compromise should be monitored in a setting equipped with medical personnel, and pulse oximetry and telemetry capabilities so that, in the event of respiratory failure, intubation will be possible. Conditions indicating severe respiratory compromise are accepted to include (Indicator 18):

- Severe dyspnea (breathing rate > 35 or accessory muscle use) despite initial bronchodilator treatment (ATS, 1995);

- Confusion or lethargy;
- Respiratory muscle fatigue as assessed subjectively, by paradoxical diaphragmatic motion, or by normalization of pH on ABG (pH < 7.42) despite continued tachypnea (breathing rate > 33) (ATS, 1995);
- Persistent or worsening hypoxemia despite supplemental oxygen (pO_2 < 60 with FiO_2 > 40 percent);
- Severe or worsening respiratory acidosis (pH < 7.3).

FOLLOW-UP

Recommendations for follow-up include many elements described previously, such as regular counseling regarding smoking cessation and yearly influenza vaccination. Some authorities recommend periodic testing of oxygen saturation at every four to six months and at least yearly follow-up of FEV_1 to estimate rate of decline (Veterans Health Administration Clinical Practice Guideline, 1997); however, frequent testing of oxygen saturation may not be necessary in patients with stable mild COPD. Moreover, frequent testing of FEV_1 is useful only if it modifies management. Therefore, although these measures may be appropriate in many cases, no indicators will be generated for follow-up.

REFERENCES

American Thoracic Society. 1995. Standards for the diagnosis and care of patients with chronic obstructive pulmonary disease. *American Journal of Respiratory Critical Care Medicine* 152: S77-S120.

Angstman G. 1992. Diagnosing COPD. *Postgraduate Medicine* 91: 61-7.

Anthonisen NR, Manfreda J, Warren CP et al. 1987. Antibiotic therapy in exacerbations of chronic obstructive pulmonary disease. *Annals of Internal Medicine* 106(2):196-204.

Anthonisen NR. 1983. Long-term oxygen therapy. *Archives of Internal Medicine* 99: 519-27.

Badgett RG, and Tanaka DJ. 1997. Is screening for chronic obstructive pulmonary disease justified? *Preventive Medicine* 26: 466-472.

Chapman K. 1996. Therapeutic approaches to chronic obstructive pulmonary disease: An emerging consensus. *American Journal of Medicine* 100: 5S-10S.

Corrado A, De Paola E, Messori A, et al. 1994. The effect of intermittent negative pressure ventilation and long-term oxygen therapy for patients with COPD. *Chest* 105: 95-99.

Ferguson G, and Cherniack R. 1993. Management of chronic obstructive pulmonary disease. *New England Journal of Medicine* 328: 1017-22.

Fletcher E, Luckett R, Goodnight-White S, Miller C, Qian W, and Costarangos-Galarza C. 1992. A double-blind trial fo nocturnal supplemental oxygen for sleep desaturation in patients with chronic obstructive pulmonary disease and a daytime PaO2 above 60 mm Hg. *American Review of Respiratory Disease* 145: 1070-1076.

Griffith D, and Kronenberg R. 1993. Chronic bronchitis. *Postgraduate Medicine* 94: 93-100.

Hagedorn S. 1992. Acute exacerbations of COPD. *Postgraduate Medicine* 91: 105-112.

Heath J. 1993. Outpatient management of chronic bronchitis in the elderly. *American Family Physician* 48: 841-8.

Hofford J. 1992. Metered dose inhaler therapy for asthma, bronchitis, and emphysema. *Journal of Family Practice* 34: 485-92.

Jacobs M. 1994. Maintenance therapy for obstructive lung disease. *Postgraduate Medicine* 95: 87-99.

Lacasse Y, Wong E, Guyatt GH, et al. 26 October 1996. Meta-analysis of respiratory rehabilitation in chronic obstructive pulmonary disease. *Lancet* 348: 1115-1119.

Listello D, and Glauser F. 1992. COPD: Primary care menagement with drug and oxygen therapies. *Geriatrics* 47: 28-38.

Littenberg B. 1988. Aminophylline treatment in sever, acute asthma: a meta-analysis. *Journal of the American Medical Association* 259 (11):1678-84.

Nesse R. 1992. Pharmacologic treatment of COPD. *Postgraduate Medicine* 91: 71-84.

Nocturnal Oxygen Therapy Trial Group. 1980. Continuous or nocturnal oxygen therapy in hypoxemic chronic obstructive lung disease. *Archives of Internal Medicine* 93: 391-8.

O'Donohue W. 1996. Home oxygen therapy. *Medical Clinics of North America* 80: 611-22.

Rosen M. 1992. Treatment of exacerbations of COPD. *American Family Physician* 45: 693-7.

Saint, S, Bent S, Vittenghoff E, et al. 22 March 1995. Antibiotics in Chronic Obstructive Pulmonary Disease Exacerbations. A meta-analysis. *Journal of the American Medical Association* 273 (12): 957-960.

The Medical Research Council Working Party. 1981. Long-term domiciliary oxygen therapy in chronic hypoxic cor pulmonale complicating chronic bronchitis and emphysema. *Lancet* 1: 681-6.

Verghese A. 1994. Acute exacerbations of chronic bronchitis. *Postgraduate Medicine* 96: 75-89.

Veterans Health Administration Clinical Practice Guideline for the Management of Persons with Chronic Obstructive Pulmonary Disease or Asthma. Version 1.0, November 17, 1997. Prepared by the COPD/Asthma Working Group.

Wrenn K, Slovis CM, Murphy F, et al. 1991. Aminophylline therapy for acute bronchospastic disease in the emergency room. Annals of Internal Medicine 115(4):241-7

RECOMMENDED QUALITY INDICATORS FOR COPD

The following indicators apply to men and women age 18 and older.

Indicator	Quality of Evidence	Literature	Benefits	Comments
Diagnosis				
1. A smoking history should be documented on the same day in patients who present with a new complaint of any of the following: • chronic cough (> 3 weeks duration); • shortness of breath; or • dyspnea on exertion.	III	Angstman, 1992; Subramanian, 1994	Improve management of symptoms. Decrease progression of COPD.	This influences likelihood of COPD diagnosis, thus directing initial therapy. Additionally, smoking cessation counseling or referral can be initiated. If smoking cessation is effective, progression of COPD will be reduced.
2. A lung exam should be documented on the same day in patients who present with a new complaint of any of the following: • chronic cough (> 3 weeks duration); • shortness of breath; or • dyspnea on exertion.	III	Angstman, 1992	Decrease symptoms through treatment of underlying condition.	By identifying physical findings that may redirect the diagnostic evaluation (which allows diagnosis of other conditions or supports diagnosis of obstructive lung disease), one may initiate the appropriate therapy and minimize inappropriate use of medications.
3. COPD patients on bronchodilator therapy[1] should have spirometry performed with and without bronchodilation within 3 months of initiation of therapy, unless spirometry was performed in the previous 12 months.	III	Angstman, 1992; Listello, 1992	Decrease symptoms by targeting appropriate treatment.	By confirming an obstructive defect and distinguishing COPD from asthma with spirometry, one can initiate the appropriate therapy, minimize inappropriate use of medications, and more properly assess future improvement or exacerbations.

Indicator	Quality of Evidence	Literature	Benefits	Comments
4. COPD patients on bronchodilator therapy should have one of the following tests within 6 months before or after initiation of therapy: • Hemoglobin; • Hematocrit; • CBC; • ABG; or • Pulse oximetry.	III	Angstman, 1992; Listello, 1992; Hagedorn, 1992	Improve survival.	Results may indicate long-term therapy and allow better evaluation of the severity of respiratory deterioration during an acute exacerbation. Detection of hypoxemia allows initiation of oxygen therapy, which has been shown to have mortality benefit in hypoxemic COPD patients.
5. COPD patients should have an ABG performed within 3 months of any of the following findings, unless hypoxemia ($PaO_2 < 55$) has been previously documented or the patient is already on chronic O_2 therapy: a. laboratory detection of erythrocytosis (Hct >55); b. notation of cyanosis or cor pulmonale in the medical record; and c. detection of $FEV_1 < 1$ liter on spirometric evaluation.	III	Angstman, 1992; Listello, 1992	Improve survival.	New factors suggesting hypoxemia should be followed by testing for hypoxemia, since oxygen treatment of this condition improves mortality.
Treatment				
6. Newly diagnosed COPD patients should be counseled or referred for smoking cessation within 3 months before or after of the new diagnosis of COPD.	III	Griffith, 1993; Heath, 1993; Listello, 1992; Chapman, 1993	Improve survival. Decrease progression of symptoms.	Smoking cessation decreases the decline in pulmonary function typically seen with sustained smoking.
7. All patients receiving pharmacologic treatment for COPD symptoms (including daily theophylline or non-PRN beta-agonists) should also be receiving ipratropium, unless intolerance is documented.	III	Griffith, 1993	Decrease shortness of breath. Limit side effects from treatment.	Ipratropium is the first choice agent because it has a higher margin of safety, fewer side effects, and bronchodilator efficacy comparable with that of beta-agonists.

110

	Indicator	Quality of Evidence	Literature	Benefits	Comments
8.	Patients newly prescribed inhaled bronchodilaters should be concurrently offered either a spacer device or instructions in proper use of a MDI.	III	Griffith, 1993; Listello, 1992	Reduce shortness of breath.	Inefficient use limits efficacy of inhaled bronchodilators. Proper delivery requires a patient who has been adequately educated in the technique.
9.	COPD patients should have a theophylline level checked within 1 week of either initiation or increase of theophylline dose.	III	Nesse, 1992	Reduce adverse medication effects.	Testing the theophylline level determines whether a new or increased dose provides appropriate serum levels, and whether a reduced dose has brought serum levels from toxic to low therapeutic range. (Note: Recommendation is to recheck in 3 to 5 days of change in dose.)
10.	In patients receiving theophylline, both of the following should occur when serum theophylline level exceeds 20 μg/ml: a. The dose should be modified within 1 day of the measurement; and b. Retesting of level should be performed within one week, unless theophylline was stopped.	III	Nesse, 1992; Listello, 1992	Prevent theophylline toxicity.	Retesting the theophylline level determines whether a modified dose provides serum levels that are neither toxic nor subtherapeutic.
11.	COPD patients should be offered home oxygen if their baseline room air oxygen saturation is <88% at rest (not during an exacerbation).	I	Listello, 1992; Chapman, 1996; Jacobs, 1994	Improve survival. Improve neuro-psychiatric function. Enhance exercise performance.	Survival increases with supplemental oxygen saturation >90%, and there is subjective improvement when patients use oxygen for 19-24 hours. Long-term oxygen therapy may increase lifespan by 6 to 7 years in patients with COPD with hypoxemia and cor pulmonale.

111

Indicator	Quality of Evidence	Literature	Benefits	Comments
Treatment: Management of Acute Exacerbations				
12. The following items should be documented in the medical record at the time of a COPD exacerbation[2]. a. Outpatient COPD medications;	III	American Thoracic Society, 1995	Reduce shortness of breath. Reduce theophylline toxicity. Assess severity.	Assessing the patient's medications helps identify other risk factors for adverse outcomes (comorbid illness). It identifies use of theophylline, indicating need to test theophylline level; identifies agents that may increase or decrease clearance of theophylline, affecting serum levels; and identifies agents such as beta blockers which may worsen bronchospasm.
b. Information on prior hospitalizations, urgent care, or ED visits for COPD (e.g., time of most recent visit or number per year);	III	American Thoracic Society, 1995		Frequent recent ED visits and hospitalizations are a marker for more severe illness and assist in severity assessment.
c. Presence or absence of new cough;	III	American Thoracic Society, 1995	Reduce shortness of breath. Provide possible survival benefit.	New productive cough in a dyspneic patient with a COPD exacerbation may signify a comorbid respiratory illness requiring treatment for resolution of symptoms (such as pneumonia). This will also guide severity adjustment, which will influence decision to hospitalize, as a worsening of a concurrent pneumonia may have serious consequences in a COPD patient.
d. Vital signs, including respiratory rate, pulse, temperature, and blood pressure; and	III	American Thoracic Society, 1995	Improve symptoms. Prevent mortality due to respiratory failure.	Vital signs guide therapy by evaluating severity of illness and identifying comorbid conditions.
e. A physical examination of the chest	III	American Thoracic Society, 1995	Prevent mortality due to respiratory failure.	A silent chest may predict more severe airway obstruction. A physical examination helps guide therapy by evaluating severity.
13. Patients admitted to the hospital for an exacerbation of COPD who have a history of coronary disease[3] should have an EKG performed within 24 hours of admission.	III	American Thoracic Society, 1995	Prevent mortality due to primary or secondary cardiac conditions.	EKG may identify concurrent ischemia (contributing to shortness of breath) and cardiac conditions associated with pulmonary disease (e.g., Multifocal Atrial Tachycardia), which may guide treatment.

112

	Indicator	Quality of Evidence	Literature	Benefits	Comments
14.	A theophylline level should be obtained for patients on theophylline who meet any of the following conditions: a. Present with an exacerbation of COPD; and b. Are hospitalized with an exacerbation of COPD.	III	American Thoracic Society, 1995	Reduce shortness of breath. Reduce theophylline toxicity	Measurement of theophylline level in a patient taking theophylline allows subtherapeutic and toxic levels to be identified. Treatment can be modified to improve symptoms or reduce toxicity from theophylline.
15.	COPD patients who present with an exacerbation should be offered inhaled bronchodilator therapy[4] if their respiratory rate is >24.	III	American Thoracic Society, 1995.	Reduce shortness of breath.	Bronchodilators are the principal treatment for COPD. They reverse the airflow obstruction, leading to improved ventilation and oxygenation, and reduction in shortness of breath.
16.	Patients presenting with COPD exacerbation should have oxygen administered if the oxygen saturation is < 88% or PO_2 is < 55 mm Hg.	III	American Thoracic Society, 1995; Fromm, 1994.	Reduce shortness of breath. Reduce complications of hypoxemia.	Oxygen should be administered to all hypoxemic patients. Inadequate oxygen leads to adverse consequences to organs including the heart and brain, and can lead to death.
17.	Patients presenting with COPD exacerbation should be offered admission to the hospital if any of the following conditions are documented in the medical record on the date of presentation: • Acute Ischemia[5]; • Pneumonia; or • Significant hypoxemia (saturation < 88%, or $PaO2$ < 55 mm Hg on room air in patients not on home oxygen).	III	American Thoracic Society, 1995.	Reduce shortness of breath. Reduce mortality.	Expert consensus identifies indications for hospital admission that consider the severity of the underlying respiratory dysfunction, progression of symptoms, response to outpatient therapies, existence of comorbid conditions, and availability of adequate home care. More severe respiratory dysfunction, progression of symptoms, or comorbid conditions imply greater risk and reduced safety of outpatient management.

113

Indicator	Quality of Evidence	Literature	Benefits	Comments
18. Patients hospitalized with a COPD exacerbation should be admitted to a monitored setting (that includes access to pulse oximetry and telemetry) while any of the following are present: • Severe dyspnea (breathing rate > 35 with accessory muscle use) despite initial therapeutic measures; • Confusion or lethargy; • Persistent or worsening hypoxemia despite supplemental oxygen (pO2 < 60 with FiO2 > 40%); or • Severe respiratory acidosis (pH < 7.3).	III		Reduce mortality.	Patients with factors indicating definite or possible near-term need for intubation require admission to an ICU or other monitored setting. A monitored setting is required for close observation of the patients' progress and allows prompt intubation -- and prevention of death from respiratory complications.
19. COPD patients hospitalized for an exacerbation should be discharged on home oxygen if the last documented oxygen saturation prior to discharge is <88%.	III	The Medical Research Council Working Party, 1981; Nocturnal Oxygen Therapy Trial Group 1980; Anthonisen, 1983; Griffith, 1993; Chapman, 1996; O'Donohue, 1996.	Improve survival. Improve neuro-psychiatric function. Enhance exercise performance.	Survival increases with supplemental oxygen to maintain saturation >90%, and there is subjective improvement when patients use oxygen for 19-24 hours. Overnight oxygen vs.improves no oxygen improves mortality in chronically hypoxic COPD patients. Continuous oxygen vs. overnight oxygen improves survival. Long-term oxygen therapy may increase lifespan 6 to 7 years in COPD patients with hypoxemia and cor pulmonale. Class I data shows mortality benefit in patients who are chronically hypoxemic; extrapolation of the data to the population who are hypoxemic on discharge (who may or may not be chronically hypoxemic) is class III.
20. Patients with a diagnosis of COPD who present with a COPD exacerbation and whose last documented oxygen[2] saturation during the exacerbation visit is < 88% should either be hospitalized or discharged on home oxygen treatment.	III	The Medical Research Council Working Party, 1981; Nocturnal Oxygen Therapy Trial Group, 1980; Anthonisen, 1983; Griffith, 1993; Chapman, 1996; O'Donohue, 1996.	Improved survival. Improve neuro-psychiatric function. Enhance exercise performance.	Benefits of oxygen therapy in hypoxemic patients include improved survival; improved neuropsychiatric function; amelioration of polycythemia, pulmonary hypertension, and cor pulmonale; and enhanced exercise performance. Class I data shows mortality benefit in patients who are chronically hypoxemic. Extrapolation of the data to the population who are hypoxemic in the acute setting (who are not known to be chronically hypoxemic) is class III.

Definitions and Examples

[1] Bronchodilator therapy: inhaled beta-agonists and/or ipratropium and/or theophylline.

[2] COPD exacerbation: subjective worsening of dyspnea or cough leading patient to seek medical help.

[3] Coronary disease: CAD, prior MI, angina, or history of angioplasty or CABG.

[4] Inhaled bronchodilator therapy: beta-agonists and/or ipratropium.

[5] Acute ischemia: (a) Physicians note of acute myocardial ischemia, accelerated angina, or unstable angina during the exacerbation, or (b) ST elevation in 2 separate leads of more than 2 mm on the day of presentation.

Quality of Evidence Codes

I	RCT
II-1	Nonrandomized controlled trials
II-2	Cohort or case analysis
II-3	Multiple time series
III	Opinions or descriptive studies

5. CIGARETTE COUNSELING[1]

Patricia Bellas, MD

In 1996, the U.S. Department of Health and Human Services published
Clinical Practice Guideline Number 18 on Smoking Cessation. This
guideline was developed by a panel convened by the Agency for Health
Care Policy and Research (AHCPR) and the Centers for Disease Control
(CDC). We relied on this document and Chapter 54 of the Guide to
Clinical Preventive Services published by the U.S. Preventive Services
Task Force (USPSTF, 1996) to construct quality indicators for the
prevention, screening and treatment of smoking. We also performed a
narrow MEDLINE literature search for review articles from 1995 to 1997
to update the literature support for the proposed indicators.

IMPORTANCE

About one-fourth of all American adults smoke tobacco. Smoking is
more common in males, persons of low socioeconomic status and those with
lower educational levels. Most smokers begin tobacco use as teenagers
(USPSTF, 1996). A majority of cancers of the lung, trachea, bronchus,
larynx, pharynx and oral cavity are attributable to tobacco use.
Smoking is also associated with cancers of the bladder, pancreas, kidney
and cervix. In the U.S., 148,000 cancer deaths per year are related to
tobacco use. Smoking is a major risk factor for coronary artery
disease, cerebrovascular disease, and peripheral vascular disease. It
causes an estimated 123,000 deaths each year from these diseases. An
additional 85,000 deaths per year from pulmonary diseases are also
attributed to tobacco use. As a result, tobacco use is the most
important modifiable cause of death in the United States. In addition,

---

[1] This chapter is a revision of one written for an earlier project
on quality of care for women and children (Q1). The expert panel for
the current project was asked to review all of the indicators, but only
rated new or revised indicators.

"second-hand" smoke affects the health of nonsmokers. In 1993, smoking-related medical care cost an estimated $50 billion (USPSTF, 1996).

Evidence from prospective cohort and case-control studies support the efficacy of reduction of health risks with cessation of smoking even among the elderly (USPSTF, 1996). Patients who stop smoking return to baseline risk profiles for coronary artery disease within three to five years (USDHHS, 1989; Rich-Edwards et al., 1995).

SCREENING

Many specialty societies and governmental organizations recommend asking patients if they smoke, including the American College of Physicians (ACP), American College of Obstetricians and Gynecologists (ACOG), American Academy of Pediatrics (AAP), and the National Cancer Institute (NCI). The AHCPR guidelines clearly emphasize the importance of systematically identifying all smokers and directs strategies at primary care providers, health care administrators, insurers, and purchasers. They encourage the implementation of office systems to ensure that all patients have their tobacco-use status identified and documented on every visit.

It is clear that routine assessment of smoking status leads to increased clinician counseling and interventions. A meta-analysis of nine trials assessing the impact of a screening system to identify smoking status found an intervention rate of 65.6 percent, versus 38.5 percent in the reference group (estimated odds ratio of 3.1, 95 percent CI 2.2-4.2). Screening systems may result in higher quit rates among patients who smoke, although this finding was not statistically significant and was based on only three studies (AHCPR, 1996). We propose that all patients be screened for tobacco use at least once (Indicator 1), and that smokers have their smoking status indicated on at least 50 percent of non-emergency visits (Indicator 2). This can be documented as part of the vital signs, or through use of special chart stickers identifying smokers or through use of computer generated reminders or in the visit assessment and plan. Repeated assessment of adults who have never smoked or have been abstinent for years is not necessary.

TREATMENT

There is limited evidence for the effectiveness of tobacco cessation counseling in improving clinical outcomes. However, there is good evidence that even brief clinician counseling has a modest impact in helping people stop smoking. In an analysis of 17 randomized controlled trials of brief advice and encouragement to stop smoking from a primary care clinician during one routine consultation, an estimated two percent (P < .001) of all smokers stopped smoking and did not relapse up to one year later as a direct consequence of this advice (Law and Tang, 1995).

Every major health care organization, including the USPSTF and the AHCPR, recommends that all smokers be counseled to stop smoking. Recognizing that clinicians may not always document advice given, our proposed indicator requires for each smoker there be documentation at least once during the course of a year that the clinician recommended smoking cessation. This documentation may be in a progress note or a specific referral for a smoking cessation program (Indicator 3).

While all smokers should be asked about their interest in quitting, specialized assessments such as the use of formal instruments are not necessary, although they may be helpful in providing information to tailor treatment (AHCPR, 1996). Successful interventions can be delivered by a variety of providers including various medical and non-medical health care providers, such as nurses, psychologists, social workers, and dentists. The greatest effect is observed when multiple providers deliver the smoking cessation interventions.

Smoking cessation interventions and counseling have the potential to improve cessation rates above that seen for brief clinician advice. Higher cessation rates have also been reported for special populations, such as pregnant women or men with known coronary artery disease or high cardiovascular risk factors (Law and Tang, 1995). There is a clear dose-response relationship between the intensity of person-to-person contact and successful cessation outcome (Table 5.1). In addition, duration (number of weeks) and number of sessions improve cessation rates (Table 5.2). Three specific content categories were associated with statistically significant increases in cessation rates. These

119

include problem solving/skills training, intratreatment social support by the clinician, and aversion smoking procedures. Therefore, all smokers who indicate they would like to quit should be offered at least one additional counseling session. This may be with the clinician, or other identified support person, group, or specialized program (Indicator 4).

Table 5.1

**Cessation Rates for Various Intensities of
Person-to-Person Contact (N = 56 studies)**

Level of Contact	Number of Study Arms	Estimated Odds Ratio (95% C.I.)	Estimated Cessation Rate (95% C.I.)
None (reference group)	49	1.0	8.8
Minimal contact (3 minutes or less)	14	1.2 (1.0-1.5)	10.7 (8.9-12.5)
Brief counseling (> 3 to <=10 minutes)	26	1.4 (1.2-1.7)	12.1 (10.0-14.3)
Counseling (>10 minutes)	60	2.4 (2.1-2.7)	18.7 (16.8-20.6)

Source: Table 12, AHCPR Guidelines #18

Table 5.2

**Cessation Rates by Number of Person-to-Person
Treatment Sessions (N = 55 studies)**

Number of Sessions	Number of Study Arms	Estimated Odds Ratio (95% C.I.)	Estimated Cessation Rate (95% C.I.)
0-1 session (reference group)	96	1.0	10.4
2-3 sessions	15	2.0 (1.6-2.4)	18.8 (15.8-21.9)
4-7 sessions	25	2.5 (2.2-2.9)	22.6 (19.9-25.3)
>7 sessions	12	1.7 (1.2-2.5)	16.7 (11.4-22.0)

Source: Table 15, AHCPR Guidelines #18

Adding nicotine replacement therapy has been found to increase cessation rates. Twelve-month cessation rates, after brief clinician counseling and multiple follow-up visits, double with the use of the nicotine patch. Use of nicotine gum may increase the success rate of counseling alone by up to one-third, particularly in heavy smokers (USPSTF, 1996). The four mg gum is preferred in heavily addicted smokers over the two mg gum. The AHCPR guidelines recommend that patients "be encouraged to use nicotine replacement therapy (patch or gum) for smoking cessation except in the presence of special circumstances." The guidelines also recommend that health care administrators, insurers and purchasers include pharmacotherapy as a paid service for all subscribers of health insurance packages. Even though both the gum and the patch are available over the counter, their cost may discourage use. Our proposed indicator states that all smokers who smoke more than five cigarettes a day be offered or counseled on the use of nicotine replacement therapy, unless there are serious medical precautions (Indicator 5). Persons who smoke five or fewer cigarettes a day may benefit from the patch, but these smokers have not been well studied (Henningfield, 1995). See Tables 5.3 and 5.4 for a summary of published meta-analyses.

Broad-based programs to stop smoking appear to be most effective. The most successful trials were more likely to employ both group and individual counseling, teams of physicians and non-physicians, multiple reinforcement sessions, and face-to-face advice. Multivariate analysis of the attributes of successful trials showed that the number of interventions was strongly associated with the smoking cessation rate (Table 5.5) (Kottke et al., 1988).

Table 5.3

Summary of Nicotine Patch Meta-analyses Efficacy Results (N = 5 meta-analyses)

Meta-analysis	Follow-up Period	Number of Trials	Efficacy Measure*
Po (1993)	6 mo	8	Odds Ratio = 2.3
Gourlay (1994)	6 mo	6	Odds Ratio = 2.2
Tang, Law, Wald (1994)	12 mo	6	Success Increment = 9%
Silagy, Mant, Fowler et al.,(1994)	12 mo	9	Odds Ratio = 2.1
Fiore, Smith, Jorenby et al.,(1994)	6 mo	16	Odds Ratio = 2.6

Source: Table 16, AHCPR Guidelines #18
* All meta-analyses used an active versus placebo patch comparison.

Table 5.4

Summary of Nicotine Gum Meta-analyses* (n = 3 meta-analyses)

Meta-analysis	Percent Abstinent (12 mo.)		Odds Ratio (95% C.I.)
	Active Gum	Control**	
Cepeda-Benito (1993)	16.9	12.5	1.4 (1.41-1.43)
Tang, Law, Wald (1994)	17.9	12.8	1.5 (1.4-1.5)
Silagy, Mant, Fowler et al.,(1994)	18.2	10.6	1.6 (1.5-1.8)

Source: Table 17, AHCPR Guidelines # 18
* Control groups are a mixture of placebo and no-gum conditions.
** Overall effect sizes are reported; Effect sizes are larger when gum is used in the context of intensive psychosocial therapy than when used with brief therapy.

Table 5.5

**Correlation of Study Characteristics with
Cessation Rates at 12 Month Follow-up**

Descriptors	Range	Mean (SD)	Correlation with Cessation Rate
No. of intervention modalities	1-6	2.1 (± 0.9)	.48*
Participant drop-out rate	0%-51%	13.8% (± 12.0%)	.05
No. of subject contacts with program	1-15	3.8 (± 4.6)	.38*
Months subject in contact with program	0-12	1.1 (± 2.1)	.55*

Source: Kottke et al., 1988.
*p<.01

FOLLOW-UP

It is generally recommended that patients who receive an intervention (such as counseling to set a quit date, nicotine replacement therapy, or intensive smoking cessation program) be assessed for abstinence. Usually this is done at the end of the intervention, or at subsequent patient visits. Most experts recommend follow-up a few days to two weeks after setting a quit date (Indicator 6). This can be done by phone or a follow-up visit. This reinforcement is important during this vulnerable time period. Persons who are unsuccessful at quitting or quickly relapse can be reassessed for continued motivation to quit smoking and need for additional interventions (AHCPR, 1996; USPSTF, 1996). Persons who continue to smoke while using nicotine replacement therapy can be counseled to stop the nicotine replacement until they re-evaluate barriers to giving up all cigarettes.

REFERENCES

Henningfield J. 1995. Nicotine medications for smoking cessation. *The New England Journal of Medicine* 133 (18): 1196-1203.

Kottke T. 1988. Attributes of successful smoking cessation interventions in medical practice. *Journal of the American Medical Association* 259 (19): 2883-2889.

Law M, and Tang J. An analysis of the effectiveness of interventions intended to help people stop smoking. *Archives of Internal Medicine* 1995 155 (18): 1933-1941.

Rich-Edwards, Janet W, Manson, JoAnn E, Hennekens, Charles H, Buring, and Julie E. 29 June 1995. The primary prevention of coronary heart disease in women. *New England Journal of Medicine* 332 (26): 1758-66.

US Department of Health and Human Services. 1989. Reducing the health consequences of smoking: 25 years of progress. A report of the Surgeon General.

US Department of Health and Human Services. 1996. Smoking Cessation. *Clinical Practice Guideline* #18

US Preventative Services Task Force. 1996. Guide to Clinical Preventative Services, 2nd ed. Baltimore: Williams & Wilkins.

RECOMMENDED QUALITY INDICATORS FOR CIGARETTE COUNSELING

These indicators apply to men and women age 18 and older. Only the indicators in bold type were rated by this panel; the remaining indicators were endorsed by a prior panel.

Indicator	Quality of Evidence	Literature	Benefits	Comments
Screening				
1. Smoking status should be documented at least once for all patients.	I, III	AHCPR, 1996	Increase the smoking cessation intervention by clinicians and the rate of cessation by patients who smoke. Decrease smoking-related morbidity and mortality.	Studies indicate that having a smoking status identification system increases rates of clinician intervention with their patients who smoke. Evidence of impact on rates of cessation is less clear.
2. Patients documented to be smokers should have their smoking status indicated on at least 50% of all non-emergency visits.	I, III	AHCPR, 1996	Increase the smoking cessation intervention by clinicians and the rate of cessation by patients who smoke. Decrease smoking-related morbidity and mortality.	Studies indicate that having a smoking status identification system increases rates of clinician intervention with their patients who smoke. Evidence of impact on rates of cessation is less clear.
Treatment				
3. There should be documentation that advice to quit smoking was given to all smokers at least once during the course of a year.[1]	I	Law and Tang, 1995; AHCPR, 1996; USPSTF, 1996	Decrease smoking-related morbidity and mortality.	Even brief physician advice to quit smoking has a modest effect on cessation rates regardless of patients motivation to quit. While clinicians are encouraged to discuss smoking at every visit, it is clear that it may not always be documented.
4. All smokers identified as attempting to quit should be offered at least one additional smoking cessation counseling visit[2] within 3 months.	I	AHCPR, 1996; Kottke ,1988	Increase smoking cessation rates. Decrease smoking-related morbidity and mortality	There is a strong dose-response relationship between the intensity (time) of person-to-person contact and successful cessation outcome.

125

	Quality of Evidence	Literature	Benefits	Comments
5. All smokers attempting to quit who smoke more than 5 cigarettes a day should be offered nicotine replacement therapy except in the presence of serious medical precautions.[3]	I	AHCPR, 1996; Law and Tang, 1995	Decrease smoking-related morbidity and mortality	Meta-analyses of nicotine replacement therapy for both patches and gum demonstrate improved cessation rates compared with control or placebo interventions. There is insufficient research on the benefit for those who smoke less than 5 cigarettes a day.
Follow-up				
6. All patients who receive a smoking cessation intervention[4] should have their abstinence status documented within 2 weeks of the completion of treatment.	III	AHCPR, 1996; USPSTF, 1996	Decrease smoking-related morbidity and mortality.	One of the common characteristics of successful counseling in the Kottke meta-analysis is reinforcement at subsequent visits.

Definitions and Examples

[1] Documentation may be in the form of progress note or billing code for smoking cessation counseling or referral for special smoking cessation services.

[2] This may be with the clinician or other identified support person, group, or specialized program. In addition to nicotine replacement therapy, clinician delivered social support and skills training are particularly effective components of smoking cessation treatment.

[3] Medical precautions include patients in the immediate (within 4 weeks) postmyocardial infarction period, those with serious arrhythmias, and those with severe or worsening angina pectoris.

[4] Smoking cessation interventions include: specific counseling sessions, an intensive program, or nicotine replacement therapy.

Quality of Evidence Codes

I	RCT
II-1	Nonrandomized controlled trials
II-2	Cohort or case analysis
II-3	Multiple time series
III	Opinions or descriptive studies

126

6. COMMUNITY-ACQUIRED PNEUMONIA

Alison Moore, MD

Several recent reviews provided the core references in developing quality indicators for the evaluation and management of community-acquired pneumonia (Campbell, 1994; Mandell, 1995; Whitson and Campbell, 1994; Brown, 1993; Bartlett and Mundy, 1995; Pomilla and Brown, 1994). Where these core references cited studies to support individual indicators, we have included the original references. We also used three guidelines regarding antimicrobial management of community-acquired pneumonia (ATS, 1993; BTS, 1993; CCAPCCG, 1993). In the following review we have excluded consideration of the evaluation and treatment of CAP in persons with HIV.

IMPORTANCE

More than four and one half million Americans develop community-acquired pneumonias (CAP) annually. Of these, about one million persons are hospitalized, generating more than $4 billion in medical expenses. CAP ranks sixth in cause-specific mortality for Americans and among the elderly, it is the fourth leading cause of death (Kovar, 1977). While attack rates are highest at the extremes of age, overall attack rates are ten to twelve cases per 1000 persons per year (Foy et al., 1973; Marrie, 1994).

The elderly and patients with chronic respiratory, cardiac, renal, or hematological illnesses suffer the greatest morbidity and mortality from CAP (Campbell, 1994; Mandell, 1995; Whitson and Campbell, 1994; Brown, 1993; Bartlett and Mundy, 1995; Pomilla and Brown, 1994; ATS, 1993; BTS, 1993; CCAPCCG, 1993). Coexisting or recent viral infection, particularly with influenza virus, continues to be an important predisposing factor for CAP. Smokers are also at increased risk. Although mortality is high among certain subgroups, such as the elderly and those with comorbid disease, 50 to 90 percent of patients with community acquired pneumonia are safely treated as outpatients (Pomilla and Brown, 1994).

127

SCREENING

There are no current recommendations in the reviewed literature on screening for pneumonia.

DIAGNOSIS

A careful history (including chronic respiratory, cardiac, hepatic or renal illnesses, diabetes, immune dysfunction, smoking status, history of recent viral illness, history of recent use of antibiotics) and physical examination (including vital signs, and a lung examination) are essential in making the diagnosis of pneumonia. CAP may have many clinical presentations. Classically, CAP is characterized by fever, cough, pleuritic chest pain, chills, increased sputum production, focal lung consolidation on physical examination and a positive chest x-ray. However, atypical presentations are common, particularly in the elderly, in whom mental status changes and tachypnea may predominate (Esposito, 1984; Venkatesh et al., 1990; Fein et al., 1990; Whitson and Campbell, 1994). Other presenting symptoms and signs may include myalgias, malaise, headache, and diarrhea, especially early in the illness. Our proposed indicator requires that, for persons suspected of having pneumonia, health care providers obtain a focused history and physical examination, including questions about onset of symptoms, nature of symptoms, coexisting illnesses, smoking status, recent use of antibiotics, recent viral illness, assessment of vital signs, and a lung examination (Indicators 1 and 2).

Chest radiography (CXR) (preferably posterior-anterior and lateral views) should be performed in all patients with signs and symptoms of pneumonia (Indicator 3). The presence of cavitation or multilobar infiltrates suggests a more complicated illness. A CXR should also be obtained in those who have fever, tachycardia, or an abnormal lung examination. These clinical findings, in the absence of asthma, have been prospectively validated and are better predictors of pneumonia in individuals than physician judgment (Heckerling et al., 1990; Emerman et al., 1991). If a pleural effusion is suspected, a lateral decubitus chest radiograph should be obtained to assess its size. A diagnostic thoracentesis should be performed if a parapneumonic effusion is present and the lateral decubitus film shows significant pleural effusion (>= 10 mm thickness in the dependent position)(Light, 1990)(Indicator 4).

The diagnostic value of a Gram stain and culture of expectorated sputum has been long debated (Niederman, 1993; Rein, 1978; ATS, 1993; BTS, 1993). This is because 10 to 30 percent of patients have a non-productive cough, 15 to 30 percent of persons get antibiotics before they are given the diagnosis of pneumonia, and negative culture results are reported for 30 to 65 percent of cultures. No studies have shown a close correlation between sputum Gram stain and results using lower respiratory tract secretions in large numbers of patients with CAP (Campbell, 1994). Given the uncertainty regarding the utility of Gram stain and culture among persons with pneumonia, we do not propose an indicator regarding the use of these tests.

Serology for specific pathogens is helpful in epidemiology studies, but diagnosis is based on a comparison of acute and convalescent sera, limiting its usefulness in directing initial therapy. Serology also lacks adequate sensitivity and specificity (Campbell, 1994).

Routine lab tests, such as complete blood count, serum electrolytes and indices of liver or renal function, are of no benefit in helping to establish a diagnosis of pneumonia, but may be helpful in identifying patients at risk for a more complicated course. The American Thoracic Society recommends inclusion of a complete blood count, serum electrolytes, hepatic enzymes, and tests of renal function in all patients with CAP who are 60 years of age or older or who have coexisting illness (ATS, 1993). The British Thoracic Society (BTS, 1993) only makes recommendations for additional tests for hospitalized persons who are suspected of having pneumonia. Blood cultures should only be obtained for persons requiring hospitalization (ATS, 1993; BTS, 1993). Consistent with the recommendations of the American Thoracic Society, our proposed indicator requires a white blood cell count, hemoglobin and hematocrit, serum electrolytes, BUN/creatinine in all patients with CAP who are 60 years of age or older, or who have coexisting illness (Indicator 5). Persons who are hospitalized with pneumonia should be offered two sets of blood cultures (Indicator 6).

An earlier RAND study on the effects of the DRG-based Prospective Payment System on quality of care for hospitalized Medicare patients developed quality indicators in this area (Kahn et al., 1992). Based on that work, we propose an indicator requiring that patients hospitalized with pneumonia have their temperature and a lung examination documented on days one and two of hospitalization (Indicator 7).

TREATMENT

By necessity, most patients are treated with an empiric antimicrobial regimen pending results from diagnostic studies as early initiation of appropriate therapy is associated with lower morbidity and mortality. Choice of any empiric regimen must take into account the spectrum of potential pathogens likely to be encountered, as no pathogen is identified in up to 50 percent of patients despite extensive testing (Fang, 1990; Berntsson, 1986).

Choosing an appropriate empiric regimen for treatment requires an understanding of the probable spectrum of pathogens encountered in a specific setting. Major variables have been identified that are believed to influence the spectrum of pathogens encountered and the decision to hospitalize in any given patient population (ATS, 1993; CCAPCCG, 1993). These variables include age, host factors[1], and severity of illness at time of initial presentation[2] (Fang, 1990; Fine, 1993; ATS, 1993; CCAPCCG, 1993, Fine, Smith, 1990; Council of the British Thoracic Society, 1987; Farr, 1991). Using these variables, the American Thoracic Society (ATS, 1993) and the Canadian Community Acquired Pneumonia Consensus Conference Group (CCAPCCG, 1993) separated CAP into four easily identifiable patient populations. Of these four groups, two are directed at outpatient treatment: one for individuals age 60 or under, without significant coexisting disease (Group 1), and another for individuals who are older than 60 years or who have

---

[1] For example, functional status, social support, coexisting illness.
[2] For example, respiratory rate > 30 breaths/min, fever > 38.3 degrees centigrade, systolic blood pressure < 90 mm Hg; diastolic pressure < 60 mm Hg, confusion, $pACO2 < 60$ OR $pACO2 > 50$ mm Hg.

coexisting illness (Group 2). The remaining two groups include patients requiring hospitalization. These groups were divided based on the severity of the pneumonia: # Group 3 for less than severe and Group 4 for severe. The definition of severe CAP was based on having respiratory failure, multilobar involvement, shock, acute renal failure, and generally includes those needing admission to an intensive care unit. Using these four groups, the most likely pathogens (and appropriate antimicrobials to treat them) were identified by reviewing the literature. Pre-established criteria were used to select pertinent clinical studies.

For Group 1, the most common pathogens included *S. pneumoniae*, *M. pneumoniae*, respiratory viruses, *C. pneumoniae*, and *H. influenzae*. Miscellaneous pathogens were sporadically noted and include Legionella species, *S. aureas*, *M. tuberculosis*, endemic fungi and aerobic gram-negative bacilli. Mortality is low (1%) in this setting and the incidence of complication arising from CAP that later requires hospitalization was less than ten percent.

Generally, the recommended treatment for persons having pneumonia and who are 60 years of age or younger and have no coexisting illnesses (Group 1) is to use a macrolide. Erythromycin is the first line agent, but one of the newer macrolides, clarithromycin or azithromycin, may also be used, especially in those intolerant of erythromycin and in smokers (to treat *H. influenzae*). Tetracycline may be used if the patient is allergic or intolerant to macrolides. However, penicillin-resistant pneumococci may be resistant to these agents (ATS, 1993; The Medical Letter, 1996) (Indicator 8).

For Group 2, the spectrum of pathogens differed from the first group by the inclusion of more virulent major pathogens, aerobic gram-negative bacilli (but not *P. aeruginosa*) and *S. aureas* and the addition of Moraxella catarrhalis among the miscellaneous group. *S. pneumoniae* remains the most common identified pathogen. Deleted from the major pathogens in Group 1 were *M. pneumoniae* and *C. pneumoniae*. Mortality among this group is three percent, but approximately 20 percent of patients initially treated as outpatients eventually required

131

hospitalization, reflecting the significance of age and coexisting illness.

The treatment recommended for persons having pneumonia who are older than 60 years and/or have comorbid conditions (Group 2) is to use a second-generation cephalosporin (e.g., cefuroxime axetil, cefaclor, loracarbef, cefpodoxime proxetil) or trimethoprim-sulfamethoxazole or a beta-lactam/beta-lactamase inhibitor (e.g., amoxicillin/clavulanic acid). Additionally, if infection with Legionalla is a concern one may add erythromycin or another macrolide to this regimen (Indicator 9).

For Group 3, those persons with CAP who require initial hospital admission, pathogens include all the major pathogens in Group 2, plus polymicrobial infection (including anaerobic bacteria), Legionella species and *C. pneumoniae*. Mortality in this group ranged from 13 to 25 percent. The treatment generally recommended for Group 3 is a second or third-generation cephalosporin or a beta-lactam/beta-lactamase inhibitor, with the possible addition of a macrolide if infection with Legionella is a concern (Indicator 10).

Group 4, those persons having severe CAP, most commonly had Legionella species and *S. pneumoniae*. Other major pathogens included aerobic gram-negative bacilli, *M. pneumoniae*, and respiratory viruses. Mortality in this group approached 50 percent. Treatment recommended for this group consists of a macrolide plus a third-generation cephalosporin with anti-pseudomonas activity or a macrolide plus another antipseudomonal agent such as imipenem/cilastin or ciprofloxacin (Indicator 11).

Clinical cure or improvement with any one of several antibiotic regimens exceeds 90 percent. The optimal length of treatment is unknown, but by convention most pneumonias are treated for ten to 14 days (Pomilla and Brown, 1994). Our proposed indicator in this area is consistent with these standards; that is, that most pneumonias should be treated for ten to 14 days, with the exception of azithromycin, which may be given for five days (ATS, 1993) (Indicator 12).

Two studies have looked at relative indications for hospitalization in patients with CAP (Fine, Smith, 1990; Black, 1991). The indications include: symptom duration less than one week or greater than four weeks, age over 65 years, immunosuppression, comorbid illness, fever greater than 38.3 degrees centigrade, multilobar involvement on CXR, aspiration or postobstructive pneumonia, pneumonia associated with *S. aureus*, or gram-negative bacilli. Other indications for hospitalization include respiratory rate greater than 30 breaths per minute, systolic blood pressure less than 90 mm Hg; diastolic pressure less than 60 mm Hg, confusion, metastatic infection, and leukopenia (Fang, 1990; Fine, 1993; Van Metre, 1954). In addition to these risk factors, the physician needs to assess whether the patient has the functional skills and social support to care for herself outside the hospital, as well as the ability to be compliant with therapy and follow-up (Fine, 1990).

As part of the Pneumonia Patient Outcomes Research Team, researchers surveyed 292 medical practitioners at four geographically separate hospitals to identify the factors clinicians considered when deciding whether or not to hospitalize CAP patients at low risk for short-term mortality (predicted probability of death of less than 4%) (Fine, 1997). Results showed that practitioners relied heavily on five clinical factors to make this decision: the patient's respiratory status, coexisting illness, clinical appearance, lung involvement of more than one lobe, and oral intake. Three patient factors were almost always associated with hospitalization: hypoxemia, inability to maintain oral intake of foods, liquids and antimicrobial medicines, and lack of patient home care support. Patients without these risk factors, but whom practitioners estimated still had more than a five percent risk of death, also were more likely to be hospitalized. Given the heterogeneity in clinical and social factors involved, we do not recommend any quality indicators for hospital admission.

FOLLOW-UP

Once antimicrobial therapy is initiated, it is important to monitor the patient for clinical response. Normally, no change in antimicrobial therapy should be considered within the first 72 hours unless initial diagnostic studies identify a pathogen not covered by original empiric therapy, a resistant pathogen is isolated from blood or another sterile site, or there is clinical deterioration (ATS, 1993). The presence of coexisting illness and advanced age is associated with delays in improvement. Patients with structural abnormalities of the respiratory tract often do not respond as readily as previously healthy patients. The virulence of the infectious agent may also delay response. Especially among patients without prior coexisting disease, fever generally disappears within two to four days, and leukocytosis resolves by the fourth or fifth day of therapy. Physical findings remain abnormal in up to 40 percent of patients at day seven. The CXR is often abnormal at four weeks.

Patients who are not improving or are deteriorating should be reevaluated for evidence of noninfectious processes, antimicrobial resistance, or unrecognized immunosuppression. Repeat microbiologic studies should be obtained, as well as an electrocardiogram to rule out unrecognized myocardial infarction (in older patients), and a chest radiograph to look for an infectious complication (Bartlett and Mundy, 1995).

The recommendations of the American Thoracic Society indicate that if clinical deterioration (e.g., no improvement or worsening in sense of well-being, continued or increased cough, decreased appetite) does occur during the first 72 hours, or no improvement is seen after 72 hours after starting antibiotics, then the ambulatory patient should be seen by the health professional for re-evaluation (ATS, 1993). Moreover, persons who are hospitalized with CAP should be seen by a health professional within six weeks of discharge to ensure that the pneumonia has completely resolved (BTS, 1993) (Indicator 13).

REFERENCES

American Thoracic Society Consensus Committee. 1993. Guidelines for the initial empiric therapy of community acquired pneumonia: proceedings of an American Thoracic Society Consensus Conference. *American Review of Respiratory Disease* 148: 1418-1426.

Bartlett JG, and Mundy LM. 1995. Community-acquired pneumonia. *New England Journal of Medicine* 333: 1618-1624.

British Thoracic Society. 1993. Guidelines for the management of community-acquired pneumonia in adults admitted to the hospital. *Brit J Hosp Med* 49: 346-350.

Brown RB. 1993. Community-acquired pneumonia: diagnosis and therapy of older adults. *Geriatrics* 148: 43-50.

Campbell GD. 1994. Overview of community-acquired pneumonia. *Med Clinics North America* 78: 1035-1048.

Emerman CL, Dawson N, Speroff T, et al. 1991. Comparison of physician judgement and decision aids for ordering chest radiographs for pneumonia in outpatients. *Annals of Emergency Medicine* 20: 1215-1219.

Esposito AL. 1984. Community-acquired bacteremic pneumococcal pneumonia: Effect of age on manifestations and outcome. *Archives of Internal Medicine* 149: 945-948.

Fein AM, Feinsilver SH, and Niederman MS. 1991. Atypical manifestations of pneumonia in the elderly. *Clin Chest Med* 12: 319-336.

Fine MJ, Hough LJ, and Medsger ARet al. 1997. The hospital admission decision for patients with community-acquired pneumonia. *Archives of Internal Medicine* 157: 36-44.

Foy HM, Cooney MK, and McMahan Ret al. 1973. Viral and mycoplasmal pneumonia in a prepaid medical care group during an eight year period. *American Journal of Epidemiology* 97: 93-102.

Heckerling PS, Tape TG, Wigton RS, et al. Clinical prediction rule for pulmonary infiltrates. *Archives of Internal Medicine* 990 (113): 664-670.

Kahn KL, Draper D, and Keeler EMet al. 1992. The effects of the DRG-based Prospective Payment System on Quality of Care for Hospitalized Medicare Patients. RAND R-3931-HCFA:

Kovar MD. 1977. Health of the elderly and the use of health services. *Public Health Rep* 92: 9-19.

Light RW, Girard WM, Jenkinson SG, et al. 1980. Parapneumonic effusions. *American Journal of Medicine* 69: 507-511.

Light RW, MacGregor MI, Luchsinger PC, et al. 1972. Pleural effusions; the diagnositc speration of transudates and exudates. *Archives of Internal Medicine* 77: 507-513.

Mandell LA. 1995. Community-acquired pneumonia: etiology, epidemiology, and treatment. *Chest* 108: 35S-42S.

Mandell LA, Niederman M, and the Canadian Community Acquired Pneumonia Consensus Conference Group. 1993. Antimicrobial treatment of community-acquired pneumonia in adults: a conference report. *Can Journal of Infectious Diseases* 4: 25-28.

Marrie TJ. 1994. Community-aquired pneumonia. *Clinical Infectious Diseases* 18: 501-515.

Pomilla PV, and Brown RB. 1994. Outpatient treatment of community-acquired pneumonia in adults. *Archives of Internal Medicine* 154: 1793-1802.

The choice of antibacterial drugs. 1996. *The Medical Letter* 38: 25-34.

Venkatesh P, Gladman J, Macfarlane JT, et al. 1990. A hospital study of community acquired pneumonia in the elderly. *Thorax* 45: 254-258.

Whitson B, and Campbell GD. 1994. Community-acquired pneumonia: new outpatient guidelines based on age, severity of illness. *Geriatrics* 49: 24-36.

INDICATORS FOR QUALITY OF CARE IN COMMUNITY-ACQUIRED PNEUMONIA

These indicators apply to men and women age 18 and older.

	Indicator	Quality of Evidence	Literature	Benefits	Comments
Diagnosis					
1.	If patient has symptoms of pneumonia,[1] on the day of admission the provider should document: a. whether the cough is productive or nonproductive; b. the presence or absence of a coexisting illness,[2] and c. the presence or absence of recent upper respiratory symptoms.[9]	III	ATS, 1993; BTS, 1993; Pomilla and Brown, 1994; Whitson and Campbell, 1994; Campbell, 1994; Bartlett and Mundy, 1995	Improves diagnosis, risk stratification and management of CAP.	Recommended by all the consensus developers and articles reviewing this topic.
2.	If patient has symptoms of pneumonia,[1] the following should be documented on the day of presentation: a. temperature; b. respiratory rate; c. heart rate; and d. lung examination.	III	ATS, 1993; BTS, 1993; Pomilla and Brown, 1994; Whitson and Campbell, 1994; Campbell, 1994; Bartlett and Mundy, 1995	Improves diagnosis, risk stratification and management of CAP.	Recommended by all the consensus developers and articles reviewing this topic.
3.	If patient has both symptoms and signs of pneumonia,[1,3] the health care provider should offer a chest radiograph (CXR) on the day of presentation.	II-3, III	ATS, 1993; BTS, 1993; Pomilla and Brown, 1994; Whitson and Campbell, 1994; Campbell, 1994; Bartlett and Mundy, 1995; Heckerling et al, 1990; Emerman et al, 1991	Improves diagnosis, risk stratification and management of CAP.	Two studies have prospectively validated clinical findings of fever, tachycardia or an abnormal lung examination and the absence of asthma as predictors of pneumonia as seen on CXR. Recommended by all the consensus developers and articles reviewing this topic.

137

	Indicator	Quality of Evidence	Literature	Benefits	Comments
4.	If a patient has both symptoms and signs of pneumonia[1,3] and suggestion of a pleural effusion on CXR[4], a lateral decubitus radiograph or ultrasound should be offered on the day of presentation to assess the size of the effusion.	III	ATS, 1993; BTS, 1993; Campbell; 1994	Allows for improved diagnosis, risk stratification and management of CAP.	Recommended by all the consensus developers and articles reviewing this topic.
5.	If a patient over 60 years of age has both symptoms and signs of pneumonia[1,3] with coexisting illness, the health care provider should offer the following blood tests on the day of presentation: a. white blood cell count; b. hemoglobin and hematocrit; c. serum electrolytes; and d. BUN or creatinine.	III	ATS, 1993	May help in identifying patients at risk for a more complicated course.	Recommended by the American Thoracic Society
6.	If patient has both symptoms and signs of pneumonia,[1,3] and is hospitalized, the health care provider should offer two sets of blood cultures on the day of hospitalization.	III	ATS, 1993; BTS, 1993	May help in identifying patients at risk for a more complicated course.	Recommended by the American Thoracic Society and the British Thoracic Society
7.	Hospitalized persons with pneumonia should have the following documented on the first and second days of hospitalization: a. temperature; and b. lung examination.	III	Kahn et al, 1992	Triage patients to match severity and treatment intensity.	These quality of care indicators were developed by an expert panel as part of a study evaluating the effects of the DRG-based prospective payment system on quality of care of hospitalized Medicare patients.
Treatment					
8.	Non-hospitalized persons <= 60 years of age diagnosed with pneumonia without a known bacteriologic etiology[5] and without coexisting illnesses[8] should be offered an oral empiric macrolide,[6] unless allergic.	III	ATS, 1993; CCAPCCG, 1993	Treat the most likely etiologic agents of CAP.	Recommended by two of the consensus developers.

138

	Indicator	Quality of Evidence	Literature	Benefits	Comments
9.	Non-hospitalized persons > 60 years of age diagnosed with pneumonia without a known bacteriologic etiology[5] and with coexisting illnesses[8] should be offered one of the following oral empiric antibiotic regimens: • a second generation cephalosporin; • trimethoprim-sulfamethoxazole; or • a beta-lactam/beta-lactamase inhibitor combination.	III	ATS, 1993; CCAPCCG, 1993	Treat the most likely etiologic agents of CAP.	Recommended by two of the consensus developers.
10.	Hospitalized persons with non-severe[7] pneumonia without a known bacteriologic etiology[5] should be offered one of the following empiric antibiotic regimens: • a second or third generation cephalosporin; or • a beta-lactam/beta-lactamase inhibitor combination.	III	ATS, 1993; CCAPCCG, 1993	Treat the most likely etiologic agents of CAP.	Recommended by two of the consensus developers.
11.	Hospitalized persons with severe pneumonia[7] without a known bacteriologic etiology[5] should be offered one of the following antibiotic regimens: • a macrolide and a third generation cephalosporin with anti-Pseudomonas activity; or • a macrolide and another anitpseudomonal agent such as imipenem/ciliastin, ciprofloxacin	III	ATS, 1993; CCAPCCG, 1993; BTS, 1993	Treat the most likely etiologic agents of CAP.	Recommended by three of the consensus developers.
12.	Persons with CAP should be offered antibiotics for 10-14 days, with the exception of azithromycin, which may be given for 5 days.	II-1,III	ATS, 1993; CCAPCCG, 1993; Pomilla and Brown, 1994	Prevent inadequate or incomplete treatment.	Recommended by two of the consensus developers and one of the review articles.

139

Indicator	Quality of Evidence	Literature	Benefits	Comments
Follow-Up				
13. Persons who have been hospitalized for pneumonia should have an appointment with a provider within 6 weeks after discharge.	III	BTS;1993	Allows health professional to determine if pneumonia has resolved.	Recommended by BTS.

Definitions and Examples

[1] Symptoms of pneumonia: Cough and at least one of the following within a two week period - dyspnea, pleuritic chest pain, rigors.

[2] Coexisting illness: The presence or absence of at least three of the following in the last two years must be documented - lung, heart, renal or liver disease, diabetes, immune dysfunction (e.g., AIDS, use of corticosteroids).

[3] Signs of pneumonia: At least one of the following within a two week period - fever, tachycardia (heart rate > 100 bpm), or abnormal respiratory findings [tachypnea (respiratory rate > 28), rales, rhonchi, decreased breath sounds].

[4] Suggestion of pleural effusion on CXR: Any one of the following - blunting of costophrenic angles, diffuse opacification, oblique angle formed by the chest wall and the margin of the pleural density.

[5] Pneumonia without a known bacteriologic etiology: Causal bacteriologic agent unknown from previous cultures.

[6] Oral empiric macrolide: Erythromycin is the first line agent, but one of the newer macrolides, clarithromycin or azithromycin, may also be used, especially in those intolerant of erythromycin and in smokers (to treat H. influenzae).

[7] Severe pneumonia: At least one of the following - respiratory rate > 30 breaths/min at admission, requirement for mechanical ventilation, requirement for vasopressors for more than 4 hours.

[8] Coexisting illnesses: Lung, heart, renal or liver disease, diabetes, immune dysfunction (e.g., AIDS, use of corticosteroids).

[9] Upper respiratory symptoms: Sore throat, pharyngitis, rhinorrhea, palatal itching, sneezing, nasal congestion, purulent nasal discharge, headache.

Quality of Evidence Codes

I	RCT
II-1	Nonrandomized controlled trials
II-2	Cohort or case analysis
II-3	Multiple time series
III	Opinions or descriptive studies

140

7. CORONARY ARTERY DISEASE - DIAGNOSIS AND SCREENING

Anthony Steimle, MD

The diagnosis of suspected coronary artery disease (CAD) is a complex topic comprising many potential clinical presentations and several diagnostic tests. Despite an abundant literature on the characteristics (such as sensitivity and specificity) of these tests in patients with CAD, few randomized trials have directly tested whether a particular diagnostic approach improves patient outcomes. Rather, the benefits of most tests must be extrapolated from combining how accurately they predict the presence and prognosis of CAD with the known effectiveness of treatments such as revascularization. Thus, the quality indicators in this chapter have largely been based on expert opinion and synthesis of this data, in the form of review articles, necessity ratings, clinical guidelines, and decision analytic models. We performed MEDLINE searches to identify English language review articles published since 1992 on coronary disease, myocardial ischemia, myocardial infarction, angina pectoris, stable angina, and unstable angina. We supplemented these sources with narrow MEDLINE searches on particular clinical scenarios and with key references from the bibliographies of review articles.

IMPORTANCE

The importance of coronary artery disease is difficult to overstate. Despite declining mortality rates, cardiovascular disease remains the leading cause of death in the United States, accounting for 45 percent of all deaths in 1988, with CAD alone responsible for 24 percent (AHA, 1991). Approximately seven million Americans are currently diagnosed with CAD (AHA 1994). In 1996, the AHA estimates that CAD in the U.S. cost society $151 billion (AHA, 1996).

SCREENING

Specialized testing to screen for CAD is not indicated for healthy adults without signs or symptoms of ischemic heart disease (Sox et al.,

1989). Screening older men who have multiple CAD risk factors may be beneficial in some cases, but specific indications for such testing are not agreed upon. A separate chapter will address hyperlipidemia screening.

DIAGNOSIS

Once a patient has presented with symptoms or signs of CAD, several specialized tests, primarily stress testing and coronary angiography, can be used to confirm the diagnosis and guide treatment. Typically, patients first undergo stress testing to predict their risk from CAD. When the results suggest a high risk, coronary angiography is then used to confirm the presence of disease and to map its anatomy. The quality indicators in this chapter focus on these two tests because they have been extensively studied, and are discrete and easily measured.

Developing concise indications for stress testing and coronary angiography is difficult for several reasons. First, the benefits of testing are not well defined. Few randomized trials have directly examined how diagnostic tests affect patient outcomes. Instead, studies have measured how well tests detect CAD and predict its prognosis. Clinicians have then combined this information with data from trials of CAD interventions such as coronary artery bypass surgery (CABS) to infer the benefits of a diagnostic strategy. Second, the same test can serve different purposes in different situations. For instance, stress testing can define a patient's likelihood of having CAD; while in a patient already known to have CAD, it can predict risk of death or myocardial infarction. Coronary angiography is a prerequisite for planning CABS or angioplasty. However, even when revascularization is not performed, angiography can confirm the diagnosis of CAD and assess prognostic factors such as left ventricular function and the number of diseased vessels.

A third reason that the indications for testing are complex is that they are intricately related to individual patient characteristics. In some patients, stress testing suggests CAD is present but that the risk for an adverse event is not high enough to warrant coronary angiography. In other patients who have a high pretest probability of disease, the diagnosis of CAD can be made based on the history and physical examination alone. If these patients are not candidates for revascularization, the physician might begin medical therapy without any diagnostic tests. The patient-specific factors which influence the need for diagnostic testing include those which predict a patient's pretest probability of disease (e.g., the CAD risk factors: age 65 or older, diabetes, hypertension, hypercholesterolemia, smoking, male gender, and family history of CAD before age 55) and those which predict risk frp, CAD (e.g., prior revascularization, prior myocardial infarctions, and reduced ejection fraction). In addition, contraindications to revascularization and/or catheterization (see definitions in Section IV of this chapter) must be considered. Thus, to validly define when diagnostic testing is necessary, quality indicators must include many of these clinical details.

The clinical presentations that require diagnostic testing for CAD can be categorized as follows: signs of CAD in asymptomatic patients, chest pain (not yet diagnosed as angina), stable angina, unstable angina, myocardial infarction, and high risk for perioperative cardiac complications.

We should note that stress testing exists in many varieties. Stress can be provided by exercise or infused medication. Ischemia can be detected by electrocardiography and/or by cardiac imaging with radionuclide scintigraphy or echocardiography. Physicians choose among these techniques based on patient characteristics. In our quality indicators, we have not specified when a particular technique should be used or when imaging is required, but only when some form stress testing is indicated. However, the technique chosen should be "diagnostic" - that is, interpretable as either positive or negative. For example, imaging should be used in patients with left bundle branch block because stress-induced ECG changes are masked.

Asymptomatic Patients

Our indicators for asymptomatic patients were based on the ratings of an expert panel on the necessity of coronary angiography (Bernstein et al., 1991) and the AHCPR clinical practice guideline for heart failure (Konstam, 1994). Diagnostic testing is not indicated in asymptomatic people unless they have signs of structural heart disease such as a reduced left ventricular ejection fraction which could be due to ischemia. A decision analytic model has estimated that stress testing for an asymptomatic 60 year-old man would prolong life-expectancy by only 12 days and would not be cost-effective (Sox et al., 1989). In contrast, because patients with CAD and reduced ejection fractions have a high mortality (25% at 5 years if LVEF is less than 0.5) (ACC/AHA, 1996) there is consensus that evaluating all patients with abnormal ejection fractions for possible CAD is beneficial and necessary (Indicators 2 and 3) (Bernstein et al., 1991). Similarly, if an asymptomatic person has had a stress test (even one which was not indicated in the first place) which suggests a high risk for death or MI, coronary angiography is considered necessary (Indicator 1) (Bernstein et al., 1991).

Stable Angina or Known CAD

The indicators for diagnosis of stable angina and known CAD were developed from the recommendations of the North of England Stable Angina Guideline Development Group (NESAGDG), the ratings of a RAND expert panel on the necessity of diagnostic testing in patients with chest pain, and the ratings of a similar panel on the necessity of coronary angiography in a variety of settings (NESAGDG, 1996; Carlisle, 1994; Bernstein, 1991). The panel ratings were adapted into indicators for those clinical scenarios which received a median necessity rating of seven or more (out of nine) and for which there was agreement among panel members.

Although the benefits of a baseline EKG in patients diagnosed with CAD have never been tested in a clinical trial, the 12-lead EKG is important in diagnosing future ischemic events and conduction defects, which influence medication choices. For these reasons, expert guidelines recommend 12-lead EKGs in the evaluation of all patients with suspected or proven CAD (NESAGDG, 1996; Braunwald, 1994; Ryan 1996) (Indicator 4). Anemia may exacerbate ischemia in patients with angina. Because anemia is usually correctable, patients with a new diagnosis of stable or unstable angina or MI should have their hemoglobin levels measured (NESAGDG, 1996) (Indicator 5).

A number of studies have examined the ability of stress testing to identify patients with CAD and patients with high-risk CAD who benefit from revascularization (Lee, 1988). A decision analysis based on such data concluded that stress testing patients with stable angina and performing coronary angiography on those with positive tests would prolong life-expectancy and be cost-effective. Stress testing 1000 men age 60 years and over with stable angina would save 62 lives at five years. Experts have thus recommended that all patients with chest pain likely to be angina or with established angina should undergo stress testing at least once unless they are not candidates for revascularization (Lee, 1988; TIMI IIIB Investigators, 1994) (Indicator 6). In contrast, decision analyses have concluded that routine coronary angiography for stable angina patients, without prior stress testing, would result in similar or worse survival at the cost of subjecting twice as many patients to an invasive procedure (Lee, 1988; Bernstein, 1991). In patients with stable coronary disease that is not high risk, the primary benefit of revascularization is control of symptoms rather than reduction in mortality. Hence, the severity of symptoms determines whether revascularization is necessary. Unfortunately, symptom severity can be difficult to glean from the medical record, making quality indicators based on angina difficult to apply.

Unstable Angina

The indicators for unstable angina were developed from the AHCPR clinical practice guideline for unstable angina and the ratings of the RAND expert panel on the necessity of coronary angiography (Braunwald, 1994; Bernstein et al., 1991). The AHCPR guideline for the management of patients being evaluated for possible unstable angina calls for a physical examination that focuses on areas of possible instability and a 12-lead ECG (Indicator 7). Patients hospitalized with unstable angina should be placed on telemetry for arrhythmia and ischemia detection (Indicator 8), should receive sequential cardiac enzyme measurements for the first 24 hours (Indicator 9) and should have a repeat ECG within 24 hours (Indicator 10).

The Thrombolysis in Myocardial Infarction (TIMI) Phase IIIB trial of 1473 patients with unstable angina and non-Q-wave MI compared routine coronary angiography to stress testing followed by coronary angiography for spontaneous or stress-induced ischemia (TIMI IIIB Investigators, 1994). The two strategies resulted in similar overall rates of death and myocardial infarction. However, routine coronary angiography was associated with shorter and fewer hospitalizations, and, for patients with non-Q-wave MIs, a trend toward fewer MIs and deaths. Based on this study, the AHCPR guideline states that early coronary angiography is a reasonable alternative to stress testing for all patients who are very likely to have true unstable angina (e.g., patients with typical symptoms at rest and transient ischemic ECG changes associated with chest pain). No randomized trials have compared medical therapy without stress testing to stress testing for patients with unstable angina. However, because of the high risk of death after an episode of unstable angina, five percent in the first month (Braunwald, 1994), the need for stress testing or coronary angiography in patients with unstable angina is widely accepted (Indicator 12).

In trials of over 100,000 MI patients, ACE inhibitors have reduced mortality by six percent in unselected patients and by 22 percent in patients with LV dysfunction (Hennekens et al., 1996). In addition, as mentioned above, patients with CAD who have depressed LV function have higher risk for mortality. Therefore, our diagnosis indicators focus on measuring LV ejection fraction, by echocardiogram, radionuclide scan, or ventriculogram, in patients with unstable angina who have other clinical features of depressed LVEF (Braunwald, 1994) (Indicator 11) and in high risk patients following an MI (Indicators 15 and 16).

Myocardial Infarction

The quality indicators for the use of diagnostic modalities in patients with MI were developed largely from guidelines by the ACP (ACP, 1989), the AHCPR (Braunwald et al., 1994), and the ACC/AHA (ACC, 1987; AHA, 1996); and from the necessity ratings of the RAND expert panel on

146

the indications for coronary angiography (Indicators 13 and 14) (Bernstein et al., 1991). In patients with acute myocardial infarction treated with thrombolysis, the TIMI II trial found that routine coronary angiography offered no advantage over stress testing. Coronary angiography was reserved only for patients with persistent signs of ischemia (TIMI Study Group, 1989). However, stress testing has not been compared to medical therapy without post-MI diagnostic testing, and the need for routine stress tests has recently been questioned, especially for patients receiving thrombolytic therapy (Stevenson et al., 1993). Nonetheless, most experts recommend such testing for all patients following MI (ACP, 1989) (Indicator 17). Their recommendations are supported by a decision analytic model which predicted that postinfarction stress testing in 55 to 64 year old men would increase quality-adjusted life-expectancy by 1.3 years at a cost of about $20,000 per quality-adjusted life-year saved (Kuntz, 1996).

Although the randomized TIMI II trial found no benefit for routine coronary angiography over stress testing in patients receiving thrombolytics (TIMI Study Group, 1989), a decision analysis has suggested that routine coronary angiography would increase life-expectancy in most post-MI patients and do so cost-effectively in those with a history of prior MI ($30,000 to $50,000 per quality-adjusted life-year saved, average one to two months gained) (Indicators 18 and 19) (Kuntz, 1996). Moreover, in the first hours of an MI, catheterization and primary PTCA instead of thrombolysis has been found to reduce mortality (4.7% versus 6.7%) (Stevenson, 1993; Grines, 1996). For these reasons, routine coronary angiography remains controversial. Thus, our quality indicators accept coronary angiography as an alternative to stress testing for all post-MI patients.

Sudden Death

The indicators for sudden death were based on the ratings of the RAND expert panel on the necessity of coronary angiography (Bernstein et al., 1991). The necessity ratings were used to develop indicators as before. Patients who have suffered sudden death or malignant ventricular dysrhythmia have a high incidence of CAD and risk of subsequent death (about 30% per year)(Braunwald, 1992). For these reasons, evaluation for CAD is considered mandatory (Indicators 20 and 21).

Age

Studies show that CAD is treated less aggressively in the elderly (Bernstein et al., 1991). We have used a cut-off of 75 years of age or less for many of our indicators because this cutoff has been used in necessity ratings for diagnostic testing (Carlisle, 1994; Bernstein et al., 1991). While it is true that the benefits of post-infarction stress testing begin to decline after age 75 because of a higher risk of complications (Kuntz, 1996), the elderly are also at the highest risk of death from CAD and have a great deal to gain from interventions that reduce mortality. Unfortunately, age is an imperfect but easily measured surrogate for poor functional status, limited life-expectancy, and risk of complications from interventions such as CABS. Thus, for the sake of simplicity, our indicators, as currently written, exclude a patient group in whom the diagnosis and treatment of CAD still has potential benefit.

Coronary Angiography

Many hospitals do not have coronary angiography on-site. Patients admitted to such hospitals are significantly less likely to to undergo coronary angiography than clinically similar patients admitted to hospitals with on-site cadiac catheterization facilities (Every et al., 1993). These hospitals should attempt to transfer patients who require coronary angiography to other facilities, unless the patient is documented to be unstable for transfer or a transfer facility is unavailable.

REFERENCES

American College of Physicians. 1989. Evaluation of patients after recent acute myocardial infarction. *Archives of Internal Medicine* 110: 485-88.

American College of Cardiology, and American Heart Association. 1986. Guidelines for exercise testing: A report of the American College of Cardiology/American Heart Association task force on assessment of cardiovascular procedures. *Journal of the American College of Cardiology* 8 (3): 725-38.

American College of Cardiology, and American Heart Association. 1987. Guidelines for coronary angiography: A report of the American College of Cardiology/American Heart Association task force on assessment of diagnostic and therapeutic cardiovascular procedures. *Journal of the American College of Cardiology* 10 (4): 935-50.

American College of Cardiology, and American Heart Association task force on practice guidelines. 1996. Guidelines for perioperative cardiovascular evaluation for noncardiac surgery. *Journal of the American College of Cardiology* 27 (4): 910-48.

American Heart Association. 1991. *1991 Heart and Stroke Facts*. American Heart Association, Dallas.

American Heart Association. 1994. *1994 Heart and Stroke Facts*. American Heart Association, Dallas.

American Heart Association. 1996. *1996 Heart and Stroke Facts*. American Heart Association, Dallas.

Bernstein SJ, et al. 1991. *Coronary angiography: A literature review and ratings of appropriateness and necessity*. RAND, Santa Monica.

Braunwald E, Editor. 1992. <u>Heart Disease: A textbook of cardiovascular medicine</u>. p.758. W.B. Saunders Company.

Braunwald E, Mark DB, Jones RH, et al. 1994. *Unstable Angina: Diagnosis and Management. Clinical Practice Guideline No. 10*. AHCPR.

Carlisle D. Unpublished RAND expert panel ratings for the necessity of diagnostic testing in patients with chest pain.

Every NR, Larson EB, Litwin PE, et al. 19 August 1993. The association between on-site cardiac catheterization facilities and the use of coronary angiography after acute myocardial infarction. Myocardial Infarction Triage and Intervention Project Investigators. *New England Journal of Medicine* 329 (8): 546-551.

Grines CL. 1996. Primary angioplasty - the strategy of choice (editorial). *New England Journal of Medicine* 335 (17): 1313-16.

Grines CL, Browne KF, Marco J, et al. 1993. A comparison of immediate angioplasty with thrombolytic therapy for acute myocardial infarction. *New England Journal of Medicine* 328: 673-9.

Konstam M, Dracup K, Baker D, et al. 1994. *Heart Failure: Evaluation and Care of Patients With Left-Ventricular Systolic Dysfunction.* Clinical Practice Guideline No. 11.

Kuntz KM, Tsevat J, Goldman L, and Weinstein MC. 1996. Cost-effectiveness of routine coronary angiography after acute myocardial infarction. *Circulation* 94: 957-65.

Lee TH, Fukui T, Weinstein MC, Tosteson ANA, and Goldman L. 1988. Cost-effectiveness of screening strategies for left main coronary artery disease in patients with stable angina. *Medical Decision Making* 8: 268-278.

North of England Stable Angina Guideline Development Group. 1996. North of England evidence based guidelines development project: summary version of evidence based guideline for the primary care of management of stable angina. *British Medical Journal* 312: 827-32.

Pilote L, Miller DP, Califf RM, et al. 1996. Derminants of the use of coronary angiography and revascularization after thrombolysis for acute myocardial infarction. *New England Journal of Medicine* 335: 1198-205.

Ryan TJ, Anderson JL, Antman EM, Braniff BA, Brooks NH, Califf RM, et al. 1996. ACC/AHA guidelines for the mangement of patients with acute myocardial infarction: a report of the American College of Cardiology/American Heart Association task force on practice guidelines. *Journal of the American College of Cardiology* 28: 1328-1428.

Sox HC, Littenberg B, and Garber AM. 1989. The role of exercise testing in screening for coronary artery disease. *Archives of Internal Medicine* 110: 456-69.

Stevenson R, Umachandran V, Ranjadayalan K, Wilkinson P, Marchant B, and Timmis AD. 1993. Reassessment of treadmill stress testing for risk stratification in patients with myocardial infarction treated by thrombolysis. *British Heart Journal* 70: 415-420.

The TIMI IIIB Investigators. 1994. Effect of tissue plasminogen activator and a comparison of early invasive and conservative strategies in unstable angina and non-Q-wave myocardial infarction: results of the TIMI IIIB trial. *Circulation* 89: 1545-1556.

The TIMI Study Group. 1989. Comparison of invasive and conservative strategies after treatment with intravenous tissue plasminogen activator in acute myocardial infarction. *New England Journal of Medicine* 320: 618-27.

Yusuf S, Zucker D, Peduzzi P, Fisher LD, Takaro T, Kennedy JW, et al. 1994. Effect of coronary artery bypass graft surgery on survival: overview of the 10-year results from randomised trials by the Coronary Artery Bypass Graft Surgery Trialists Collaboration. *Lancet* 344: 563-70.

RECOMMENDED QUALITY INDICATORS FOR CORONARY ARTERY DISEASE - DIAGNOSIS AND SCREENING

These indicators apply to men and women age 18 and older.

Indicator	Quality of Evidence	Literature	Benefits	Comments
With or Without Symptoms of CAD				
1. Patients 40-75 years old who have a high risk stress test[1] should be offered coronary angiography within 4 weeks of the stress test (unless they have contraindications to revascularization[2] or have had coronary angiography within 2 years of the stress test).	III	Konstam et al., 1994	Decrease mortality.	
2. Patients 40-75 years old who have two or more CAD risk factors[3] and a newly diagnosed low LVEF[4] ($\leq$ 0.45) should be offered stress testing or coronary angiography within 3 months of the diagnosis of low LVEF (unless an etiology of LV dysfunction other than CAD is documented in the medical record or they have contraindications to revascularization or they have had stress testing or coronary angiography within the 2 years prior to the diagnosis of low LVEF).	III	AHA, 1996	Decrease mortality.	RCTs show CABS prolongs life in CAD with low LVEF, but benefits of testing are unproven.
3. Patients 40-75 years old who have an ejection fraction $\leq$ 0.45 and a positive stress test[5] should be offered coronary angiography within 4 weeks of the stress test (unless they have contraindications to revascularization or have had coronary angiography within 2 years of the stress test).	III	AHA, 1996	Decrease mortality.	

152

Indicator	Quality of Evidence	Literature	Benefits	Comments
Stable Angina or Known CAD[6]				
4. Patients < 75 years old with newly diagnosed CAD should have a 12-lead ECG within 3 months of diagnosis.	III	Braunwald, 1992; Grines , 1996; Yusuf, 1994	Decease morbidity and mortality from conduction defects. Decrease morbidity from future cardiovascular events.	A baseline ECG may help diagnose underlying conduction defects and signs of possible LV dysfunction (LBBB), and serve as a baseline for future ischemic events.
5. Patients < 75 years old with any of the conditions listed below should have a hemoglobin and/or hematocrit measured within 1 week of diagnosis: a. angina[7]; b. unstable angina, or c. MI[8]	III	Braunwald, 1992	Decease morbidity and mortality.	Anemia may exacerbate ischemia and is potentially correctable.
6. Patients 40-75 years old newly diagnosed with stable angina or CAD should be offered stress testing or coronary angiography within 3 months of the diagnosis (unless they have contraindications to revascularization[2]).	III	AHA, 1996; Bernstein, 1991	Decease morbidity and mortality.	
Unstable Angina				
7. Patients < 75 years old being evaluated for "unstable angina" or "rule out unstable angina" should have an examination at the time of evaluation documenting all of the following: a. temperature; b. blood pressure; c. heart rate; d. heart exam; e. lung exam, and f. a 12-lead ECG.	III	Grines, 1996	Decrease complications . Decease morbidity.	Good face validity, but no trial data. Recommended by experts.
8. Patients < 75 years old admitted with unstable angina should be placed on cardiac monitoring (i.e., telemetry).	III	Grines, 1996	Decrease mortality.	

153

	Indicator	Quality of Evidence	Literature	Benefits	Comments
9.	Patients < 75 years old admitted with unstable angina should have cardiac enzymes[9] measured every 6 to 8 hours for the first 24 hours of admission.	III	Grines, 1996	Increase diagnostic accuracy. Decrease mortality.	
10.	Patients < 75 years old admitted with unstable angina should have a repeat ECG 12-36 hours after admission.	III	Grines, 1996	Increase diagnostic accuracy. Decrease mortality.	
11.	Patients < 75 years old admitted with unstable angina who have any one of the conditions below should have a measurement of LVEF by echocardiogram, radionuclide scan, or ventriculogram during their hospitalization or within 10 days of discharge unless a prior LVEF is documented in the past year: a. a history of prior MI; b. left bundle branch block on their resting ECG; c. cardiomegaly by examination; d. cardiomegaly on chest X-ray, or e. a diagnosis of heart failure.	III	Grines, 1996	Decease morbidity. Decrease mortality.	Finding of a low ejection fraction should change management plan and could thereby decrease mortality.
12.	Patients 40-75 years old with a discharge diagnosis of "unstable angina" should be offered stress testing or coronary angiography prior to or within 7 days of hospital discharge (unless they have contraindications to revascularization or have had stress testing or coronary angiography within two years prior to discharge).	III	Grines, 1996	Decrease mortality.	

154

Indicator	Quality of Evidence	Literature	Benefits	Comments
Myocardial Infarction				
13. Patients < 75 years old hospitalized for the diagnosis of an MI or "rule out MI" should have a physical examination documenting all of the following: a. temperature, b. blood pressure, c. heart rate, d. heart exam, and e. lung exam.	III	Grines, 1996	Decrease complications. Decrease mortality.	Detect complications of MI- CHF, shock, VSD, MR, acute MI, heart block.
14. Patients < 75 years old hospitalized for the diagnosis of an MI or "rule out MI" should have a 12-lead ECG within 20 minutes of presentation.	III	Grines, 1996	Decrease mortality.	An ECG will identify patients with ECG criteria for thrombolysis
15. Patients < 75 years old hospitalized with an MI should have an assessment of LVEF prior to discharge if they have any risk factors for low LVEF[13] (unless it is noted during hospitalization that prior to admission LVEF was < 0.45).	III	ACC/AHA, 1987	Decrease mortality.	These factors are associated with decreased EF.
16. Patients < 75 years old hospitalized with an MI who have a history of prior MI, but no risk factors for low LVEF[13], should have an assessment of LVEF during the hospitalization or within 2 weeks of discharge (unless it is noted during hospitalization that prior to admission LVEF was < 0.45).	III	ACC/AHA, 1987	Decrease mortality.	
17. Patients with an MI should be offered symptom-limited stress testing or coronary angiography within 8 weeks after the MI (unless they have contraindications to revascularization[2] or have had coronary angiography within two years of the MI).	III	Grines, 1993; ACC/AHA, 1986; Lee, 1988	Decrease mortality.	

155

Indicator	Quality of Evidence	Literature	Benefits	Comments

18. Patients < 75 years old hospitalized with an MI who have any of the following conditions after discharge but within 8 weeks of the MI should be offered coronary angiography within 2 weeks of the diagnosis of the condition (unless they have contraindications to revascularization[2] or have had coronary angiography within two years of the MI):
 	
  a. a high risk stress test;
  b. new heart failure;
  c. LVEF ≤ 0.45;
  d. new severe mitral regurgitation,[10,]
  e. new ventricular septal defect;
  f. sustained ventricular tachycardia[11] or ventricular fibrillation which occurs ≥ 48 hr. after onset of the MI;
  g. angina at rest lasting ≥15 min., or
  h. shock[12].
	III	Grines, 1993; ACC/AHA 1987; Konstam, 1994; Lee, 1988; NESAGDG, 1996	Decrease mortality.	

156

Indicator	Quality of Evidence	Literature	Benefits	Comments

19. Patients < 75 years old who are hospitalized with an MI complicated by any of the following should be offered coronary angiography prior to discharge (unless they have contraindications to revascularization[2] or have had coronary angiography within two years of the MI):
  a. a high risk stress test;
  b. new heart failure;
  c. LVEF ≤ 0.45;
  d. new severe mitral regurgitation;
  e. new ventricular septal defect;
  f. sustained ventricular tachycardia or ventricular fibrillation ≥ 48 hr. after onset of the MI;
  g. > 5 min. of angina at rest occurring ≥24 hr. after the onset of the MI;
  h. shock, or
  i. pulmonary edema requiring intubation.
	III	Konstam, 1994	Decrease mortality.	

Sudden Death				
20. Patients < 75 years old admitted after cardiac arrest should be offered a stress test or coronary angiography before discharge (unless they have contraindications to revascularization[2] or have had coronary angiography within two years of the MI)	III	Konstam, 1994	Decrease mortality.	Cardiac arrest patients have a high mortality.
21. Patients < 75 years old admitted after cardiac arrest and who have a positive stress test during hospitalization should be offered coronary angiography before discharge (unless they have contraindications to revascularization or have had coronary angiography within two years of the MI).	III	Konstam, 1994	Decrease mortality.	

Definitions and Examples

[1] High risk stress test: A test read as positive or suggestive of ischemia with one of the following - ECG positive for ischemia at a workload of < 5 METs or at a heart rate of <= 120, two or more stress-induced (reversible) radionuclide defects or echocardiographic wall motion abnormalities, a peak exercise systolic blood pressure < 110 mm Hg with HR > 150, a decrease in systolic blood pressure by > 20 mm Hg during exercise, or a decrease in LVEF of 10% or more during exercise. Reversible radionuclide defects or echocardiographic wall motion abnormalities occur with stress but improve at rest. Stress imaging tests which show fixed radionuclide defects or wall motion abnormalities with only small areas of reversibility should not be considered positive for the purposes of our indicators (although such tests may be associated with a high risk of adverse events, they are generally viewed as suggesting that revascularization might be of little benefit).

[2] Contraindications to Revascularization and Catheterization:

a. Terminal illness (malignancy, severe COPD, AIDS, hepatic cirrhosis).
b. Intracranial pathology contraindicating systemic anticoagulation (e.g., stroke within 1 month).
c. Advanced dementia.
d. Bedbound (i.e. severe impairment in ability to perform basic activities of daily living).
e. Anaphylaxis to contrast material.
f. Digitalis intoxication.
g. Progressive renal insufficiency.
h. Active gastrointestinal bleeding
i. Ejection fraction less than 25% or left ventricular end-diastolic dimension > 7.5 cm.
j. Active infection, sepsis, or fever which may be due to infection.
k. Patient refusal of catheterization or of both PTCA and CABS.
l. Coronary anatomy documented in the medical record not to favor revascularization - often evidenced by a prior coronary angiogram which revealed multivessel coronary disease but did not result in revascularization.
m. In unstable patients, lack of a cardiac catheterization laboratory or a cardiac surgical team in the hospital. Attempts should be made to stabilize such patients with medical therapy so that they may be transferred.
n. Two or more prior CABS operations.
o. Stress radionuclide or echocardiographic imaging which reveals only small areas of reversible radionuclide defects or echocardiographic wall motion abnormalities, that is only small areas of ischemia.

(NOTE: any patient described in the medical record as not a candidate for CABS or PTCA should be considered to have a contraindication to revascularization).

[3] CAD risk factors: age ≥ 65, male gender, diabetes mellitus, cigarette smoking, hypertension, hypercholesterolemia, and family history of CAD before the age of 55.

[4] LVEF: left ventricular ejection fraction, also termed "left ventricular function", may be described as a percentage or qualitatively (e.g. normal, mildly reduced, moderately reduced, severely reduced). An LVEF < 0.45 is equivalent to moderately reduced (or if not qualified, "reduced").

[5] Positive stress test: (Includes high risk stress tests.) A test read as positive or suggestive of ischemia with or without a high risk feature. Examples of positive but not high risk tests include those with good peak workloads (> 4 METs) and < 2 mm flat or downsloping ST segment depression or a single reversible exercise-induced radionuclide defect or echocardiographic wall motion abnormality. When the stress ECG is positive but the stress imaging is normal or negative, the entire stress test is negative unless the official report interprets it as positive.

[6] Known CAD : known coronary artery disease, includes the diagnoses of angina, stable angina, unstable angina, myocardial infarction, coronary artery disease, ischemic heart disease, prior CABS, or prior PTCA.

[7] Angina: Any symptom resulting from myocardial ischemia. Most often manifest as chest discomfort or dyspnea but numerous other symptoms have been described. Whether a symptom is "angina", that is, due to myocardial ischemia, is a subjective judgment on the part of the clinicians caring for a patient.

158

[8] MI: myocardial infarction.

[9] Cardiac enzymes: creatine kinase, troponin, lactate dehydrogenase (LDH), or myoglobin.

[10] Severe Mitral Regurgitation: regurgitation or insufficiency of the mitral valve assessed on echocardiogram or ventriculogram as "severe" or 4 (on a 1 to 4 scale).

[11] Sustained ventricular tachycardia: ventricular tachycardia lasting > 30 seconds or causing pulselessness or loss of consciousness. Includes torsades de pointes.

[12] Shock - systolic blood pressure < 80 mm Hg for one hour or more.

[13] Risk factors for low ejection fraction include any of the following during hospitalization:
   a. heart failure
   b. pulmonary edema
   c. chest x-ray reported as pulmonary congestion or pulmonary edema
   d. chest x-ray reported as cardiomegaly
   e. systolic BP < 90 (on more than half of the determinations).

Quality of Evidence Codes

I	Randomized Controlled Trial (RCT)
II-1	Nonrandomized controlled trials
II-2	Cohort or case analysis
II-3	Multiple time series
III	Opinions or descriptive studies

159

8. CORONARY ARTERY DISEASE - PREVENTION AND TREATMENT

Anthony Steimle, MD

Because treatments for coronary artery disease (CAD) have been particularly well studied, many of the quality indicators for this chapter are directly supported by randomized controlled trials (RCTs). RCTs have shown that several medications - including lipid lowering drugs, aspirin, beta-blockers, ACE inhibitors, and thrombolytic agents - prolong survival for a broad spectrum of CAD patients. Other studies have found that coronary artery bypass surgery (CABS) benefits subgroups of patients with the most extensive disease. To develop our quality indicators for CAD treatment, we performed MEDLINE searches to identify English language articles published since 1992 on treatment for each of the following: coronary disease, myocardial ischemia, myocardial infarction (MI), angina pectoris, stable angina, and unstable angina. We also searched for articles on coronary artery bypass surgery and percutaneous transluminal coronary angioplasty (PTCA). We supplemented these searches with key references from the bibliographies of review articles. Our proposed quality indicators draw heavily from several particularly well-done overviews (Braunwald et al., 1994; Ryan et al., 1996; Hennekens et al., 1996; and Yusuf et al., 1988).

IMPORTANCE

The public health importance of CAD was described in the preceding chapter on screening and diagnosis. Although it remains the leading cause of death in the United States, mortality from coronary heart disease decreased 34 percent between 1980 and 1990. Models estimate that 43 percent of this reduction is due to improvements in the treatment of patients with known CAD (as opposed to primary prevention or lifestyle changes) (Hunick et al., 1997). Despite this progress, surveys reveal that the management of CAD in the United States does not yet conform with ideal practices as suggested by clinical trials (Rogers et al., 1994) and that the quality of treatment can be improved further.

PREVENTION

Randomized trials in people without known CAD have examined the effects of both aspirin and lipid-lowering drugs on cardiovascular outcomes. However, the use of these agents for primary prevention remains controversial. In two trials of U.S. and British physicians, aspirin reduced the risk of nonfatal myocardial infarction, slightly increased the risk of hemorrhagic stroke, and had no impact on total vascular mortality (Yusuf et al., 1988). Thus, aspirin has not been routinely recommended for people without clinical CAD, although it may be appropriate for those at particularly high risk for myocardial infarction. The role of lipid-lowering drugs in primary prevention is discussed in Chapter 10.

TREATMENT

Stable Angina and Known CAD

This category comprises patients with known CAD not currently suffering from one of the two acute ischemic syndromes, acute myocardial infarction or unstable angina. These patients have a history of angina, MI, CABS, PTCA, or angiographically proven CAD. Several medications have been shown to be beneficial in these patients.

Clinical trials have found that aspirin benefits most patients with clinically apparent vascular disease, including patients with acute MI, prior MI, prior stroke or transient ischemic attack (TIA), prior CABS or PTCA, and prior unstable angina. In these patients, aspirin reduces nonfatal MI by about 30 percent, nonfatal stroke by 30 percent, and death by 17 percent (Ryan et al., 1996). Thus, practice guidelines recommend aspirin for all people with known CAD as well those with other vascular disease (Braunwald et al., 1994; Ryan et al., 1996; NESAGDG, 1996) (Indicators 1 and 2).

Beta-blockers have been shown to prolong survival in patients with stable angina and either silent ischemia or recent MI (Braunwald et al., 1994). The role of beta-blockers in asymptomatic CAD patients who have never had an infarction is less clear. However, the North of England expert panel recommends beta-blockers as first line agents (over nitrates and calcium channel blockers) for all patients with CAD who require chronic antianginal medications (NESAGDG, 1996). It is also reasonable to use beta-blockers as first-line antihypertensives in this population. Unfortunately, it is difficult to identify through chart review those patients who need antianginal treatment or who might have already failed a trial of beta-blockade for hypertension or angina.

Cholesterol reduction in patients with CAD is discussed in Chapter 10.

Cigarette smoking is an important modifiable risk factor for CAD (USDHHS, 1989). Persons who stop smoking reduce their risk of myocardial infarction and death from coronary artery disease (USPSTF, 1996) and patients who have had an MI who stop smoking reduce their risk of mortality (Ryan, 1996) (Indicator 3). Smoking cessation counseling is discussed in Chapter 5.

Unstable Angina

Four RCTs in over 3000 patients with unstable angina have shown that aspirin reduces both death and MI by about 70 percent at seven days and by about 50 percent between three and 18 months (Braunwald et al., 1994; Theroux et al., 1988). In a trial of 479 patients meeting strict criteria for unstable angina (> 20 minutes rest pain with ischemic ECG changes), heparin has been shown to reduce fatal and nonfatal MIs by 88 to 96 percent at one week (Theroux et al., 1988). In this trial, the addition of aspirin to heparin resulted in no additional benefit. However, because heparin is beneficial early while aspirin has long-term benefits, the AHCPR unstable angina clinical practice guideline (Braunwald et al., 1994) recommends using both drugs (Indicators 4 and 5).

Beta-blockers have been shown to reduce the progression of unstable angina to MI. Although they have never been proven to reduce mortality in unstable angina, they have been shown to do so for acute MI, recent MI, and in stable angina with silent ischemia (Braunwald et al., 1994). Thus, the weight of evidence supports treating unstable angina with beta-blockers in addition to heparin. However, patients admitted with the diagnosis "unstable angina" include many at low risk who are unlikely to have acutely unstable CAD and do not require intensive heparin and beta-blocker therapy. In order to separate these lower risk patients, often called "soft rule-outs", from those with true unstable angina, we have adapted criteria from the TIMI IIIB study (> 5 minutes of rest pain associated with ST-segment depression or T-wave inversion) (TIMI IIIB Investigators, 1994). Unfortunately, these strict criteria exclude many patients with bona fide unstable angina (Indicator 6).

Nitroglycerin has no proven effect on mortality in unstable angina but is indicated for the relief of symptoms (Braunwald et al., 1994). Since symptoms are difficult to assess retrospectively through chart review, our quality indicators do not specify indications for nitroglycerin.

The TIMI IIIB trial (TIMI IIIB Investigators, 1994) of 1473 patients found no benefit from thrombolytic therapy in patients with unstable angina who do not have ST elevation or LBBB, the ECG criteria for acute infarction (Ryan et al., 1996; TIMI IIIB Investigators, 1994). Our quality indicators do not specify that thrombolytics are contraindicated for unstable angina because surveys suggest that thrombolytics are underused for MI rather than overused for unstable angina (Rogers et al., 1994), and MI and unstable angina can be difficult to distinguish at presentation. In the future, new enzyme markers may allow for the rapid identification of subsets of patients with unstable angina who would benefit from thrombolytic therapy.

The AHCPR unstable angina guideline (Braunwald et al., 1994) recommends acute revascularization for patients with ongoing and refractory angina who are found on coronary angiography to have either a greater than 95 percent stenosis of a "culprit" vessel or multi-vessel disease with depressed LV function. Early revascularization has been studied in patients with unstable angina in the TIMI IIIB trial (TIMI IIIB Investigators, 1994). However, both arms of this study managed patients with refractory ischemia invasively, so revascularization was not compared to medical therapy. Because the decision to revascularize acutely is complex and the benefits unproven, we have not developed quality indicators for revascularization specific to unstable angina. Rather, we have developed indicators for catheterization specific to unstable angina (see Chapter 7), and revascularization indicators that apply to all patients with CAD (see "Revascularization", below).

Myocardial Infarction

RCTs in over 40,000 patients have demonstrated that thrombolytic agents given early in acute MI reduce mortality. Mortality at 35 days is reduced by about 26 percent when a thrombolytic agent is given within six hours after symptom onset and by about 18 percent when given within 12 hours (Indicator 8) (Ryan et al., 1996; Yusuf et al., 1988). The mortality benefit persists at least four years (Ryan et al., 1996) and results in about 20 lives saved per 1000 treated. Over age 75, the relative reduction in mortality is less and the complications of thrombolytic agents greater so that only ten lives are saved per 1000 treated (Ryan et al., 1996). For this reason, the ACC/AHA MI practice guidelines cautiously recommend thrombolytic therapy in the elderly but acknowledge that the supporting evidence is weaker (Ryan et al., 1996).

Recently, RCTs have compared coronary angioplasty to thrombolytic therapy for acute MI and have found that in expert hands angioplasty can reduce mortality, reinfarction, strokes, and length of hospital stay (Grines et al., 1993). However, most hospitals are not equipped to perform primary angioplasty, and observational data suggest that, when performed in the community setting, primary angioplasty may be equivalent to thrombolysis (Every et al., 1996). For these reasons, our indicator for reperfusion in acute MI allows for either thrombolytic therapy or angioplasty (Indicator 8).

Randomized trials have tested the effects of aspirin in approximately 20,000 post-MI patients. In patients with MI, aspirin reduces the risk of vascular death by approximately 15 percent, of nonfatal MI by 30 percent, and of nonfatal stroke by 40 percent. Benefit is seen both during an infarction, whether thrombolytsis was given or not, and following an MI as part of secondary prevention (Indicators 7 and 14) (Ryan et al., 1996; Antman et al., 1996; Yusuf et al., 1990).

The benefits of heparin for patients not receiving thrombolytic therapy have not been tested since routine therapy with aspirin, beta -

blockers, nitrates, and ACE inhibitors became available. Nonetheless, an overview of randomized trials from the pre-thrombolytic era in which patients did not receive these other therapies found a 17 percent reduction in mortality and a 22 percent reduction in reinfarction. In patients who do receive thrombolytic therapy, recommendations for heparin depend on the agent used. For patients treated with tissue plasminogen activator, an overview of randomized trials found an 18 percent reduction in mortality. In contrast, when agents which result in systemic anticoagulation are used, an added benefit for heparin has not been demonstrated in randomized trials (Ryan et al., 1996)(Indicator 9).

In trials of over 50,000 patients with acute MI, beta-blockers have reduced mortality by 13 percent in the first week (with a 25 percent reduction in the first two days) and by 23 percent over the following months to years (Hennekins et al., 1996; Yusuf et al., 1988; Yusuf et al., 1990). Early treatment with beta-blockers has also been shown to reduce nonfatal reinfarction by 19 percent and nonfatal cardiac arrests by 16 percent (Yusuf et al., 1990). In trials of over 100,000 MI patients, ACE inhibitors have reduced mortality by six percent in unselected patients and by 22 percent in patients with LV dysfunction (Hennekens et al., 1996). For most patients with MI, recent reviews recommend beginning beta-blockers within 12 hours and adding ACE inhibitors within 24 hours for in the absence of contraindications (e.g., if blood pressure is adequate) (Ryan et al., 1996; Hennekens et al., 1996). Experts recommend ACE inhibitors most strongly for patients with LV dysfunction, clinical CHF, and large anterior infarctions, because these patients derive the greatest benefit (Ryan et al., 1996) (Indicators 11 and 16). Whether some MI patients should receive beta-blockers and others ACE inhibitors, or all whether patients should receive both is unknown. Because of these uncertainties, our indicators accept either beta-blockers or ACE inhibitors as first-line therapy after MI (Indicators 10, 11 and 15).

In numerous randomized trials, calcium channel blockers have not reduced mortality during or after acute MI, and in certain subgroups, they may have increased mortality (Ryan et al., 1996 and Yusuf et al.,

1990). Thus, calcium channel blockers are not recommended for the routine treatment of MI. A meta-analysis of 16 trials found that short-acting nifedipine increased mortality 16 percent during and after myocardial infarction (Hennekens et al., 1996). In the Multicenter Diltiazem Postinfarction Trial (MDPIT), post-hoc subgroup analysis found a 41 percent increase in death and nonfatal reinfarction in patients with pulmonary congestion (MDPIT, 1988). Thus, the American College of Cardiology and American Heart Association recommend that short-acting nifedipine be avoided in all post-MI patients (Indicator 12) and diltiazem and verapamil be avoided in those with LV dysfunction or CHF (Ryan et al., 1996) (Indicator 13).

Prior to the advent of thrombolytics, early trials suggested that nitrates reduced mortality after MI by 20 to 35 percent (Ryan et al., 1996). However, in very large recent trials (ISIS-4 and GISSI-3), nitroglycerin had only small, statistically insignificant effects on mortality (Ryan et al., 1996). Thus, we have not included an indicator for nitrates, although most experts still recommend them for the treatment of MI (Ryan et al., 1996).

Treatment of elevated cholesterol in patients following MI is discussed in Chapter 10.

Revascularization

Seven trials between 1972 and 1984 randomized 2649 patients with one, two, and three-vessel CAD to either CABS or medical therapy. A meta-analysis of these trials (Yusuf et al., 1994) found that surgery significantly reduced mortality in all patients by 39 percent, in patients with three-vessel disease by 40 percent, and in patients with left main disease by 70 percent. Other patients may also benefit from revascularization, particularly those with severe angina or with proximal LAD stenosis. However, it is difficult to retrospectively assess many of the subjective factors such as symptom severity which can make surgery necessary for less extensive CAD. Thus, we have confined our quality indicators to patients with left main disease or three-vessel disease plus low left ventricular ejection fraction (LVEF) (Indicators 17 and 18). These patients' mortality benefit is so great that revascularization should almost always be offered regardless of other factors.

More recently, six trials have compared CABS to multivessel PTCA in 4200 patients. Meta-analyses of these trials (Pocock et al., 1995; BARI Investigators, 1996) found comparable mortality with both procedures. However, only a minority of subjects screened with multivessel CAD were candidates for angioplasty while nearly all were eligible for CABS. In addition, CABS relieved angina better, improved functional status more, led to fewer repeat procedures, and was equally cost-effective compared to PTCA (Hlatky et al., 1997). Finally, the mortality benefit of multivessel PTCA has never been directly compared to medical therapy. Despite these caveats, our quality indicator accepts either PTCA or CABS for three-vessel CAD. Because mortality may be similar for selected patients, their choice of procedure often rightly depends on individual and physician preferences.

REFERENCES

Antman EM, Lau J, Kupelnick B, Mostellar F, and Chalmers TC. 1992. A comparison of results of meta-analyses of randomized control tirals and recommendations of clinical experts: treatments for myocardial infarction. *Journal of the American Medical Association* 268: 240-248.

Braunwald E, Mark DB, Jones RH, et al. 1994. *Unstable Angina: Diagnosis and Management. Clinical Practice Guideline No. 10*. AHCPR.

Bypass angioplasty revascularization investigation (BARI) investigators Comparison of coronary bypass surgery with angioplasty in patients with multivessel disease. 1996. *New England Journal of Medicine* 335: 217-25.

Every NR, Parsons LS, Hlatky M, et al. 1996. A comparison of thrombolytic therapy with primary coronary angioplasty for acute myocardial infarction. *New England Journal of Medicine* 335: 1253-60.

Grines CL, Browne KF, Marco J, et al. 1993. A comparison of immediate angioplasty with thrombolytic therapy for acute myocardial infarction. *New England Journal of Medicine* 328: 673-9.

Hennekens CH, Albert CM, Godfried SL, Gaziano JM, and Burning JE. 1996. Adjunctive drug therapy of acute myocardial infarction - evidence from the clinical trials. *New England Journal of Medicine* 335: 1660-67.

Hlatky MA, Rogers WJ, Johnstone I, et al. 1997. Medical care costs and quality of life after randomization to coronary angioplasty or coronary bypass surgery. *New England Journal of Medicine* 336: 92-9.

Hunick MGM, Goldman L, Tosteson ANA, et al. 1997. The recent decline in mortality from coronary heart disease, 1980-1990: the effect of secular trends in risk factors and treatment. *Journal of the American Medical Association* 277: 535-542.

Multicenter diltiazem post infarction trial research group. 1988. The effect of dilitiazem on mortality and reinfarction after myocardial infarction. *New England Journal of Medicine* 319: 385-392.

National Cholesterol Education Program. 1994. National Cholesterol Education Program: second report of the expert panel on detection, evaluation, and treatment of high blood cholesterol in adults. *Circulation* 89: 1333-1445.

169

North of England Stable Angina Guideline Development Group. 1996. North of England evidence based guidelines development project: summary version of evidence based guideline for the primary care of management of stable angina. *British Medical Journal* 312: 827-32.

Pocock SJ, Henderson RA, Rickards AF, et al. 1995. Meta-analysis of randomised trials comparing coronary angioplasty with bypass surgery. *Lancet* 346: 1184-89.

Post Coronary Artery Bypass Graft Trial Investigators. 1997. The effect of aggressive lowering of low-density lipoprotein cholesterol levels and low-dose anticoagulation on obstructive changes in saphenous-vein coronary-artery bypass grafts. *New England Journal of Medicine* 336: 153-62.

Rogers WJ, Bowlby LJ, Chandra NC, et al. 1994. Treatment of myocardial infarction in the United States (1990 to 1993): observations from the National Registry of Myocardial Infarction. *Circulation* 90: 2103-2114.

Ryan TJ, Anderson JL, Antman EM, Braniff BA, Brooks NH, Califf RM, et al. 1996. ACC/AHA guidelines for the mangement of patients with acute myocardial infarction: a report of the American College of Cardiology/American Heart Association task force on practice guidelines. *Journal of the American College of Cardiology* 28: 1328-1428.

Sacks FM, Pfeffer MA, Moye LA, et al. 1996. The effect of pravastatin on coronary events after myocardial infarction in patients with average cholesterol levels. *New England Journal of Medicine* 335: 1001-9.

Scandinavian Simvastatin Survival Study Group. 1994. Randomized trial of cholesterol loweing in 4444 patients with coronary heart disease: the Scandinavian Simvastatin Survival Study (4S). *Lancet* 344: 1383-9.

Theroux P, Ouimet H, McCans J, et al. 1988. Aspirin, heparin, or both to treat acute unstable angina. *New England Journal of Medicine* 319: 1105-11.

TIMI IIIB Investigators. 1994. Effect of tissue plasminogen activator and a comparison of early invasive and conservative strategies in unstable angina and non-Q-wave myocardial infarction: results of the TIMI IIIB trial. *Circulation* 89: 1545-1556.

US Department of Health and Human Services. 1989. *Reducing the Health Consequences of Smoking; 25 Years of Progress: A Report of the Surgeon General-1989*. U.S. Department of Health and Human Services, Rockville, MD.

US Preventive Services Task Force. 1996, 2nd ed. Guide to Clinical
Preventive Services,Baltimore, MD: Williams and Wilkins.

Yusuf S, Sleight P, Held P, and McMahon S. 1990. Routine medical
management of acute myocardial infarction: lessons from overviews
of recent randomized controlled trials. *Circulation* 82 (supplI):
II-117-II-134.

Yusuf S, Wittes J, and Friedman L. 1988. Overview of result of
randomized clinical trials in heart disease. *Journal of the
American Medical Association* 260: 2259-63.

Yusuf S, Zucker D, Peduzzi P, Fisher LD, Takaro T, Kennedy JW, et al.
1994. Effect of coronary artery bypass graft surgery on survival:
overview of the 10-year results from randomised trials by the
Coronary Artery Bypass Graft Surgery Trialists Collaboration.
Lancet 344: 563-70.

RECOMMENDED QUALITY INDICATORS FOR CORONARY ARTERY DISEASE - PREVENTION AND TREATMENT

The following criteria apply to men and women age 18 and older.

Indicator	Quality of Evidence	Literature	Benefits	Comments
Stable Angina or known CAD				
1. Patients newly diagnosed with CAD should be offered aspirin (at a dose of at least 81 mg/day continued indefinitely) within one week of the diagnosis of CAD unless they have a contraindication to aspirin.[1]	I	Braunwald, 1994; NESAGDG, 1996; Ryan et al., 1996; Yusuf et al., 1988	Reduce mortality, recurrent MIs, strokes, bypass graft closure.	Aspirin reduces mortality in patients with CAD.
2. Patients with a prior diagnosis of CAD who are not on aspirin and do not have contraindications to aspirin[1] should be offered aspirin (at a dose of at least 81 mg/day continued indefinitely) within one week of any visit to a provider in which CAD was addressed.	I	Braunwald, 1994; NESAGDG, 1996; Ryan et al., 1996; Yusuf et al., 1988	Reduce mortality, recurrent MIs, strokes, bypass graft closure.	
3. Patients newly diagnosed with CAD who smoke should have documentation of counseling on smoking cessation within 3 months of the diagnosis of CAD.	I	Braunwald, 1994; NESAGDG, 1996; Ryan et al., 1996; Yusuf et al., 1988	Reduce mortality, reinfarction.	Smoking cessation reduces mortality post MI, but relapse is rate is high.
Unstable Angina				
4. Patients admitted with the diagnosis of unstable angina[2] should receive aspirin within 24 hours of admission.	I	Braunwald et al., 1994; Theroux et al., 1988	Reduce mortality.	

172

Indicator	Quality of Evidence	Literature	Benefits	Comments

5. Patients admitted with the diagnosis of definite unstable angina[3] who do not have contraindications to heparin[4] should receive:
 	
  a. heparin within 2 hours of the initial ECG that demonstrates ischemic changes; and
 	
  b. continuous heparin infusion for at least 24 hours (or until 26 hours after the ECG with ischemic changes).
	I	Braunwald et al., 1994; Theroux et al., 1988	Reduce mortality.	

6. Patients < 75 years old admitted with the diagnosis of unstable angina who have angina > 5 minutes at rest associated with ischemic ST segment changes should receive beta-blockers within 4 hours (unless they have contraindications to beta-blockers[5]).	I	Braunwald et al., 1994; Yusuf et al., 1988	Reduce progression to MI.	
Myocardial Infarction				
7. Patients presenting with acute myocardial infarction should receive at least 160 mg of aspirin within 12 hours of presentation unless they have contraindications to aspirin.[1]	I	Ryan et al., 1996; Yusuf et al., 1988	Reduce mortality, recurrent MIs and ischemia, strokes.	

8. Patients <75 years old presenting with an acute myocardial infarction who are within 12 hours of the onset of MI symptoms[12] and who do not have contraindications to thrombolysis[6] or revascularization[7] should receive a thrombolytic agent within 1 hour of the time their ECG initially shows either of the following findings:
 	
  a. ST elevation > 0.1 mV in 2 or more contiguous leads, or
 	
  b. a LBBB not known to be old
	I	Ryan et al., 1996; Yusuf et al., 1988	Reduce mortality, reinfarction, infarct size, improve LVEF.	Under age 75, 18 lives saved per 1000 treated; over age 75, 10 lives saved per 1000 treated.

173

Indicator	Quality of Evidence	Literature	Benefits	Comments
9. Patients admitted within 12 hours of the onset of acute myocardial infarction who do not have contraindications to heparin[1,4] should receive heparin (subcutaneously or IV) for at least 24 hours unless they have received streptokinase, APSAC, or urokinase.	III	Ryan et al., 1996	Reduce reinfarction and mortality.	The ACC/AHA MI guidelines recommend heparin for all patients with MI (except those receiving certain thrombolytic agents) while noting that the evidence supporting this recommendation is not definitive. The majority of experts also make this recommendation.
10. Patients admitted with acute myocardial infarction whose LVEF[8] is either unknown at admission or >= 45%, should receive either a beta-blocker or an ACE inhibitor or both within 12 hours of admission (unless they have contraindications to both beta-blockers[5] and ACE inhibitors[9]).	I	Ryan et al., 1996; Hennekens et al., 1996	Reduce mortality, infarct size, reinfarction.	It is unclear which patients should receive beta-blockers and which should receive ACE inhibitors. Subgroup data from trials suggest benefits are additive and that some patients should receive both.
11. Patients admitted with acute myocardial infarction and are known to have a LVEF <= 45% at admission should receive an ACE inhibitor within the first 24 hours of admission (unless they have contraindications to ACE inhibitors[9]).	I	Ryan et al., 1996; Hennekens et al., 1996	Reduce mortality, reinfarction.	ACE inhibitors may be used in place of beta-blockers in any MI patient; however, their benefit appears to be greatest in patients with LV dysfunction or large anterior infarctions.
12. Patients admitted with acute myocardial infarction should NOT receive short-acting nifedipine during the hospitalization.	I	Ryan et al., 1996; Hennekens et al., 1996	Avoid increased mortality.	
13. Patients admitted with acute myocardial infarction should NOT receive any calcium channel blocker if they have a reduced LVEF (< 45%) or heart failure during the hospitalization.	I	Ryan et al., 1996; Hennekens et al., 1996	Avoid increased mortality.	In very rare cases, diltiazem or verapamil may be indicated in these patients for relief of ongoing ischemia or control of rapid atrial fibrillation when all other agents have failed.
14. Patients discharged after an acute myocardial infarction who do not have contraindications to aspirin[1] should be discharged on aspirin at a dose of at least 81 mg/day.	I	Ryan et al., 1996	Reduce mortality.	

174

	Indicator	Quality of Evidence	Literature	Benefits	Comments
15.	Patients discharged after an acute myocardial infarction who have either an LVEF>=45% documented during hospitalization or an unknown LVEF, should be discharged on a beta-blocker or an ACE inhibitor or both (unless they have contraindications to both beta-blockers[5] and ACE inhibitors[9]).	I	Ryan et al., 1996; Hennekens et al., 1996	Reduce mortality.	
16.	Patients discharged after an acute myocardial infarction who have an LVEF<= 45% documented at any time during the hospitalization should receive ACE inhibitors at discharge (unless they have contraindications to ACE inhibitors[9]).	I	Ryan et al., 1996; Hennekens et al., 1996	Reduce mortality.	

Revascularization

	Indicator	Quality of Evidence	Literature	Benefits	Comments
17.	Patients < 75 years old with CAD who do not have contraindications to revascularization[7] should be offered PTCA or CABS[10] within 1 month of coronary angiography if they have 3 vessel CAD[11] and an LVEF < 45%.	I	Yusuf et al., 1994	Reduce mortality, relieve angina.	Most patients with 3 vessel CAD are more appropriately treated with CABS than with PTCA. PTCA/CABS also benefits many patients with less severe CAD by relieving angina.
18.	Patients < 75 years old with CAD who do not have contraindications to revascularization[7] should be offered CABS within 1 month of coronary angiography if they have left main stenosis > 50%.	I	Yusuf et al., 1994	Reduce mortality, relieve angina.	Most patients with 3 vessel CAD are more appropriately treated with CABS than with PTCA. PTCA/CABS also benefits many patients with less severe CAD by relieving angina .

Definitions And Examples

[1] Contraindications to aspirin:
  a. Hypersensitivity/allergy to salicylate (rare)
  b. Bleeding within the past 4 weeks (including gastrointestinal bleeding, melena, epistaxis, any bleeding requiring transfusion; excluding occult hemoglobin in stools and menses).

[2] Angina: Any symptom resulting from myocardial ischemia. Most often manifest as chest discomfort or dyspnea but numerous other symptoms have been described. Whether a symptom is "angina", that is, due to myocardial ischemia, is a subjective judgment on the part of the clinicians caring for a patient.

[3] Definite Unstable Angina: angina > 5 minutes at rest associated with ischemic ECG changes (either dynamic T wave inversions or = 1 mm ST-segment depression or elevation in two contiguous leads).

[4] Potential contraindications to heparin:

   a. Previous hemorrhagic stroke at any time or non-hemorrhagic stroke within 1 month
   b. Known intracranial neoplasm, mass, or other intracerebral pathology (e.g., aneurysm, abscess)
   c. Bleeding within the past 4 weeks (including gastrointestinal bleeding, melena, epistaxis, any bleeding requiring transfusion; excluding occult hemoglobin in stools and menses)
   d. Suspected aortic dissection
   e. Current use of anticoagulants in therapeutic doses (e.g. coumadin with INR = 2)
   f. Bleeding diathesis (e.g., dysfunctional platelets, Von Willebrand's disease, thrombocytopenia, clotting factor deficiency, hemophilia
   g. Received streptokinase, APSAC, or urokinase during the current admission.

[5] Relative Contraindications to Beta Blockers:

   a. Heart rate < 60 bpm.
   b. Systolic blood pressure < 100 mm Hg
   c. Heart failure
   d. PR interval (on ECG) > 0.24 seconds
   e. Second or third-degree AV block
   f. Bifasicular block
   g. Chronic obstructive pulmonary disease
   h. History of asthma
   i. Peripheral vascular disease
   j. Insulin dependent diabetes mellitus.

[6] Potential contraindications to thrombolytics:

   a. Previous hemorrhagic stroke at any time; other strokes or cerebrovascular events within one year.
   b. Known intracranial neoplasm, mass, or other intracerebral pathology (e.g., aneurysm, abscess)
   c. Bleeding within the past 4 weeks (including gastrointestinal bleeding, melena, epistaxis, any bleeding requiring transfusion; excluding occult hemoglobin in stools and menses).
   d. Suspected aortic dissection
   e. Blood pressure >180/110
   f. Current use of anticoagulants in therapeutic doses (e.g. coumadin with INR = 2).
   g. Bleeding diathesis (e.g., dysfunctional platelets, Von Willebrand's disease, thrombocytopenia, clotting factor deficiency, hemophilia.
   h. Trauma within 4 weeks (head trauma, concussion, bone fracture)
   i. CPR within 4 weeks
   j. Surgery with 4 weeks (excluding cataract sugery)
   k. Pregnancy.

[7] Contraindications to Revascularization and Catheterization:

   a. Terminal illness (malignancy, severe COPD, AIDS, hepatic cirrhosis).
   b. Intracranial pathology contraindicating systemic anticoagulation (e.g., stroke within 1 month)
   c. Advanced dementia
   d. Bedbound (i.e. severe impairment in ability to perform basic activities of daily living)
   e. Anaphylaxis to contrast material
   f. Digitalis intoxication
   g. Progressive renal insufficiency

h. Severe anemia (HCT < 30) or active gastrointestinal bleeding

i. Ejection fraction less than 25% or left ventricular end-diastolic dimension > 7.5 cm

j. Active infection, sepsis, or fever which may be due to infection

k. Patient refusal of catheterization or of both PTCA and CABS

l. Coronary anatomy documented in the medical record not to favor revascularization - often evidenced by a prior coronary angiogram which revealed multivessel coronary disease but did not result in revascularization

m. In unstable patients, lack of a cardiac catheterization laboratory or a cardiac surgical team in the hospital. Attempts should be made to stabilize such patients with medical therapy so that they may be transferred

n. Two or more prior CABS operations

o. Stress imaging which reveals fixed radionuclide defects or echocardiographic wall motion abnormalities with only small areas of reversibility.

[8] LVEF: left ventricular ejection fraction, also termed "left ventricular function"; may be described as a percentage or qualitatively (e.g. normal, mildly reduced, moderately reduced, severely reduced). An LVEF < 0.45 is equivalent to moderately reduced (or if not qualified, "reduced").

[9] Contraindication to angiotensin converting enzyme (ACE) inhibitors:

    a. Systolic blood pressure < 100 mm Hg

    b. Creatinine > 2.0

    c. Bilateral renal artery stenosis

    d. Allergy to ACE inhibitors

    e. Serum potassium > 5.5.

[10] CABS: coronary artery bypass surgery.

[11] Three vessel CAD: 70% narrowing of all three major coronary arteries or one of their first order branches (left anterior descending or one its branches the diagonals, the circumflex or one of its branches to obtuse marginals, and the right coronary artery or its branch the posterior descending artery). Three vessel CAD will also be defined by the catheterization report stating "three vessel" CAD. (NOTE: any patient described in the medical record as not a candidate for CABS or PTCA should be considered to have a contraindication to revascularization).

[12] Patients who receive cardiac cathertization within 90 minutes of these findings are not eligible for this indicator.

Quality of Evidence Codes

I   Randomized controlled trials

II-1   Nonrandomized controlled trials

II-2   Cohort or case analysis

II-3   Multiple time series

III   Opinions or descriptive studies

177

9. HEART FAILURE

Arleen Brown, MD

The quality indicators for heart failure were developed using the AHCPR Clinical Practice Guideline Number 11, "Heart Failure: Evaluation and Care of Patients With Left-Ventricular Systolic Dysfunction" (Konstam, 1994), and the guideline from a joint task force of the American College of Cardiology and American Heart Association (ACC/AHA Task Force, 1995). These guidelines were supplemented by recent reviews of heart failure (Packer, 1992; Cohn, 1996). Where these core references cited studies to support individual indicators, we have referenced the original sources. We also performed MEDLINE searches of the medical literature from 1985 to 1995 to supplement these references for particular indicators.

IMPORTANCE

Heart failure is a common disease with high associated morbidity and mortality. Over two million people in the United States are affected by this syndrome, and there are over 400,000 new cases of heart failure diagnosed annually (Smith, 1985). In addition it is the only cardiovascular disease that is increasing in prevalence (MMWR, 1994). In the Framingham study, the five-year mortality after congestive heart failure (CHF) developed was approximately 60 percent in men and 45 percent in women (McKee, 1971). In the past two decades, there has been significant improvement in the pharmacologic management of patients with heart failure secondary to left ventricular systolic dysfunction. However, despite these advances, annual mortality exceeds 20 percent overall (Schocken, 1992), and may reach 26 percent over six months for those with severe disease (CONSENSUS, 1987).

Heart failure is also a costly diagnosis. In 1992, over $10 billion were spent on physician visits, medications, nursing home stays, and other health care expenditures, with more than $7 billion of this amount spent on hospitalizations. Because Medicare reimbursements were only half of the actual charges, these hospitalizations represent an important source of uncompensated medical care.

Heart failure is a clinical syndrome characterized by intravascular and interstitial volume overload and inadequate tissue perfusion. The most common etiology of heart failure in the United States is coronary artery disease, which is the underlying cause in approximately two-thirds of persons with heart failure. Other causes of heart failure are dilated cardiomyopathy (often viral or secondary to toxins such as alcohol), chronic hypertension, valvular disease, and hypertrophic cardiomyopathy. Heart failure may also be divided into systolic dysfunction and diastolic dysfunction. Systolic dysfunction, the impairment of the ventricle's ability to pump blood forward, is defined by a low ventricular ejection fraction and may result in both congestion and hypoperfusion. Diastolic dysfunction is defined as impaired ventricular relaxation or distention during diastole. It is increasingly recognized as an important cause of heart failure, and may occur in up to 40 percent of patients with heart failure. The left-ventricular ejection fraction may be normal (as in patients with left ventricular hypertrophy) or elevated (as in patients with hypertrophic cardiomyopathy). Combined systolic and diastolic dysfunction is also common.

This chapter will emphasize management of patients with left-ventricular systolic dysfunction. It will not cover guidelines for heart failure due to diastolic dysfunction because there are limited data on therapies known to be effective, nor will it cover heart failure due to valvular disease, aneurysm, or myocardial disease (such as amyloidosis or sarcoidosis).

SCREENING

The prevention of clinical heart failure, through prevention of coronary disease and control of hypertension, is crucial to decreasing the morbidity and mortality associated with this syndrome. Primary prevention measures for coronary disease and control of hypertension are discussed in Chapters 10 and 11, respectively. Additionally, there is a significant role for preventing progression to symptomatic heart failure in asymptomatic patients with an ejection fraction under 40 percent. These patients have been shown to benefit from the use of angiotensin converting enzyme (ACE) inhibitors. The Studies of Left Ventricular Dysfunction (SOLVD) trial showed that enalapril, titrated to 10 mg twice daily, reduced the development of symptomatic heart failure from 30 percent in the placebo group to 21 percent in the treatment group at the three year follow-up (SOLVD Investigators, 1992). Treatment with ACE inhibitors in this population is discussed further below.

DIAGNOSIS

Symptoms that suggest heart failure include paroxysmal nocturnal dyspnea (PND); orthopnea; dyspnea on exertion; lower extremity edema; reduced exercise tolerance; unexplained confusion, altered mental status, or fatigue in an elderly person; and abdominal symptoms associated with ascites and/or hepatic engorgement (such as nausea or abdominal pain). However, most of these symptoms have limited specificity and/or sensitivity for heart failure (Konstam, 1994).

Many patients with a severely reduced ejection fraction will be asymptomatic. One study found that 20 percent of patients with ejection fraction less than 40 percent had no clinical criteria for heart failure (Marantz, 1988), while another found that only 42 percent of patients with an ejection fraction under 30 percent had dyspnea on exertion (Mattleman, 1983).

Of the symptoms that suggest heart failure, dyspnea on exertion is often the presenting symptom, and the combination of orthopnea, paroxysmal nocturnal dyspnea, and progressive dyspnea on exertion are relatively specific for heart failure. In addition, patients with a history of previous myocardial infarction, poorly controlled hypertension, or other heart disease, who also have any of the suggestive symptoms, should be evaluated for heart failure (Konstam, 1994).

Because heart failure may be precipitated or exacerbated by several other clinical conditions, patients with symptoms suggestive of heart failure or with documented new heart failure should be asked about (Kostam, 1994; ACC/AHA Task Force, 1995)(Indicator 2):

- prior myocardial infarction;
- angina or anginal equivalents;
- current complaint of fatigue or dyspnea;
- current complaint of edema or recent weight gain;
- other cardiac history, such as murmur, failure, arrhythmia, pacemaker, rheumatic heart disease, enlarged heart;
- hypertension;
- diabetes;
- renal disease;
- pulmonary disease;
- thyroid disease;
- gastrointestinal disease;
- medications;
- alcohol use.

The physical examination is important, both to the initial evaluation of patients with symptoms suggestive of heart failure and in follow-up evaluation. Many patients with early symptoms of heart failure or with moderate-to-severe left ventricular systolic dysfunction have no physical findings suggestive of heart failure. However, there are several findings on the physical exam that suggest heart failure (Indicator 3):

- Elevated jugular venous pressure or positive hepatojugular reflux;
- A third heart sound;
- Laterally displaced apical impulse;
- Pulmonary rales that do not clear with cough;
- Peripheral edema not due to venous insufficiency.

The third heart sound is the most sensitive physical finding, and in one study was found in 68 percent of patients with EF below 30 percent (Mattleman, 1983). A laterally displaced apical impulse was found in 42 percent of patients, while rales were found in 37 percent of patients (Harlan, 1977). Data on the specificity of the examination in heart failure are limited; however, the most specific signs are elevated jugular venous pressure and the third heart sound. In addition, rales in a patient with other symptoms and no known pulmonary disease are highly suggestive of heart failure (Konstam, 1994). In studies of the overall utility of the clinical exam for detecting an ejection fraction under 50 percent, sensitivity has ranged from 66 to 95 percent and specificity from 29 to 76 percent (Sanford, 1982; Mattleman, 1983; Cease, 1986; Eagle, 1988; McNamara, 1988; Gadsboll, 1989).

In order to provide a baseline for monitoring treatment response and address potential hypertensive control issues, the initial physical examination of a patient with suspected or documented heart failure should include documentation of weight and blood pressure (Indicator 6).

Because many patients with heart failure do not manifest any signs, the sensitivity of even careful physical examination is limited. In addition, intra- and inter-rater reliability of the clinical exam in heart failure patients is variable. For the physical examination, interrater agreement ranged from 0.6 for the third heart sound to 0.92 for hepatojugular reflux (Butman, 1993). Agreement was lower, 0.48, for cardiomegaly on chest x-ray. Therefore, some patients with symptoms that are highly suggestive of heart failure, especially those who are treated with medications for heart failure, should undergo echocardiography or radionuclide ventriculography to measure ejection fraction even in the absence of physical examination findings (Indicators 1 and 5)(ACC/AHA Task Force, 1995; Konstam, 1994; Retchin and Brown, 1991). Assessment of left ventricular function helps to evaluate not only the presence of heart failure, but also may indicate its etiology and assist in management of the condition. Echocardiogram and/or radionuclide angiography may help to distinguish systolic from diastolic dysfunction. In addition, these studies may help to distinguish heart failure from other disease states such as pulmonary disease, venous insufficiency, and obesity, with similar signs and symptoms, yet different management strategies. Echocardiography and radionuclide ventriculography are both acceptable means of assessing left ventricular function and can be used to distinguish between systolic or diastolic dysfunction. Although each test has relative advantages and disadvantages in assessing left ventricular function, the proposed indicators do not favor one diagnostic mode over the other (Indicators 1 and 5).

Several other diagnostic tests are recommended by experts for the evaluation of causative, precipitating, or complicating causes of new heart failure. A chest radiograph should be performed to evaluate for cardiomegaly, to distinguish between cardiac and pulmonary causes of dyspnea, and to provide information on chamber size and valvular disease. A chest radiograph without cardiomegaly argues against the diagnosis of heart failure except when pulmonary hyperinflation may mask an enlarged heart (Echeverria, 1983; Dougherty, 1984). An electrocardiogram should also be performed to evaluate the patient for causes of congestive heart failure such as myocardial ischemia, atrial fibrillation, bradyarrhythmias, prior myocardial infarction, low voltage, and left ventricular hypertrophy (Indicator 4).

Several laboratory tests are indicated in the evaluation and management of heart failure. A complete blood count should be performed to evaluate for heart failure due to anemia. A hematocrit below 25 may result in signs and symptoms of heart failure in the absence of underlying cardiac abnormalities. Because renal disease may cause volume overload that can mimic or exacerbate heart failure, an evaluation of renal function should be performed. This should include a urinalysis and serum creatinine. In addition, electrolytes, blood urea nitrogen (BUN), and creatinine should be evaluated to assist in subsequent management, such as determining whether and when an ACE inhibitor should be started (Indicators 4 and 7).

TREATMENT

Diuretic Therapy

Patients with heart failure and symptoms or signs of volume overload should be treated with a thiazide and/or loop diuretic (Whight, 1974; Kupper, 1986). Symptoms of volume overload include orthopnea, PND, and dyspnea on exertion. The signs of volume overload include pulmonary rales, a third heart sound, jugular venous distention, hepatic engorgement, ascites, peripheral edema, and pulmonary vascular congestion or pulmonary edema on chest radiograph.

Potassium depletion is common in patients treated with diuretics (although patients who are taking ACE inhibitors concomitantly may not have significant potassium depletion). Even though serum potassium may be an unreliable indicator of total body potassium, experts recommend that all patients starting diuretics should have their serum potassium checked within one week of the start of treatment (Indicator 10). In addition, heart failure patients in whom diuretic dose is increased should have a potassium level checked within one week of the increase in dose (Kostam, 1994) (Indicator 12).

Although diuretics provide hemodynamic and symptomatic benefits in persons with heart failure with pulmonary or peripheral edema, they have potential toxicity, due in part to activation of the renin-angiotensin system, and limited efficacy, as patients on diuretics alone have high rates of clinical deterioration (Captopril-Digoxin Multicenter Research Group, 1983). Other medications may be indicated, as reviewed below.

ACE Inhibitors

Mortality benefit has been demonstrated from the use of the ACE inhibitor enalapril in patients with heart failure. In the SOLVD study, patients with heart failure who had reduced left ventricular ejection fractions had a reduction in four-year mortality from 40 percent on placebo to 35 percent on enalapril, with median survival increased by six months (SOLVD Investigators, 1992). The CONSENSUS trial of patients with NYHA Class IV heart failure found a mortality reduction from 52 percent with placebo to 36 percent for those on enalapril (CONSENSUS, 1987). In addition, in the Veterans Affairs Cooperative Vasodilator-Heart Failure Trial II, enalapril reduced mortality in heart failure patients more than the combination of isosorbide dinitrate and hydralazine (Cohn, 1991).

Several studies have also shown improvement in functional status (SOLVD Investigators, 1992; CONSENSUS, 1987; Bussmann, 1987; Captopril-Digoxin Multicenter Research Group, 1983; Franciosa, 1985; Jennings, 1984; Kleber, 1991; Magnani, 1986; McGrath BP, 1985; Remes, 1986; Sharpe, 1984), physical functioning (Chalmers, 1987; Lewis, 1989; Riegger, 1990; Riegger, 1991), and a reduction in hospitalizations (SOLVD Investigators, 1992) among patients with heart failure and reduced left-ventricular ejection fraction who are taking ACE-inhibitors. It is not clear whether the favorable effects of ACE inhibitors can be attributed to hemodynamic effects, the reduction in the level of angiotensin II in plasma or in tissue, increased plasma concentrations of bradykinin or nitric oxide, and/or inhibition of the central nervous system.

Side effects associated with the use of ACE inhibitors include hypotension, increases in serum creatinine and potassium, cough, and less commonly, dizziness and angioedema (Kjekshus, 1988; Frank, 1989; Packer, 1989; Hasford, 1991). In the SOLVD and CONSENSUS trials, the changes in blood pressure and serum chemistries were relatively small (CONSENSUS, 1987; SOLVD Investigators, 1992), and it has been suggested that relatively low blood pressure, moderate renal insufficiency, and mild hyperkalemia are not absolute contraindications to the initiation or continued use of ACE inhibitors (Konstam, 1992). Because some patients with blood pressure lower than 90 mm Hg can be safely started and maintained on ACE inhibitors, the AHCPR guideline recommends that physicians who are uncomfortable starting or maintaining this therapy in patients with low systolic blood pressure at baseline refer such patients to a clinician with expertise in treating heart failure, rather than discontinue the use of ACE inhibitors or other vasodilators.

Potassium-sparing diuretics should be discontinued in patients on ACE inhibitors, regardless of the serum potassium, and potassium supplements should be withheld unless the patient has a low serum potassium. All patients with renal insufficiency who are on ACE inhibitors should be carefully monitored and doses titrated upward cautiously. Patients with serum creatinine of 3.0 mg/dL or greater were excluded from major trials of these agents, so the risks and benefits of ACE inhibitors in these patients are not known. Because cough is common in heart failure (SOLVD, 1992; Cohn, 1991), patients ACE inhibitors who report coughing should be evaluated for pulmonary congestion as the cause before considering discontinuation of the medication. Dizziness and angioedema are usually mild and do not require discontinuation of the drug; however, angioedema of the oropharyngeal region is an absolute contraindication to further use of the ACE inhibitor (Indicator 10).

The AHCPR clinical practice guidelines recommend that patients with heart failure due to left ventricular systolic dysfunction receive a trial of ACE inhibitors unless they have one or more of the following specific contraindications (Konstam, 1994)(Indicator 8):

1. A history of intolerance or adverse reaction to ACE inhibitors;

2. Serum potassium greater than 5.5 mEq/L that cannot be reduced;

3. Symptomatic hypotension (SBP < 100 mm Hg)

Even after a myocardial infarction and the development of left ventricular systolic dysfunction (EF < 40%), treatment with ACE inhibitors can slow or prevent progression to symptomatic heart failure. The Survival and Ventricular Enlargement (SAVE) trial, which evaluated the use of captopril in patients with myocardial infarction in the preceding three to 16 days and ejection fractions of 40 percent or lower, found 20 percent mortality in captopril-treated patients compared to 25 percent mortality in those on placebo over two to five years follow-up (Pfeffer, 1992). In addition, the proportion of patients hospitalized for heart failure fell from 17 percent to 14 percent. The Cooperative New Scandinavian Enalapril Survival Study (CONSENSUS) II found a reduction in incidence of symptomatic heart failure with enalapril, from 30 percent to 27 percent, but no reduction in mortality (CONSENSUS, 1987).

Based on these data, two categories of asymptomatic patients should undergo screening for left ventricular dysfunction. Persons who have a history of Q-wave infarction without a record of a post-infarction ejection fraction measurement should have an ejection fraction measured. In addition, patients hospitalized for a myocardial infarction should have an ejection fraction determined unless they are at low risk for moderate to severe systolic dysfunction. Indicators for the determination of the ejection fraction in patients with new myocardial infarction can be found in the Chapter 7.

Patients should be seen within one week of initiation of an ACE inhibitor to monitor blood pressure, renal function, and serum potassium (Indicator 9). Doses of ACE inhibitors should be titrated upward slowly. Treatment should be modified if:

1. There is an increase in serum creatinine of 0.5 mg/dL or more;

2. There is a serum potassium of 5.5 mEq/L or higher;

3. The patient reports symptomatic hypotension (with a documented SBP < 100 mm Hg).

Digoxin

Cardiac glycosides have been used to treat heart failure for two centuries, yet their use remains controversial (Konstam, 1994; Cohn, 1996). Although digoxin is the preferred agent in patients with heart failure and atrial fibrillation with rapid ventricular response, it is not clear that it is of benefit in patients in sinus rhythm. A meta-analysis of seven randomized, placebo-controlled trials of digoxin found less research study withdrawal due to clinical deterioration among digoxin-treated patients compared to those on placebo (Jaeschke et al., 1990). The Captopril-Digoxin Multicenter Research Group found a trend toward fewer emergency department visits or hospital admissions for heart failure in patients treated with digoxin compared to those who received placebo and a diuretic (Captopril-Digoxin Multicenter Research Group, 1988). In the RADIANCE trial, patients withdrawn from digoxin while continuing to receive diuretics and an ACE inhibitor were nearly six times more likely to have clinical deterioration than patients who continued to take digoxin (Packer et al., 1993). However, there are still questions about when digoxin should be initiated. In addition, the effects of digoxin on mortality are not clear. Retrospective studies have suggested an adverse effect on survival (Bigger, 1985). However, the Digitalis Investigation Group (DIG, 1997) study, found that, compared to placebo, digoxin had no significant effect on mortality, but was associated with a reduction in hospitalization rates.

Direct-Acting Vasodilators

Hydralazine/isosorbide dinitrate has been shown to reduce mortality in heart failure. The absolute mortality was 12 percent for hydralazine/isosorbide dinitrate compared to 19 percent for placebo at one year and 36 percent versus 47 percent respectively at three years (Cohn, 1986). However, in direct comparison with enalapril, there was similar improvement in exercise capacity but hydralazine/isosorbide dinitrate had a lower absolute mortality reduction than did the ACE inhibitor (Cohn, 1991). The side effects of hydralazine/isosorbide dinitrate led to discontinuation of the agent in 18 to 33 percent of study participants due to headache, palpitations, and nasal congestion.

Based on these data, it has been recommended that hydralazine/isosorbide dinitrate be used in patients with moderate to severe heart failure who are intolerant to or have contraindications to ACE inhibitor use (Konstam, 1994; ACC/AHA Task Force, 1995; Cohn, 1996) (Indicator 13). More recently, angiotensin receptor inhibitors (such as losartan) have been used in some heart failure patients who are unable to take ACE inhibitors, but there are currently no randomized controlled trial data to support this use.

Beta Blockers

Although several studies suggest that careful titration of beta-blockers may be beneficial for selected patients with heart failure, the routine use of these agents for heart failure is still experimental (Konstam, 1994).

Anticoagulation

There has never been a controlled trial of anticoagulation in heart failure, and routine anticoagulation is controversial (Konstam, 1994).

Revascularization

See Chapter 8 for a discussion of revascularization in patients with CAD.

Weight Loss and Other Non-Pharmacologic Management

Recent studies show that regular exercise can improve the functional status and symptoms of patients with heart failure. Therefore, experts recommend that all patients with stable heart failure should be encouraged to exercise (Sullivan, 1989; Coats, 1990; Kellermann, 1990; Konstam, 1994; ACC/AHA Task Force, 1995; Cohn, 1996). Expert consensus also supports dietary sodium restriction, though evidence for the efficacy of this recommendation is lacking (Konstam, 1994) (Indicator 14).

FOLLOW-UP

Follow-up for patients on diuretics or ACE inhibitors was discussed in the section on treatment.

Because readmission for heart failure is common and costly, attention has focused on interventions to reduce rehospitalization (Gooding, 1985; Rich, 1995). A recent randomized controlled trial consisting of a multidisciplinary, nurse-directed intervention demonstrated improved quality of life, fewer hospitalizations, and a trend toward improved survival in elderly patients with heart failure (Rich, 1995). Additional analyses showed an improvement in medication adherence (Rich, 1996).

Management after hospitalization should include a visit in the outpatient clinic or a home visit no later than one week after discharge (Retchin and Brown, 1991). This visit should include a check of electrolytes, BUN, and creatinine unless they have been done since hospital discharge. Other goals of the post-discharge visit should be to assess adherence to medications and to dietary restrictions, if any; to ensure that the patient's weight is stable; to adjust medication dosages as indicated; and to ensure that patient, family, and caregivers understand how and when to contact the practitioner (Kostam, 1994; ACC/AHA Task Force, 1995) (Indicators 15, 16 and 17).

REFERENCES

American College of Cardiology, and American Heart Association Task Force on Practice Guidelines (Committee on Evaluation and Management of Heart Failure). 1995. Guidelines for the evaluation and management of heart failure. *Circulation* 92: 2764-84.

Bigger JT, Fleiss JL, Rolnitzky LM, et al. 1985. Effect of digitalis treatment on survival after myocardial infarction. *American Journal of Cardiology* 55: 623-30.

Bussmann WD, Storger H, Hadler D, et al. 1987. Long-term treatment of severe chronic heart failure with captopril: a double-blind, randomized, placebo-controlled, long-term study. *Journal of Cardiovascular Pharmacology* 9 Suppl 2: S50-60.

Butman SM, et al. 1993. Bedside cardiovascular examination in patients with severe chronic heart failure: importance of rest or inducible jugular venous distention. *Journal of the American College of Cardiology* 22: 968-974.

Captopril-Digoxin Multicenter Research Group. 1988. Comparative effects of captopril and digoxin in patients with mild to moderate heart failure. *Journal of the American Medical Association* 259: 539-44.

Captopril Multicenter Research Group. 1983. A placebo-controlled trial of captopril in refractory chronic congestive heart failure. *Journal of the American College of Cardiology* 2 (4): 755-63.

Cease KM, and Nicklas JM. 1986. Prediction of left ventricular ejection fraction using simple quantitative clinical information. *American Journal of Medicine* 81: 429-436.

Chalmers JP, West MJ, Cyran J, et al. 1987. Placebo-controlled study of lisinopril in congestive heart failure: a multicentre study. *Journal of Cardiovascular Pharmacology* 9 (Suppl 3): S89-97.

Coats AJ, Adamopoulos S, Meyer TE, Conway J, and Sleight P. 1990. Effects of physical training in chronic heart failure [see comments]. *Lancet* 335 (8681): 63-6.

Cohn JN. 1996. The management of chronic heart failure. *New England Journal of Medicine* 335 (7): 490-8.

Cohn JN, Archibald DG, Ziesche S, et al. 1986. Effect of vasodilator therapy on mortality in chronic congestive heart failure. Results of a Veterans Administration Cooperative Study. *New England Journal of Medicine* 314 (24): 1547-52.

Cohn JN, Johnson G, Ziesche S, et al. 1991. A comparison of enalapril with hydralazine-isosorbide dinitrate in the treatment of chronic congestive heart failure. *New England Journal of Medicine* 325 (5): 303-10.

Coronary artery surgery study (CASS). 1983. A randomized trial of coronary artery bypass surgery. Survival data. *Circulation* 68 (5): 939-50.

Dougherty AH, Naccarelli GV, Gray EL, Hicks CH, and Goldstein RA. 1984. Congestive heart failure with normal systolic function. *American Journal of Cardiology* 54 (7): 778-82.

Eagle KA, Quertermous T, Singer DE, et al. 1988. Left ventricular ejection fraction. Physician estimates compared with gated blood pool scan measurements. *Archives of Internal Medicine* 148 (4): 882-5.

Echeverria HH, Bilsker MS, Myerburg RJ, and Kessler KM. 1983. Congestive heart failure: echocardiographic insights. *American Journal of Medicine* 75 (5): 750-5.

Franciosa JA, Wilen MM, and Jordan RA. 1985. Effects of enalapril, a new angiotensin-converting enzyme inhibitor, in a controlled trial in heart failure. *Journal of the American College of Cardiology* 5 (1): 101-7.

Frank GJ. 1989. The safety of ACE inhibitors for the treatment of hypertension and congestive heart failure. *Cardiology* 76 (Suppl 2): 56-67.

Gadsboll N, Hoilund-Carlsen PF, Nielsen GG, et al. 1989. Interobserver agreement and accuracy of bedside estimation of right and left ventricular ejection fraction in acute myocardial infarction. *American Journal of Cardiology* 63 (18): 1301-7.

Gooding J, and Jette AM. 1985. Hospital readmissions among the elderly. *Journal of the American Geriatric Society* 33 (9): 595-601.

Hasford J, Bussmann WD, Delius W, Koepcke W, Lehmann K, and Weber E. 1991. First dose hypotension with enalapril and prazosin in congestive heart failure. *Int J Cardiol* 31 (3): 287-93.

Jaeschke R, Oxman AD, and Guyatt GH. 1990. To what extent do congestive heart failure patients in sinus rhythm benefit from digoxin therapy? Asystemic overview and meta-analysis. *American Journal of Medicine* 88: 279-286.

Jennings G, Kiat H, Nelson L, Kelly MJ, Kalff V, and Johns J. 1984. Enalapril for severe congestive heart failure. A double-blind study. *Medical Journal of Australia* 141 (11): 723-6.

Kannel WB. 1989. Epidemiological aspects of heart failure. *Cardiol Clin* 7 (1): 1-9.

Kannel WB, Hjortland M, and Castelli WP. 1974. Role of diabetes in congestive heart failure: the Framingham study. *American Journal of Cardiology* 34 (1): 29-34.

Kellermann JJ, Shemesh J, Fisman EZ, et al. 1990. Arm exercise training in the rehabilitation of patients with impaired ventricular function and heart failure. *Cardiology* 77 (2): 130-8.

Kjekshus J, and Swedberg K. 1988. Tolerability of enalapril in congestive heart failure. *American Journal of Cardiology* 62 (2): 67A-72A.

Kleber FX, Niemoller L, Fischer M, and Doering W. 1991. Influence of severity of heart failure on the efficacy of angiotensin-converting enzyme inhibition. *American Journal of Cardiology* 68 (14): 121D-126D.

Konstam M, Dracup K, Baker D, et al. June 1994. *Heart failure: evaluation and care of patients with left-ventricular systolic dysfunction. Clinical Practice Guideline No. 11.* Agency for Health Policy and Research, Public Health Service, U.S. Department of Health and Human Services, Rockville, MD.

Kupper AJ, Fintelman H, Huige MC, Koolen JJ, Liem KL, and Lustermans FA. 1986. Cross-over comparison of the fixed combination of hydrochlorothiazide and triamterene and the free combination of furosemide and triamterene in the maintenance treatment of congestive heart failure. *European Journal of Clinical Pharmacology* 30 (3): 341-3.

Lewis GR. 1989. Comparison of lisinopril versus placebo for congestive heart failure. *American Journal of Cardiology* 63 (8): 12D-16D.

Magnani B, and Magelli C. 1986. Captopril in mild heart failure: preliminary observations of a long-term, double-blind, placebo-controlled multicentre trial. *Postgraduate Medical Journal* 62 (Suppl 1): 153-8.

Marantz PR, Tobin JN, Wassertheil-Smoller S, et al. 1988. The relationship between left ventricular systolic function and congestive heart failure diagnosed by clinical criteria. *Circulation* 77 (3): 607-12

Mattleman SJ, Hakki AH, Iskandrian AS, Segal BL, and Kane SA. 1983. Reliability of bedside evaluation in determining left ventricular function: correlation with left ventricular ejection fraction determined by radionuclide ventriculography. *Journal of the American College of Cardiology* 1 (2 Pt 1): 417-20.

McGrath BP, Arnolda L, Matthews PG, et al. 1985. Controlled trial of enalapril in congestive cardiac failure. *British Heart Journal* 54 (4): 405-14.

McKee PA, Castelli WP, McNamara PM, and Kannel WB. 1971. The natural history of congestive heart failure: the Framingham study. *New England Journal of Medicine* 285 (26): 1441-6.

McNamara RF, Carleen E, Moss AJ, and and the Multicenter Postinfarction Research Group. 1988. Estimating left ventricular ejection fraction after myocardial infarction by various clinical parameters. *American Journal of Cardiology* 62: 192-196.

MMWR. 1994. Mortality from congestive heart failure--United States, 1980-1990. *Morbidity and Mortality Weekly Report* 43 (5): 77-81.

Packer M. 1989. Identification of risk factors predisposing to the development of functional renal insufficiency during treatment with converting-enzyme inhibitors in chronic heart failure. *Cardiology* 76 (Suppl 2): 50-5.

Packer M. 1992. Treatment of chronic heart failure. *Lancet* 340: 92-95.

Packer M, Gheorghiade M, Young JB, et al. 1 July 1993. Withdrawal of digoxin from patients with chronic heart failure treated with angiotensin-converting-enqyme inhibitions. RADIANCE Study. *New England Journal of Medicine* 329 (1): 1-7.

Pfeffer MA, Braunwald E, Moye LA, et al. 1992. Effect of captopril on mortality and morbidity in patients with left ventricular dysfunction after myocardial infarction. Results of the survival and ventricular enlargement trial. *New England Journal of Medicine* 327 (10): 669-77.

Remes J, Nikander P, Rehnberg S, et al. 1986. Enalapril in chronic heart failure, a double-blind placebo-controlled study. *Ann Clin Res* 18 (3): 124-8.

Retchin SM, and Brown B. 1991. Elderly patients with congestive heart failure under prepaid care. *American Journal of Medicine* 90: 236-242.

Rich MW, Beckham V, Wittenberg C, Leven CL, Freedland KE, and Carney RM. 1995. A multidisciplinary intervention to prevent the readmission of elderly patients with congestive heart failure. *New England Journal of Medicine* 333 (18): 1190-5.

Rich MW, Gray DB, Beckham V, Wittenberg C, and Luther P. 1996. Effect of a multidisciplinary intervention on medication compliance in elderly patients with congestive heart failure. *American Journal of Medicine* 101 (3): 270-6.

Riegger GA. 1990. The effects of ACE inhibitors on exercise capacity in the treatment of congestive heart failure. *Journal of Cardiovascular Pharmacology* 15 (Suppl 2): S41-6.

Riegger GA. 1991. Effects of quinapril on exercise tolerance in patients with mild to moderate heart failure. *European Heart Journal* 12 (6): 705-11.

Sanford CF, Corbett J, Nicod P, et al. 1982. Value of radionuclide ventriculography in the immediate characterization of patients with acute myocardial infarction. *American Journal of Cardiology* 49: 637-644.

Schocken DD, Arrieta MI, Leaverton PE, and Ross EA. 1992. Prevalence and mortality rate of congestive heart failure in the United States. *Journal of the American College of Cardiology* 20 (2): 301-6.

Sharpe DN, Murphy J, Coxon R, and Hannan SF. 1984. Enalapril in patients with chronic heart failure: a placebo-controlled, randomized, double-blind study. *Circulation* 70 (2): 271-8

Smith WM. 1985. Epidemiology of congestive heart failure. *American Journal of Cardiology* 55 (2): 3A-8A.

The SOLVD Investigators. 1991. Effect of enalapril on survival in patients with reduced left ventricular ejection fractions and congestive heart failure. *New England Journal of Medicine* 325 (5): 293-302.

The SOLVD Investigators. 1992. Effect of enalapril on mortality and the development of heart failure in asymptomatic patients with reduced left ventricular ejection fractions. *New England Journal of Medicine* 327 (10): 685-91

Sullivan MJ, Higginbotham MB, and Cobb FR. 1989. Exercise training in patients with chronic heart failure delays ventilatory anaerobic threshold and improves submaximal exercise performance. *Circulation* 79 (2): 324-9.

The CONSENSUS Trial Study Group. 1987. Effects of enalapril on mortality in severe congestive heart failure. Results of the Cooperative North Scandinavian Enalapril Survival Study (CONSENSUS). *New England Journal of Medicine* 316 (23): 1429-35.

The Digitalis Investigators Group. 1997. The effect of digoxin on mortality and morbidity in patients with heart failure. *New England Journal of Medicine* 336: 525-33.

Whight C, Morgan T, Carney S, and Wilson M. 1974. Diuretics, cardiac failure and potassium depletion: a rational approach. *Medical Journal of Australia* 2 (23): 831-3.

RECOMMENDED QUALITY INDICATORS FOR HEART FAILURE

These indicators apply to men and women age 18 and older.

Indicator	Quality of Evidence	Literature	Benefits	Comments
Diagnosis				
1. Patients newly diagnosed with heart failure[1] who are beginning medical treatment should receive an evaluation of their ejection fraction[2] within 1 month of the start of treatment.	III	Konstam, 1994; Marantz, 1988	Improve function; reduce symptoms.	No data for the time interval.
2. Patients newly diagnosed with heart failure should have a history at the time of the diagnosis documenting the presence or absence of all of the following: a. Prior myocardial infarction or cardiac disease; b. Current symptoms of chest discomfort or angina; c. History of hypertension; d. History of diabetes; e. Current medications; and f. Alcohol use.	III	Retchin, 1991; Konstam, 1994; ACC/AHA Task Force, 1995	Reduce symptoms; reduce mortality.	Rule out reversible/treatable causes or precipitants of heart failure.
3. Patients with a new diagnosis of heart failure should have the following elements of the physical examination documented at the time of presentation: a. Weight; b. Blood pressure; c. Lung exam; d. Cardiac exam; e. Abdominal exam; and f. Lower extremity examination.	III	Retchin, 1991	Reduce symptoms.	Physical exam findings are of limited sensitivity and specificity.

Indicator	Quality of Evidence	Literature	Benefits	Comments
4. Patients with a new diagnosis of heart failure should be offered all of the following studies within 1 month of the diagnosis (unless performed within the prior 3 months): a. Chest x-ray; b. EKG; c. Complete blood count; d. Serum sodium, potassium, and bicarbonate; e. Serum creatinine; and f. Urinalysis.	III	Retchin, 1991; Kostam, 1994	Detect underlying causes for heart failure; reduce symptoms.	There is no evidence for the time periods for any of these tests. The choice of tests is based more on clinical judgment and opinion than on trials showing improved outcomes
5. Patients with a diagnosis of heart failure who are being treated with medications for their heart failure should have one of the following documented in the medical record at least every two years: • a previously measured ejection fraction, or • a new evaluation of their ejection fraction.	III	Retchin, 1991; Konstam, 1994; ACC/AHA Task Force, 1995	Decrease mortality.	Assessment of left ventricular function may indicate the etiology of the heart failure and assist in condition management.[2]
6. Patients who are hospitalized for symptoms of heart failure should have all of the following elements of the physical examination documented on the day of hospitalization: a. Weight; b. Blood pressure; c. Lung exam; d. Cardiac exam; e. Abdominal exam; and f. Lower extremity examination.	III	Retchin, 1991	Guide management decisions; reduce symptoms.	No data on time interval. This indicator applies only to patients admitted primarily for heart failure.

197

Indicator	Quality of Evidence	Literature	Benefits	Comments
7. Patients who are hospitalized for heart failure should have the following performed within one day of hospitalization: a. Serum electrolytes; and b. Serum creatinine.	III	Mattleman, 1983; Echeverria, 1983; Dougherty, 1984; Aguirre, 1989; Aronow, 1990; Godsboll, 1989; Eagle, 1988	Improve symptoms; decrease complications of hyper- or hypo-kalemia and renal insufficiency.	No data on time intervals
Treatment				
8. Patients with a diagnosis of heart failure who have an ejection fraction of less than 40% and no contraindications to ACE inhibitors should be receiving an ACE inhibitor.	I	Captopril-Digoxin Multicenter Research Group, 1983; Jennings, 1984; Sharpe, 1984; McGrath, 1985; Magnani, 1986; Remes, 1986; Chalmers, 1987; CONSENSUS, 1987; Bussman, 1987; Lewis, 1989; Riegger, 1990; Riegger, 1991; Cohn, 1991; SOLVD Investigators, 1992.	Reduce mortality; decrease symptoms; improve functional status.	SOLVD trial showed that enalapril (titrated to 10 mg bid) reduced the development of symptomatic heart failure from 30% in the placebo group to 21% in the treatment group at 3 year follow-up.
9. Patients with the diagnosis of heart failure who are started on an ACE inhibitor should have a potassium checked within 1 week of starting the ACE inhibitor	III	Konstam, 1994; ACC/AHA Task Force, 1995; Cohn, 1996;	Reduce complications of hyperkalemia.	Serum potassium must be monitored closely in patients on ACE inhibitors. There are no data for the time interval.
10. Patients with the diagnosis of heart failure who are on an ACE inhibitor should have the following checked every year: a. Serum potassium; and b. Serum creatinine.	III	Konstam, 1994; ACC/AHA Task Force, 1995; Cohn, 1996	Reduce complications of hyperkalmia and renal failure.	There are no data for the time interval.

198

	Indicator	Quality of Evidence	Literature	Benefits	Comments
11.	Patients with the diagnosis of heart failure who are started on a diuretic should have a potassium level checked within 1 week of the start of treatment	III	Konstam, 1994	Reduce hypokalemic complications.	There are no data for the time interval.
12.	Patients with the diagnosis of heart failure in whom diuretic dose is increased should have a potassium level checked within 1 week of the increase in dose.	III	Konstam, 1994	Reduce hypokalemic complications.	There are no data for the time interval.
13.	Patients with the diagnosis heart failure and an ejection fraction of less than 40% who are not on ACE inhibitors should be on hydralzine/isosorbide dinitrate, in the absence of contraindications.[3]	I	Cohn, 1986; Cohn, 1991; Konstam, 1994; ACC/AHA Task Force, 1995; Cohn, 1996	Reduce mortality.	Hydralzine/isosorbide dinitrate has been shown to reduce mortality in heart failure, though the absolute mortality reduction is less than that for ACE inhibitors. There is similar improvement in exercise capacity compared to ACE inhibitors.
14.	Patients with a new diagnosis of heart failure who are started on medical treatment for heart failure should have dietary counseling [4] within 1 month of the start of medical treatment.	II-1, II-2	Konstam, 1994	Reduce symptoms; improve medical management.	Recent studies show that regular exercise can improve the functional status and symptoms of patients with heart failure. No studies have evaluated a specific dietary sodium restriction.
Follow-up					
15.	Patients who have been hospitalized for heart failure should have follow-up contact within 4 weeks of discharge.	I, III	Retchin, 1991; Rich, 1995	Prevent worsening of symptoms; prevent toxicity from medications.	There are no data on the time interval. Recent randomized controlled trial data showed improved quality of life, fewer hospitalizations, and a trend toward improved survival in elderly patients with heart failure who participated in a multidisciplinary nurse-directed intervention.
16.	Patients who have been hospitalized for heart failure should have the following physical examination elements performed during the first post-discharge visit: a. Weight; b. Blood pressure; c. Lung exam; d. Cardiac exam; e. Abdominal exam; and f. Lower extremity examination.	III	Retchin, 1991	Prevent worsening of symptoms; prevent toxicity from medications.	

199

17.	Patients who have been hospitalized for heart failure should have the following laboratory tests performed within 4 weeks of discharge:
	
	  a. Creatinine; and
	  b. Potassium.
		III	Retchin, 1991	Prevent worsening of symptoms; prevent toxicity from medications.

Definitions and Examples

[1] Medical treatment for congestive heart failure: medications prescribed to treat symptomatic systolic dysfunction, including diuretics (e.g., thiazide and loop diuretics), ACE inhibitors, hydralazine/isosorbide dinitrate, and digoxin.

[2] Evaluation of ejection fraction: Tests evaluating ejection fraction include echocardiogram, MUGA and left heart catheterization.

[3] Contraindications to hydralazine/isosorbide:
- Systolic blood pressure < 100 mm Hg
- Allergy to hydralazine/isosorbide
- Lupus

[4] Dietary counseling: Any mention in the medical record of counseling regarding diet, fluid intake, or salt intake, or a referral to a dietician or nutritionist.

Quality of Evidence Codes

I	Randomized Controlled Trial (RCT)
II-1	Nonrandomized controlled trials
II-2	Cohort or case analysis
II-3	Multiple time series
III	Opinions or descriptive studies

200

10. HYPERLIPIDEMIA

Beatrice Golomb, MD, PhD

The development of quality indicators for screening and treatment of hyperlipidemia was initially based on current guidelines and review articles on hyperlipidemia. Strong emphasis was placed on guidelines from the National Cholesterol Education Panel (NCEP) and American College of Physicians (ACP), which represent, respectively, more aggressive and more conservative perspectives on the management of hyperlipidemia. Additional articles identified through MEDLINE literature searches were used, with information culled from review articles, guidelines and, in particular, randomized trials and meta-analyses demonstrating significant effects of cholesterol-lowering treatment on mortality.

IMPORTANCE

Approximately seven million Americans currently have heart disease. Each year, 1.5 million people sustain heart attacks, of which roughly one-third die (McBride and Davis, 1992). The costs for care of cardiovascular disease were approximately $109 billion in 1992 (McBride and Davis, 1992). Despite a reduction in age-adjusted mortality rates over recent decades, coronary artery disease remains the leading cause of mortality in the U.S. (Harris-Hooker, 1994). Because of the prevalence of cardiovascular disease, with the attendant health and economic consequences, public health efforts have targeted modifiable risk factors such as hyperlipidemia. Data from animal studies, and from ecological, epidemiological, and clinical trials in humans indicate a relation of cholesterol to heart disease, and to initiation and progression of atherosclerotic disease (Stensvold et al., 1992; Tunstall-Pedoe, 1988; O'Keefe et al., 1995). Data also indicate a relationship between cholesterol reduction and a reduction in atherosclerotic progression (Kroon et al., 1996); release of endothelium-derived relaxing factor leading to nonspecific widening of coronary arteries (Keaney et al., 1994; van Boven et al., 1994); reduced coronary events and reduced coronary mortality; and reduced overall mortality in high-risk populations with preexisting heart disease, as reported by the Scandinavian Simvastatin Survival Study Group (The "4S" Group, 1994).

Concerns about hyperlipidemia are compounded by the fact that it affects large segments of the population: two-thirds of middle-aged adults have lipids above the designated desirable range (Anderson et al., 1987). Cholesterol screening and treatment have substantial economic consequences; for example, among people aged 20 to 74 years who are screened, an estimated 41 percent will require a second screening test to assess lipoproteins (Sempos et al., 1989). Annual costs of screening for hyperlipidemia by NCEP guidelines have been projected at up to $10 billion (Froom, 1989). Using these same guidelines, minimal annual costs for combined screening and treatment of hypercholesterolemia in asymptomatic individuals over age 65 have been projected at $1.6 to $16.8 billion (Kaiser, 1993). For the total population aged 20 to 74, it is estimated that 36 percent, or 60 million people, would merit drug treatment if NCEP guidelines were uniformly applied (Sempos et al., 1989). In this case, expenditures for drug treatment would greatly exceed the current expenditures of $5 billion in 1995 for one class of lipid-lowering drugs alone, the HMG-CoA reductase inhibitors (Heinrichs, 1996). Therefore, decisions regarding cholesterol screening and management have potentially profound public health and economic ramifications.

SCREENING AND PREVENTION

Prevention of Hypercholesterolemia

Although recommended by many agencies, the use of diet to control cholesterol remains controversial. Diets that are tolerable to patients, and are low in total and saturated fats, do not lead to substantial reductions in serum cholesterol levels (ACP, 1996). Moreover, they do not reduce mortality from cardiovascular or other diseases. The Canadian Task Force on Periodic Health Examination (CTF) describes the evidence for general dietary advice on lowering total fat, saturated fat and cholesterol intake in the routine care of men age 30

202

to 69, as "fair." It also found insufficient evidence for such advice in other populations (CTF, 1993). Due to lack of consensus in this area, there are no indicators regarding dietary treatment to lower total and saturated fat.

There are data supporting dietary advice to consume fatty fish as a secondary prevention measure; one study documented a significant 30 percent reduction in overall mortality (Burr et al., 1989) These results are comparable to those achieved with statins in the "4S" trial (The "4S" Group, 1994); however, counseling regarding fish consumption is not widespread and is not an element of most guidelines. Moreover, fish consumption does not exert its benefit through cholesterol reduction, although it is often discussed in the context of cholesterol (Harris, 1989; Simopoulos, 1990; Schmidt and Dyerberg, 1994).

Screening and Primary Prevention

Guidelines for screening cholesterol are in agreement only for a restricted subset of patients at high risk. The NCEP and ACP guidelines can be taken to reflect two major divergent perspectives.

The NCEP guidelines recommend screening total cholesterol and HDL at least every five years in all adults over age 20 (Expert Panel on Detection Evaluation and Treatment of High Blood Cholesterol in Adults, 1993). This is in sharp contrast with the ACP guidelines, which do not specify any minimum age for screening in those without previously diagnosed atherosclerotic disease. The ACP's position, in which no screening is mandated in primary prevention, stems from the absence of demonstrated benefit of hyperlipidemia treatment for primary prevention of coronary artery disease (CAD).

In those without previously diagnosed atherosclerotic disease, no study to date has shown significantly increased survival with cholesterol reduction. The same is true for studies of cholesterol reduction and cardiac mortality, although one mixed secondary and high-risk primary prevention study came close to demonstrating mortality benefit (Shepherd et al., 1995). The largest primary prevention study unexpectedly showed a significant 30 percent increase in overall mortality in those assigned to treatment (Committee of Principal

203

Investigators, 1978). Several meta-analyses of single and multiple risk factor intervention studies involving lipids have also demonstrated a trend toward increased overall mortality in low-risk populations assigned to treatment (McCormick and Skrabanek, 1988; Muldoon et al., 1990; Davey Smith et al., 1993). One such study suggests that harm or benefit is probably a function of baseline level of risk, with those at highest risk benefiting, and those at lowest risk placed at greater risk for overall mortality, which is consistent with divergent findings for primary and secondary prevention populations (Davey et al., 1993).

With regard to cholesterol screening, guidelines of the American Academy of Family Physicians and the American College of Obstetricians and Gynecologists are similar to those of the NCEP, whereas guidelines of the CTF more closely mirror those of the ACP (CTF, 1993; U.S. Public Health Service, 1995). In New Zealand, Britain, the Netherlands, and Europe in general, printed guidelines and consensus statements favor an approach to screening and treatment that is more conservative than that of the NCEP, with none advocating universal screening, and some maintaining that drug treatment is rarely indicated unless cholesterol exceeds 300 mg/dl (Rossner et al., 1993).

While many would agree that screening of lipids in individuals (at least in men over age 35 and women over age 45) with two or more risk factors for cardiovascular disease is appropriate, even in the absence of identified atherosclerotic disease, there is no consensus that such screening is mandatory (ACP, 1996). Due to the lack of demonstrated mortality benefit with treatment of hyperlipidemia in the primary prevention population, no indicators are directed at screening in this group.

Screening for Hypercholesterolemia in Patients With Preexisting Coronary Heart Disease

In contrast to primary prevention, mortality benefit has been demonstrated for cholesterol reduction in men with preexisting heart disease. The "4S" trial (The "4S" Group, 1994) showed HMG-CoA reductase inhibitors to produce a 30 percent reduction in relative risk of overall mortality with simvastatin treatment in a high-risk secondary prevention group of 4444 patients with CAD and high cholesterol, consisting primarily of men with prior myocardial infarction (MI). Benefit to overall mortality in the older population within this study (age 60 to 70) was smaller but remained significant (The "4S" Group, 1994). In support of the "4S" study finding, meta-analysis has shown a reduction in overall mortality with cholesterol-lowering treatment in high-risk individuals, primarily men with preexisting heart disease (Davey Smith et al., 1993). Experts agree that lipid screening -- including HDL and total cholesterol -- should be performed in men with identified atherosclerotic disease (particularly coronary disease), and perhaps also after stroke or carotid occlusion and peripheral vascular disease (ACP, 1996). It is also believed that treatment to lower cholesterol should be initiated in this group if an elevated cholesterol (LDL greater than 130) is identified. For this reason, our screening and treatment indicators are directed at screening for hyperlipidemia in men under age 70 with prior vascular disease.

Frequency of Screening

Because reductions in mortality have been shown with treatment of hyperlipidemia in men under age 70 with preexisting heart disease, men with heart disease who do not have identified hyperlipidemia should nonetheless have lipid measurements periodically to allow prompt initiation of treatment when indicated. Although there is no direct evidence supporting the opinion, a frequency of every five years is often cited as reasonable for cholesterol screening in men with heart disease who do not currently require cholesterol-lowering treatment (ACP, 1996) (Indicator 1).

Timing of Screening in Secondary Prevention

The timing of cholesterol measurement in secondary prevention is complicated by the fact that MI and surgery, including bypass surgery, can lower the serum cholesterol concentration substantially, giving a false impression that treatment of hyperlipidemia is not warranted. In most cases, the cholesterol begins to drop the first 48 hours after the event (Ryder et al., 1984), and then returns to baseline levels three months later (Brugada et al., 1996). Thus, a cholesterol level below the treatment threshold cannot exclude the need for lipid-lowering treatment if the measurement was done more than 48 hours and less than three months after the cardiac event. Because it may take three months for a sound cholesterol value to be determined after the diagnosis of CAD (particularly if CAD is discovered through a cardiac event or is concurrent with a need for surgery), our indicator permits a four-month window after the diagnosis of CAD in which cholesterol measurement may be done (Indicator 2).

Women

No study or meta-analysis has independently shown a reduction in overall mortality in any category of women assigned to cholesterol-lowering treatment (ACP, 1996). Although women were included in the "4S" study, independent mortality benefit for this group was not demonstrated (The "4S" Group, 1994). In the absence of demonstrated treatment benefit, guidelines from both the CTF and the ACP view the evidence for care of hyperlipidemia in women as insufficient (CTF, 1993; Garber et al., 1996). Therefore, although treatment of high cholesterol in women at high risk may be appropriate, because of lack of consensus and lack of evidence of mortality benefit with cholesterol lowering treatment for women, neither screening nor treatment for high cholesterol in women will be included as an indicator.

The Elderly

In men age 60 to 70 with existing heart disease (primarily those with a prior MI), overall mortality was shown to decline with cholesterol reduction using HMG-CoA reductase inhibitors in the "4S" study; however, the benefit was less pronounced than that for younger individuals (The "4S" Group, 1994). This finding cannot be extrapolated to older individuals. Cholesterol alone is a weak predictor of coronary heart disease mortality in the elderly and not consistently predictive after age 75 (U.S. Preventive Services Task Force, 1995). Indeed, higher cholesterol values appear to be associated with *increased* survival in individuals over age 80 (CTF, 1993; Kaiser, 1993; Kronmal et al., 1993). For this reason we restrict our screening and treatment indicators to the population in whom benefit has been demonstrated, that is, men under age 70.

DIAGNOSIS

Screening for hyperlipidemia focuses on levels of serum total cholesterol and HDL; however, treatment is currently predominantly guided by the LDL cholesterol level (Expert Panel on Detection Evaluation and Treatment of High Blood Cholesterol in Adults, 1993). In men under age 70 with preexisting coronary disease, for whom treatment would be clearly indicated in the presence of high LDL, a measurement of LDL should be done within three months after a total serum cholesterol value exceeding 200 mg/dl is documented, unless an earlier measure of LDL is documented within the prior two years (Indicator 3).

Marked fluctuations in cholesterol result from differences in laboratory technique, and from such types of biological variability as infection, surgery, emotional stress, or parturition, as well as diurnal variation, postural variation, and variation with the time of tourniquet placement. For this reason, the ACP (1996) recommends that the pharmacological treatment of a patient for hyperlipidemia be based on the average of at least two cholesterol or LDL measurements, to prevent the side effects and economic costs associated with unnecessary treatment (Indicator 4).

Although our indicator requires a record of at least two cholesterol measurements before initiating anti-hyperlipidemic treatment, an exception is made for patients with identified heart disease. For these patients, prompt initiation of treatment may be more important than the need to confirm a cholesterol value with a second measurement. Nonetheless, absence of a second measurement will complicate assessment of the true effect of the treatment for hyperlipidemia, even in those with previously identified heart disease.

TREATMENT

Dietary and Pharmacological Treatment in Patients With Preexisting Coronary Disease

Dietary Treatment

If cholesterol is elevated, the NCEP recommends initiation of a Step I diet. In such a diet, total and saturated fat consumption accounts for no more than 30 percent and ten percent, respectively, of all caloric intake. If this is not effective, a Step II diet is recommended before beginning pharmacological therapy to reduce cholesterol. The exception to this is individuals with established heart disease, in whom a Step II diet should be tried only briefly before pharmacological therapy is initiated. However, studies have shown that a low-fat diet alone leads to limited cholesterol reductions in patients assigned to dietary treatment as compared with controls. Because diets, such as a Step I diet, reduce cholesterol by an average of only two percent, recommendations for dietary treatment are not universal (ACP, 1996). For this reason we do not propose an indicator requiring that dietary treatment precede initiation of drug treatment.

Pharmacological Therapy

The section on screening describes the data on mortality benefit and indications for both screening and treatment with cholesterol-lowering treatment. To recapitulate, mortality benefit from cholesterol-lowering treatment has been demonstrated in men under age 70 with preexisting coronary disease who have "high" cholesterol. While the LDL cutoff at which benefit is derived from cholesterol-lowering treatment is a subject of continued study, it is generally agreed that cholesterol-lowering treatment should be initiated within three months of an LDL measurement exceeding 130 mg/dl in those who are not already on dietary or pharmacological treatment (Indicator 5). Evidence of mortality benefit has only been demonstrated with pharmacological therapy. Therefore, men under age 70 with preexisting heart disease who continue to have an LDL above 130 mg/dl after six months of dietary treatment should begin receiving pharmacological treatment or have LDL rechecked promptly (Indicator 6).

We define "pharmacological therapy" as any approved drug for treatment of hyperlipidemia. We have chosen not to generate indicators restricting drug choice on the grounds that expert agreement would likely be possible only for selected lipid profiles that refer to a minority of patients, limiting the utility of the indicator.

FOLLOW-UP

All patients for whom cholesterol-lowering pharmacological treatment has been initiated, or for whom the dose has been modified, should have their cholesterol value rechecked after four months to ensure that cholesterol is being successfully reduced (Indicator 7). Based on the repeat measurements, the medication dose may be further modified, or a different lipid-lowering drug may be substituted to achieve the desired lipid reduction. There are no firm data to indicate the optimum timing of reevaluation, which may vary with the pharmacological agent used. We have allowed four months for retesting in our indicator (Indicator 8).

REFERENCES

American College of Physicians. 1996. Guidelines for using serum cholesterol, high-density lipoprotein cholesterol, and triglyceride levels as screening tests for preventing coronary heart disease in adults. *Archives of Internal Medicine* 124: 515-517.

Anderson K, W Castelli, et al. 1996. Cholesterol and mortality: 30 years of follow-up from the Framingham study. *Journal of the American Medical Association* 257 (16): 2176-80.

Brugada R, N Wenger, et al. 1996. Changes in plasma cholesterol levels after hospitalization for acute coronary events. *Cardiology* 87 (3): 194-9.

Burr M, A Fehily, et al. 1989. Effects of changes in fat, fish and fibre intakes on death and myocardial reinfarction: Diet and Reinfarction Trial (DART). *Lancet* II: 757-61.

Canadian Task Force on the Periodic Health Examination. Periodic health examination, 1993 update: 2. Lowering the blood total cholesterol level to prevent coronary heaert disease. *Canadian Medical Association Journal* 148 (4): 521-538.

Committee of Principal Investigators. 1989. WHO Clofibrate Trial: A cooperative trial in the primary prevention of ischaemic heart disease using clofibrate. *British Heart Journal* 40: 1069-1118.

Davey Smith G, F Song, et al. 1993. Cholesterol lowering and mortality: the importance of considering initial level of risk. *British Medical Journal* 306: 1367-73.

Expert Panel on Detection Evaluation and Treatment of High Blood Cholesterol in Adults. 1993. Summary of the Second Report of the National Cholesterol Education Program (NCEP) Expert Panel on Detection, Evaluation, and Treatment of High Blood Cholesterol in Adults (Adult Treatment Panel II). *Journal of the American Medical Association* 269 (23): 3015-20.

Froom J. 1989. Selections from current literature: The cholesterol controversy. *Family Practice* 6 (3): 232-7.

Garber A, W Browner, et al. 1996. Cholesterol screening in asymptomatic adults, revisited. *Archives of Internal Medicine* 124 (5): 518-531.

Harris W. 1989. Fish oils and plasma lipid and lipoprotein metabolism in humans -- a critical review. *J Lipid Res* 30: 785-807.

Harris-Hooker S, and S GL. Lipids, lipoproteins and coronary heart disease in minority populations. *Atherosclerosis* 108 (Suppl): S83-104.

Kaiser F. Cholesterol and the older adult. *Southern Medical Journal* 86 (10): 2S11-2S14.

Keaney JJ, J Gaziano, et al. Low-dose alpha-tocopherol improves and high-dose alpha-tocopherol worsens endothelial vasodilator function in cholesterol-fed rabbits. *Journal of Clinical Investigation* 93 (2): 844-5.

Kronmal R, K Cain, et al. 1993. Total serum cholesterol levels and mortality risk as a function of age: A report based on the Framingham data. *Archives of Internal Medicine* 153: 1065-1073

Kroon A, W Aengevaeren, et al. 1996. LDL-Apheresis Atherosclerosis Regression Study (LAARS). Effect of aggressive versus conventional lipid lowering treatment on coronary atherosclerosis. *Circulation* 93 (10): 1826-35.

McBride P, and J Davis. 1992. Cholesterol and cost-effectiveness: Implications for practice, policy, and research. *Circulation* 85 (5): 1939-41.

McCormick J, and P Skrabanek. 1988. Coronary heart disease is not preventable by population interventions. *Lancet* ii: 839-41.

Muldoon M, S Manuck, et al. 1990. Lowering cholesterol concentrations and mortality: a review of primary prevention trials. *Br Med J* 301: 309-14.

O'Keefe JJ, CJ Lavie, et al. 1995. Insights into the pathogenesis and prevention of coronary artery disease. *Mayo Clinic Proceedings* 70 (1): 69-79.

Rossner W, W Palmer, et al. 1993. An international perspective on the cholesterol debate. *Family Practice* 10 (4): 431-438.

Ryder R, T Hayes, et al. 1984. How soon after myocardial infarction should plasma lipid values be assessed? *British Medical Journal* 289: 1651-3.

Scandinavian Simvastatin Survival Study Group. 1994. Randomised trial of cholesterol lowering in 4444 patients with coronary heart disease: The Scandinavian Simvastatin Survival Study (4S). *Lancet* 344: 1383-9.

Schmidt E, and J Dyerberg. 1994. Omega-3 fatty acids: current status in cardiovascular medicine. *Drugs* 47: 405-24.

Sempos C, R Fulwood, et al. 1989. The prevalence of high blood cholesterol levels among adults in the United States. *J Am Med Assoc* 262: 45-52.

Shepherd J, S Cobbe, et al. 1995. Prevention of coronary heart disease with pravastatin in men with hypercholesterolemia. *New England Journal of Medicine* 333 (20): 1301-7.

Simopoulos A. 1990. Diet and new lesions of the coronary arteries. *Journal of the American Medical Association* 254: 1251.

Stensvold I, P Urdal, et al. 1992. High-density lipoprotein cholesterol and coronary, cardiovascular and all cause mortality among middle-aged Norwegian men and women. *European Heart Journal* 13 (9): 1155-63.

Tunstall-Pedoe H. 1988. Epidemiology and pathogenesis of ischaemic heart disease. *Current Opinion in Cardiology* 3: 550-60.

US Preventive Services Task Force Screening for high blood cholesterol and other lipid abnormalities. 15-37.

US Public Health Service. 1995. Cholesterol screening in adults. *American Family Physician* 51 (1): 129-136.

Van Boven A, J Jukema, et al. 1994. Endothelial dysfunction and dyslipidemia: possible effects of lipid lowering and lipid modifying therapy. *Pharmacological Research* 29 (3): 261-72.

RECOMMENDED QUALITY INDICATORS FOR HYPERLIPIDEMIA

These indicators apply to men and women age 18 and older, except where otherwise noted.

Indicator	Quality of Evidence	Literature	Benefits	Comments
Screening				
1. Men under age 70 with preexisting heart disease[2] who are not on pharmacological therapy for hyperlipidemia[5] should have cholesterol level documented at least every 5 years.	III	4S, 1994	Improve survival.	Cholesterol lowering reduces mortality in hyperlipidemic men under age 70 with identified heart disease (4S, class I evidence). Identification of hyperlipidemia in these men is therefore important, and screening should be repeated periodically. A 5-year period is often cited as reasonable interval for rescreening, although no data support any particular interval.
2. Men under age 70 with newly diagnosed coronary disease[1] should have had total cholesterol documented within 2 years before or within 4 months after the diagnosis is first noted in the medical record.	III	ACP, 1996	Decrease mortality.	Mortality benefit has been shown with cholesterol reduction in hyperlipidemic men under age 70 with prior heart disease (4S, 1994). Because MI or surgery can lower the cholesterol value, thereby obscuring a true high cholesterol, some recommend against measurement within the first 3 months after MI or surgery. A high value in this time will dictate need for treatment; thus an expanded 4 month window is given.
Diagnosis				
3. Men under age 70 with preexisting coronary disease[2] who have a total cholesterol level exceeding 200 mg/dl should have a measure of their LDL cholesterol[3] documented within 2 years before or 3 months after the 200 mg/dl level.	III	NCEP, 1993	Decrease mortality.	LDL cholesterol is used to guide need for treatment.

213

Indicator	Quality of Evidence	Literature	Benefits	Comments
4. Patients without preexisting coronary disease[2] who are started on pharmacological treatment for hyperlipidemia should have had at least 2 measurements of their cholesterol (total or LDL) documented in the year before the start of pharmacological treatment.	III	ACP, 1996	Prevent morbidity associated with unnecessary treatment.	High variability in cholesterol measurements renders unjustified pharmacological treatment of hyperlipidemia based on a single measurement. Ideally, two measurements should exceed the physician's treatment threshold prior to institution of lipid-lowering treatment, though some will accept the average of the two. For subjects with identified cardiac disease, prompt initiation of treatment may be viewed as a higher priority than the need to corroborate a cholesterol value with a second measurement. This could be justified on the grounds that benefit of cholesterol reduction to cardiac outcomes has been shown in those with heart disease even in the presence of "normal" cholesterol.
Treatment				
5. Men under age 70 with preexisting coronary disease[2] who have an untreated LDL cholesterol level >130 mg/dl should begin diet[4] or drug therapy[5] within 3 months of the high LDL measurement.	I	NCEP, 1993; 4S, 1994; ACP, 1996	Reduce mortality.	Mortality benefit with pharmacological therapy has been shown in this group. Treatment with HMG-CoA reductase inhibitors is preferred, since significant mortality benefit during the time of treatment has been demonstrated only with simvastatin.
6. Men under age 70 with preexisting coronary disease[2] who have an LDL level >130 mg/dl after 6 months of dietary cholesterol-lowering treatment[4] should receive one of the following within 2 months: • pharmacological therapy[5] for hyperlipidemia; or • a repeat LDL measurement.	III	4S, 1994; ACP 1996	Reduce mortality.	In patients with preexisting coronary disease, a maximum of 6 months of dietary treatment is recommended before drug treatment is started, unless cholesterol is brought below 130 mg/dl with diet alone. Drug treatment has been shown to reduce mortality in this group (4S, class I evidence), whereas dietary therapy has not.

214

Indicator	Quality of Evidence	Literature	Benefits	Comments
Follow-up				
7. Patients in whom pharmacological therapy for hyperlipidemia[5] has been initiated should have their cholesterol rechecked within 4 months.	III	4S, 1994	Prevent morbidity from treatment side effects. Improve survival.	Ineffective cholesterol-lowering treatment poses risks without benefits. Therefore cholesterol measurements should be obtained after adding or changing a cholesterol-lowering drug to ensure that treatment is effective and to allow treatment modification if it is not. Additionally, effective lipid reduction improves mortality in men under age 70 with heart disease (class I evidence, 4S). Therefore mortality may be improved by assuring that therapy given is effective.
8. Patients receiving pharmacological therapy for hyperlipidemia[5] who have had a dosage or medication change should have cholesterol rechecked within 4 months of the change.	III	4S, 1994	Prevent morbidity from treatment side effects. Improve survival.	Ineffective cholesterol-lowering treatment poses risks without benefits. Therefore cholesterol measurements should be obtained after adding or changing a cholesterol-lowering drug to ensure that treatment is effective and to allow treatment modification if it is not. Additionally, effective lipid reduction improves mortality in men under age 70 with heart disease (class I evidence, 4S). Therefore mortality may be improved by assuring that therapy given is effective.

Definitions and Examples

[1] Newly diagnosed coronary disease: New diagnosis of CAD mentioned in chart, admission for myocardial infarction, admission for unstable angina.

[2] Prexisting heart disease: History of myocardial infarction, angioplasty, cardiac bypass surgery, or a physician's note of CAD or angina.

[3] Either LDL cholesterol or both HDL and triglycerides to allow calculation of LDL.

[4] Dietary therapy: Includes any mention of diet counseling in the medical record (either by a physician, nurse, physician assistant, dietitian or nutritionist).

[5] Pharmacological (drug) therapy: May include HMG-CoA reductase inhibitors (simvastatin, lovastatin, fluvastatin, pravastatin, atorvastatin or other statins), niacin, gemfibrozil, cholestyramine, colestipol, or a combination of agents.

Quality of Evidence Codes

I	RCT
II-1	Nonrandomized controlled trials
II-2	Cohort or case analysis
II-3	Multiple time series
III	Opinions or descriptive studies

215

11. HYPERTENSION[1]

Steven Asch, MD, MPH and Kenneth Clark, MD, MPH

We depended mainly on five sources in constructing quality
indicators for hypertension. For screening for hypertension, we used
three organizations' published guidelines: the Canadian Task Force on
the Periodic Health Examination (CTF), the United States Preventive
Services Task Force (USPSTF) and the American College of Physicians
(ACP) (CTF, 1984; USPSTF, 1996; Hayward et al., 1991; Littenberg et al.,
1991, in Eddy, 1991; Littenberg, 1995). For indicators of treatment and
follow-up care we relied upon the Fifth Report of the Joint National
Committee on Detection, Evaluation, and Treatment of High Blood Pressure
(JNC V) and a recently published meta-analysis of 14 studies of the
treatment of hypertension (NHBPEP, 1993; Collins et al., 1990). The JNC
V has been endorsed by more than 30 medical specialty organizations.
When these core references cited studies to support individual
indicators, we have referenced the original source. When the core
references were unclear in their support for a particular indicator, we
performed a focused MEDLINE search for articles addressing that topic.

IMPORTANCE

Hypertension is one of the most common medical conditions. It is
present in an estimated 43 million Americans (USPSTF, 1996). Most of
the morbidity from hypertension derives from the damage it does to
target organs. It is a leading risk factor for coronary artery disease,
congestive heart failure, renal disease and stroke (USPSTF, 1996).
Hypertension often goes undetected and even when detected may be
inadequately treated. The second National Health and Nutrition
Examination Survey (NHANES II) found that among hypertensive adults, 54
percent were aware of their condition, 33 percent took medications for

---

[1] This chapter is a revision of one written for an earlier project on quality of
care for women and children (Q1). The expert panel for the current project was asked to
review all of the indicators, but only rated new or revised indicators.

it, and only 11 percent were under control (NHBPEP, 1985). Hypertension is also a costly disease; patients under treatment spend about $900 to $1,400 annually for drugs, laboratory tests, and provider visits (Hilleman et al., 1994).

SCREENING

No randomized trials or observational studies have directly evaluated screening unselected patients for hypertension. Nonetheless, based on the demonstrated efficacy of treatment (see below), several widely accepted guidelines have been promulgated. The USPSTF recommends that all adults undergo blood pressure screening every two years for those with diastolic and systolic blood pressures below 85 mm Hg and 140 mm Hg, respectively, and every year for those with diastolic blood pressures of 85 to 89 mm Hg. The ACP makes no recommendations about the frequency of blood pressure measurement, but urges screening of all patients presenting for care. The CTF recommends that blood pressure be measured at every medical visit (USPSTF, 1996; Littenberg et al., 1991, in Eddy, 1991; Hayward et al., 1991; Littenberg, 1995; CTF, 1984)(Indicator 1).

Estimates of the cost-effectiveness of screening patients for hypertension vary widely. While the screening test itself poses little risk to the patient's health, incorrectly labeling a patient as hypertensive may. Searching for secondary causes of hypertension may entail some invasive procedures and pharmacologic therapy may have side effects. Cost-effectiveness studies have supported case finding (the measurement of blood pressure in patients presenting for care for other reasons) over mass screening, finding that each quality-adjusted life-year saved costs about $15,000 (Weinstein, 1976). More recent studies have estimated the cost-effectiveness of screening middle-aged women to be in the range of $23,000 per quality-adjusted life-year (Eddy, 1991; Littenberg, 1995).

DIAGNOSIS

Measurement Technique

The measurement of systolic and diastolic blood pressure using a mercury sphygmomanometer cuff is one of the oldest objective measures in medicine. Because its use predated modern experimental design, it is difficult to assess its efficacy. Studies have shown some difficulties in cuff measurements of the blood pressure of obese and elderly patients when compared to more invasive and impractical intra-arterial measurements, but virtually all studies of the natural history and treatment of the disease have been based on cuff measurements.

Classification

The JNC V introduced a new diagnostic staging system based on the degree of elevation of cuff measurements, which is shown in Table 11.1.

Table 11.1

High Blood Pressure Diagnostic Staging System

Category	Systolic (mm Hg)	Diastolic (mm Hg)
Normal	<130	<85
High normal	130-139	85-89
Stage 1 (mild)	140-159	90-99
Stage 2 (moderate)	160-179	100-109
Stage 3 (severe)	180-209	110-119
Stage 4 (very severe)	>210	>120

Source: National High Blood Pressure Education Program, 1993.

Natural history studies of mild hypertension and the placebo arms of interventional studies have shown extreme variability in the blood pressures of Stages 1 to 2 hypertensives (Management Committee of the Australian National Blood Pressure Study, 1980; Medical Research Council Working Party, 1985). For that reason, the JNC V recommends using the

219

average of three measurements documented over the course of several weeks to confirm the diagnosis (Indicators 2 and 3).

Initial History and Physical

The initial history and physical of the newly diagnosed hypertensive patient searches for secondary causes, target organ disease and additional cardiac risk factors. A focused literature search revealed no direct evaluation of the value of the history and physical in preventing complications or death, so we have relied upon expert opinion. We modified the recommendations in the JNC V consensus statement to produce our quality indicators (Indicator 4).

Initial Laboratory Examination

Like the initial history and physical, initial laboratory tests search for secondary causes, target organ damage, and other cardiac risk factors. In addition, these tests may serve as a baseline for monitoring the side effects of pharmacotherapy. A focused literature review again revealed no direct evaluation of routine testing, so we again modified the JNC V recommendations when constructing our indicators (Indicator 6).

Secondary Hypertension Due to Drugs

Clinical trials have associated many drugs with the development of hypertension, including oral contraceptives, steroids, nasal decongestants, appetite suppressants, cyclosporine, erythropoietin, tricyclic antidepressants, and monamine oxidase inhibitors. The JNC V recommends the discontinuation of these drugs (at least temporarily) to determine if they are the cause of the patient's hypertension (Indicator 5).

TREATMENT

Lifestyle Changes

Most experts recommend nonpharmacological lifestyle changes (e.g., weight reduction, low sodium diet, physical activity, alcohol avoidance) as the first line of treatment in Stage 1-3 hypertension. The evidence for such recommendations is fairly solid. An observational trial of 301

220

obese patients revealed significant declines in blood pressure in those who successfully lost weight (Schotte and Stunkard, 1990). A randomized trial of 878 Stage 1-2 patients who were more than ten percent above their ideal body weight showed that weight loss enhances the antihypertensive effect of medication (Langford et al., 1991). Avoiding dietary sodium reduces systolic blood pressure by an average of 4.9 mm Hg and diastolic blood pressure by 2.6 mm Hg according to a meta-analysis of 23 randomized trials with 1536 subjects (Cutler et al., 1991). Patients with low levels of physical fitness, as measured by treadmill, developed hypertension one and a half times more often in a cohort of 4820 men and 1219 women observed for four years (Blair et al., 1984). Epidemiological studies have linked excessive alcohol consumption and hypertension. In addition, a randomized controlled trial of 41 heavy drinkers supports this association. Though this randomized trial was plagued by a high dropout rate, it demonstrated that physicians simply advising patients to reduce their alcohol consumption resulted in an average drop of more than 5 mm Hg in systolic blood pressure (Maheswaran et al., 1991) (Indicators 7 and 8).

Pharmacotherapy

If nonpharmacologic measures do not lower the blood pressure to normal levels or if the patient has Stage 4 disease, the JNC V recommends the addition of medication to the patient's regimen. A meta-analysis of 14 randomized trials has demonstrated a 42 percent reduction in strokes, a 14 percent reduction in coronary heart disease and a 12 percent reduction in all-cause mortality over four to six years of follow-up (Collins et al., 1990; Hebert et al., 1988) (Indicators 9 and 10). These studies have predominantly used middle-aged or elderly men as subjects (Anastos et al., 1991). The benefits of pharmacologic treatment are most pronounced among those with Stage 4 hypertension, increasing five-year survival from close to zero to 75 percent (Hansson, 1988).

Choice of Pharmacologic Agent

Although many classes of drugs (e.g., angiotensin-converting enzyme inhibitors, calcium channel blockers, direct vasodilators, centrally acting alpha antagonists) have been proven effective at lowering blood pressure, only beta blockers and diuretics have demonstrated in randomized controlled trials that they effectively lower mortality. Indeed, recent observational data have given rise to the suspicion that calcium channel blockers may increase overall mortality (Psaty et al., 1995). All 14 trials cited in the above meta-analysis used beta blockers or diuretics to lower the blood pressure of the intervention group. While awaiting data expected in 2001 from ALLHAT (Antihypertensive and Lipid-Lowering Treatment to Prevent Heart Attack), a randomized trial evaluating ACE inhibitors, calcium channel blockers, centrally acting agents and cardiovascular morbidity and mortality, the JNC V recommended initial pharmacologic therapy with either a diuretic or a beta blocker.

Concomitant Disease

The presence of concomitant disease may alter this JNC V recommendation. Both beta blockers and thiazide diuretics are associated with mild increases in serum lipids, though this effect has not been shown to persist (Grimm et al., 1981). For that reason, some experts recommend avoiding these agents in patients with known hyperlipidemia. Similarly, some diabetics should avoid beta blockers because of the masking of hypoglycemic symptoms. Several randomized trials have shown that ACE inhibitors and calcium channel blockers delay the progression of diabetic nephropathy (Lederle, 1992; Baba et al., 1986; Bjorck et al., 1986; Marre et al., 1988; Hommel et al., 1986). The Systolic Hypertension in the Elderly Program (SHEP) clinical trial showed that low-dose diuretic-based (chlorthalidone) treatment is effective in preventing major cerebral and cardiovascular events in diabetic and nondiabetic older patients with isolated systolic hypertension (Curb et al., 1996) (Indicator 11). Asthmatic patients should avoid beta blockers due to their bronchoconstrictive effect (Barker et al., 1991). Many thiazide diuretics increase uric acid and should thus be avoided as initial therapy for patients with gout (Barker et al., 1991). Patients with known coronary artery disease but no dilated cardiomyopathy should receive beta blockers preferentially over diuretics as initial therapy. Several randomized controlled trials have demonstrated that beta blockers reduce mortality in such patients (First International Study of Infarct Survival Collaborative Group, 1988).

FOLLOW-UP

No studies directly address the optimal follow-up period for hypertensive patients. The JNC V recommends two visits each year. The goal of antihypertensive therapy is to lower the blood pressure to normal levels. If hypertension persists despite treatment, most experts recommend altering the patient's regimen. However, there is no consensus as to the optimal algorithm for modifying the regimen. Increasing the dose, changing to another class of agents, adding an agent from another class, reducing the frequency of administration to improve compliance, and renewed efforts at lifestyle modification are all acceptable strategies.

REFERENCES

Anastos K, Charney P, Charon RA, et al. Hypertension in women: What is really known? *Archives of Internal Medicine* 115 ((4)): 287-93.

Baba T, T Ishizaki, Y Ido, et al. November 1986. Renal effects of nicardipine, a calcium entry blocker, in hypertensive type II diabetic patients with nephropathy. *Diabetes* 35: 1206-14.

Barker LR. 1991. Hypertension. In *Principles of Ambulatory Medicine*, Third Ed. Baltimore, MD: Williams and Wilkins.

Bjorck S, Nyberg G, Mulec H, et al. 23 August 1986. Beneficial effects of angiotensin converting enzyme inhibition on renal function in patients with diabetic nephropathy. *British Medical Journal* 293: 471-4.

Blair SN, NN Goodyear, LW Gibbons, et al. 27 July 1984. Physical fitness and incidence of hypertension in healthy normotensive men and women. *Journal of the American Medical Association* 252 (4): 487-90.

Canadian Task Force on the Periodic Health Examination. 15 May 1984. The periodic health examination: 2. 1984 update. *Canadian Medical Association Journal* 130 ((10)): 1278-85.

Collins R, R Peto, S MacMahon, et al. 1990. Blood pressure, stroke, and coronary heart disease. Part 2, short-term reductions in blood pressure: Overview of randomised drug trials in their epidemiological context. *Lancet* 335: 827-38.

Curb JD, Pressel SL, Cutler JA, et al. 18 December 1996. Effect of Diuretic-Based Antihypertensive Treatment on Cardiovascular Disease Risk in Older Diabetic Patients with Isolated Systolic Hypertension. *Journal of the American Medical Assocation* 276 (23): 1886-1892.

Cutler JA, D Follmann, P Elliott, et al. 1991. An overview of randomized trials of sodium reduction and blood pressure. *Hypertension* 17 ((Suppl. 1)): I27-I33.

First International Study of Infarct Survival Collaborative Group. 23 April 1988. Mechanisms for the early mortality reduction produced by beta-blockade started early in acute myocardial infarction: ISIS-1. *Lancet* 1 (8591): 921-3.

Grimm RH, AS Leon, DB Hunninghake, et al. January 1981. Effects of thiazide diuretics on plasma lipids and lipoproteins in mildly hypertensive patients. *Archives of Internal Medicine* 94 (1): 7-11.

Hansson L. 10 February 1988. Current and future strategies in the treatment of hypertension. *The American Journal of Cardiology* 61 (2C-7C):

Hayward RSA, EP Steinberg, DE Ford, et al. 1 May 1991. Preventive care guidelines: 1991. *Archives of Internal Medicine* 114 (9): 758-83.

Hebert PR, NH Fiebach, KA Eberlein, et al. 1988. The community-based randomized trials of pharmacologic treatment of mild-to-moderate hypertension. *American Journal of Epidemiology* 127 (3): 581-90.

Hilleman DE, SM Mohiuddin, BD Lucas Jr, et al. 1994. Cost-minimization analysis of initial antihypertensive therapy in patients with mild-to-moderate essential diastolic hypertension. *Clinical Therapeutics* 16 (1): 88-102.

Hommel E, H Parving, E Mathiesen, et al. 23 August 1986. Effect of captopril on kidney function in insulin-dependent diabetic patients with nephropathy. *British Medical Journal* 293: 467-70.

Langford HG, Davis BR, D Blaufox, et al. 1991. Effect of drug and diet treatment of mild hypertension on diastolic blood pressure. *Hypertension* 17 (2): 210-7.

Lederle, and RM. 1992. The effect of antihypertensive therapy on the course of renal failure. *Journal of Cardiovascular Pharmacology* 20 (Suppl. 6): S69-S72.

Littenberg B. 15 June 1995. A practice guideline revisited: Screening for hypertension. *Archives of Internal Medicine* 122 (12): 937-9.

Littenberg B, AM Garber, and and HC Sox. 1991. Screening for hypertension. *Common Screening Tests*. Eddy DM, 22-47 & 397. Philadelphia, PA: American College of Physicians.

Maheswaran R, M Beevers, and and DG Beevers. 1992. Effectiveness of advice to reduce alcohol consumption in hypertensive patients. *Hypertension* 19 (1): 79-84.

Management Committee of the Australian National Blood Pressure Study. 14 June 1980. The Australian therapeutic trial in mild hypertension. *Lancet* 1: 1261-7.

Marre M, G Chatellier, H Leblanc, et al. 29 October 1988. Prevention of diabetic nephropathy with enalapril in normotensive diabetics with microalbuminuria. *British Medical Journal* 297 (6656): 1092-5.

Medical Research Council Working Party. 13 July 1985. MRC trial of treatment of mild hypertension: Principal results. *British Medical Journal* 291: 97-104.

National High Blood Pressure Education Program. 25 January 1993. The fifth report of the Joint National Committee on Detection, Evaluation, and Treatment of High Blood Pressure (JNC V). *Archives of Internal Medicine* 153: 154-83.

National High Blood Pressure Education Program. 1985. Hypertension prevalence and the status of awareness, treatment, and control in the United States: Final report of the Subcommittee on Definition and Prevalence of the 1984 Joint National Committee 1985. *Hypertension* 7 (3): 457-68.

Psaty BM, SR Heckbert, TD Koepsell, et al. 1 February 1995. The risk of incident myocardial infarction associated with anti-hypertensive drug therapies. *Circulation* 91 (3): 925.

Schotte DE, and and AJ Stunkard. August 1990. The effects of weight reduction on blood pressure in 301 obese patients. *Archives of Internal Medicine* 150: 1701-4.

U.S. Preventive Services Task Force. 1989. *Guide to Clinical Preventive Services: An Assessment of the Effectiveness of 169 Interventions*. Baltimore, MD: Williams and Wilkins.

Weinstein, M. 1976. *Hypertension: A Policy Perspective*. Cambridge, MA: Harvard University Press.

RECOMMENDED QUALITY INDICATORS FOR HYPERTENSION

These indicators apply to men and women age 18 and older. Only the indicators in bold type were rated by this panel; the remaining indicators were endorsed by a prior panel.

Indicator	Quality of Evidence	Literature	Benefits	Comments
Screening				
1. Systolic and diastolic blood pressure should be measured on patients otherwise presenting for care at least once each year.	III	USPSTF, 1996; Hayward et al., 1991; Littenberg et al., 1991, in Eddy, 1991; Littenberg, 1995; CTF, 1984	Decrease hypertensive complications.[1]	Blood pressure measurement has been recommended by 3 widely accepted guidelines. Increased detection of asymptomatic hypertensives prompts treatment.
Diagnosis				
2. All patients with average blood pressures of >140 systolic and/or >90 diastolic as determined on at least 3 separate visits should have a diagnosis of hypertension documented in the record.	III	JNCV, 1993	Decrease hypertensive complications.	Timely diagnosis of hypertension prompts treatment.
3. Patients with a new diagnosis of stage 1-3 hypertension should have at least 3 measurements on different days with a mean SBP>140 and/or a mean DBP>90.	III	Management Committee of the Australian National Blood Pressure Study, 1980; Medical Research Council Working Party, 1985	Prevent medication side effects such as orthostatic hypotension, fatigue, and impotence.	Observational studies have shown variability in the blood pressure of patients with mild to moderate hypertension. False labeling of patients as hypertensive can lead to unnecessary treatment and potential medication side effects.

227

Indicator	Quality of Evidence	Literature	Benefits	Comments
4. Initial history and physical of patients with hypertension should document assessment of at least 2 items from each of the following groups by the third visit: • History: Family or personal history of premature CAD, CVA, diabetes, hyperlipidemia; • Medication and substance abuse: Personal history of tobacco abuse, alcohol abuse, or taking of medications that may cause hypertension;[2] • Physical examination: Examination of the fundi, heart sounds, abdomen for bruits, peripheral arterial pulses, neurologic system.	III	NHBPEP, 1993	Reduce or eliminate medication side effects. Prevent other symptoms from the underlying disease (e.g., renal failure from renal artery stenosis). Decrease synergistic risk of cardiovascular complications.[1] Prevent hypertensive complications.[1]	No controlled trials directly examine the elements of quality in the history and physical for hypertensives. These minimum recommendations from JNC V search for secondary causes, other cardiac risk factors, and target organ damage. Identification of secondary causes can eliminate the need for therapy. Staging of target organ damage should prompt more aggressive control of hypertension for advanced disease.
5. Stage 1 hypertensive patients taking drugs that may cause hypertension[2] should have the drug discontinued (at least temporarily) before pharmacotherapy is initiated.	I	NHBPEP, 1993	Prevent or reduce medication side effects.	Clinical trials have associated many drugs with hypertension. The JNC V recommends discontinuation of the implicated drugs to determine if they are causing hypertension. Drugs known to cause hypertension include: oral contraceptives, steroids, nasal decongestants, appetite suppressants, cyclosporine, monamine oxidase inhibitors, tricyclic antidepressants, and erythropoietin.

228

Indicator	Quality of Evidence	Literature	Benefits	Comments
6. Initial laboratory tests should include at least 5 of the following: • Urinalysis; • Serum, plasma, or blood glucose; • Serum potassium; • Serum creatinine; • Serum cholesterol; or • Serum triglyceride.	III	NHBPEP, 1993	Reduce or eliminate medication side effects. Prevent other symptoms from the underlying disease (e.g., renal failure from renal artery stenosis). Decrease synergistic risk of cardiovascular complications.[1] Prevent hypertensive complications.[1]	No clinical trials directly examine the efficacy of initial laboratory testing for hypertensive patients. These minimum recommendations from JNC V search for secondary causes, other cardiac risk factors, and end organ damage.
Treatment				
7. First-line treatment for Stage 1-2 hypertension is lifestyle modification. The medical record should indicate counseling for at least 1 of the following interventions prior to initiating pharmacotherapy: • weight reduction if obese; • increased physical activity if sedentary; • low sodium diet, or • alcohol intake reduction if alcohol drinker.	I-II	Schotte and Stunkard, 1990; Langford, 1991; Blair et al., 1984; Cutler et al., 1991; Maheswaran et al., 1991	Avoid side effects of medical therapy. Decreases hypertensive complications.	Cohort data from 301 obese patients showed weight loss reduces blood pressure, and a randomized trial of 878 obese patients showed that weight loss enhances antihypertensive pharmacotherapy. A meta-analysis of 23 randomized trials showed that lowering dietary sodium lowers blood pressure. Cohort observational data indicates that sedentary patients develop hypertension more frequently. A randomized trial showed that advising alcoholics to reduce their drinking reduced their blood pressure.

229

Indicator	Quality of Evidence	Literature	Benefits	Comments
8. First-line treatment for Stage 3 hypertension is lifestyle modification. The medical record should indicate counseling for at least 1 of the following interventions: • weight reduction if obese; • increased physical activity if sedentary; • low sodium diet, or • alcohol intake reduction if alcohol drinker.	I-II	Schotte and Stunkard, 1990; Langford, 1991; Blair et al., 1984; Cutler et al., 1991; Maheswaran et al., 1991	Avoid side effects of medical therapy. Decreases hypertensive complications.	Cohort data from 301 obese patients showed weight loss reduces blood pressure and a randomized trial of 878 obese patients showed that weight loss enhances antihypertensive pharmacotherapy. A meta-analysis of 23 randomized trials showed that lowering dietary sodium lowers blood pressure. Cohort observational data indicate that sedentary patients develop hypertension more frequently. A randomized trial showed that advising alcoholics to reduce their drinking reduced their blood pressure.
9. Stage 1-2 hypertensives whose blood pressure remains Stage 1-2 after 6 months lifestyle modification should receive pharmacotherapy, if not already on it.	I	Collins, 1990; Hebert, 1988; JNC V, 1993	Decrease hypertensive complications.	A meta-analysis of 14 randomized trials using pharmacotherapy in hypertension showed a 42% reduction in stroke, a 14% reduction in coronary heart disease, and a 12% reduction in mortality.
10. Stage 3 hypertensives should receive pharmacotherapy.	I	Collins, 1990; Hebert, 1988; JNC V, 1993	Decrease hypertensive complications.	A meta-analysis of 14 randomized trials using pharmacotherapy in hypertension showed a 42% reduction in stroke, a 14% reduction in coronary heart disease, and a 12% reduction in mortality.
11. First-line pharmacotherapy for diabetics should include an ACE inhibitor, a calcium channel blocker, or a thiazide diuretic.	I	Lederle, 1992; Baba, 1987; Bjorck, 1986; Marre, 1988; Hommel, 1986; Curb, 1996	Decrease hypertensive complications (particularly nephropathy).	Randomized trials have shown these agents to reduce progression of proteinuria and diabetic nephropathy.
Follow-up				
12. Hypertensive patients should visit the provider at least once each year.	III	NHBPEP, 1993	Reduce hypertensive complications and medication side effects.	JNC V recommends twice each year, but original panel changed to once.

230

		III	NHBPEP, 1993	Decrease hypertensive complications.	JNC V recommendations.
13.	Hypertensive patients with consistent average SBP>160 or DBP>90 over 6 months should have one of the following interventions recorded in the medical record: • Change in dose or regimen of antihypertensives; or • Repeated education regarding lifestyle modifications				

Definitions and Examples

[1]. Hypertensive complications include: Cardiovascular disease, cerebrovascular disease, retinopathy and nephropathy. Cardiovascular disease can result in chest pain, shortness of breath, claudication, fatigue, and death. Cerebrovascular disease can result in neurologic symptoms (e.g., aphasia, paralysis) and death. Retinopathy can result in visual field defects and blindness. Nephropathy can result in edema, arrhythmias, nausea, vomiting, fatigue, dialysis, and death.

[2]. Drugs known to cause hypertension include: oral contraceptives, steroids, nasal decongestants, appetite suppressants, cyclosporine, monamine oxidase inhibitors, tricyclic antidepressants, and erythropoietin.

NOTE: Stages 1-4 hypertension are defined as listed below. See Table 11.1 for the complete high blood pressure diagnostic staging system.

Stage of Hypertension	Systolic (mm Hg)	Diastolic (mm Hg)
Stage 1 (mild)	140-159	90-99
Stage 2 (moderate)	160-179	100-109
Stage 3 (severe)	180-209	110-119
Stage 4 (very severe)	>210	>120

Quality of Evidence Codes

I	RCT
II-1	Nonrandomized controlled trials
II-2	Cohort or case analysis
II-3	Multiple time series
III	Opinions or descriptive studies

231

12. UPPER RESPIRATORY INFECTIONS[1]

Eve A. Kerr, MD, MPH and Kenneth A. Clark, MD, MPH

We conducted a MEDLINE search of the medical literature for all English-language review articles published between 1990 and 1997 for the following topics: pharyngitis, common cold, influenza, rhinovirus, bronchitis, cough, and rhinitis. We selected articles from the MEDLINE results and references from the review articles were obtained in areas of controversy. In addition, we consulted two medical texts (Panzer et al., 1991; Barker et al., 1991) for general clinical approaches to respiratory infections. This section first outlines our findings on the general importance of URIs and then discusses five common clinical subcategories: pharyngitis, bronchitis, influenza, nasal congestion, and sinusitis.

Respiratory tract infections account for more than ten percent of all office visits to the primary care physician (Perlman and Ginn, 1990). According to the 1993 National Health Interview Survey (NHIS), over 250 million cases of respiratory infections occur in the U.S. yearly (National Center for Health Statistics [NCHS], 1994). Respiratory infections include the common cold, influenza, pharyngitis, sinusitis, bronchitis, and pneumonia. Influenza and the common cold account for the majority of cases.

---

[1] This chapter is a revision of one written for an earlier project on quality of care for women and children (Q1). The expert panel for the current project was asked to review all of the indicators, but only rated new or revised indicators.

ACUTE PHARYNGITIS

IMPORTANCE

According to the National Ambulatory Medical Care Survey: 1991 Summary, acute pharyngitis ranked tenth as a reason for visit in the ambulatory care setting. It accounted for 1.6 percent of all visits.

SCREENING

There are no current recommendations on screening for acute pharyngitis in asymptomatic patients.

DIAGNOSIS

Multiple bacterial and viral organisms may cause acute pharyngitis (Barker et al., 1991). In evaluating acute pharyngitis, the critical clinical decision is whether or not to use antibiotics, or to culture, for group A streptococcal infection. Group A streptococcus is the causative agent of rheumatic fever, which can result in serious renal and cardiac disease. The incidence of rheumatic fever is currently low, and has been decreasing independent of antibiotic use (Little and Williamson, 1994). In fact, over 78,000 persons would be required in an RCT to show convincingly a 50 percent reduction in the attack rate of rheumatic fever with antibiotics (Shvartzman, 1994). The benefit of prescribing antibiotics for pharyngitis must be weighed against the costs. Little and Williamson (1994) estimate that if every case of pharyngitis were treated with antibiotics, the average general practitioner in the United Kingdom would have roughly a one in three chance of having a patient die from anaphylaxis after treatment for sore throat. This is slightly higher than the chances of nephritis or rheumatic fever developing post-pharyngitis, neither of which have a high death rate.

Komaroff (1986) has helped define pretest probabilities and diagnostic strategies for pharyngitis (Panzer et al., 1991). Based on prospective studies estimating sensitivity and specificity of clinical findings with respect to confirmed diagnosis of Group A streptococcal infection, Komaroff has determined that in adult patients who have a sore throat but do not have a fever, tonsillar exudate, or anterior cervical adenopathy, the probability of streptococcal pharyngitis is less than three percent (Indicator 1). On the other hand, when all three of these findings are present, the probability of streptococcal pharyngitis is at least 40 percent.

Diagnostic tests that are useful to determine the presence of group A streptococcus include throat culture and rapid streptococcal antigen tests. Throat cultures are shown to be falsely negative in approximately ten percent of patients (Panzer et al., 1991). Rapid antigen tests are highly specific, but variably sensitive (80 to 95 percent) (Panzer et al., 1991).

According to Komaroff (1986) and based on the prospective studies of persons with sore throat, a reasonable diagnostic strategy is as follows:

1. Patients with pharyngitis who have a low probability of streptococcal infection (lack of fever, cervical adenopathy, and tonsillar exudate) do not require a throat culture or treatment with antibiotics. The exceptions to this are: persons with a history of rheumatic fever, documented streptococcal exposure in the past week, and residence in a community in which there is a current streptococcal epidemic.

2. Persons with an intermediate probability of streptococcal infection (presence of one or two of the following: fever, cervical adenopathy, or tonsillar exudate) should receive a throat culture. Whether to treat immediately or await culture results is left to the discretion of the clinician.

3. Persons with a high probability of streptococcal pharyngitis (presence of all three of the following: fever, cervical adenopathy, and tonsillar exudate) should be treated immediately with antibiotics. Throat culture is not required for confirmation (Indicators 2 and 4).

4. In young persons, the diagnosis of mononucleosis, especially for pharyngitis of greater than one week's duration (Wood et al., 1980) should also be entertained.

TREATMENT

For documented or presumed group A streptococcus, treatment with penicillin or erythromycin is appropriate. Treatment should be for ten days with penicillin V or erythromycin, or with a single intramuscular injection of 1.2 million units of penicillin B benzathine (Indicator 3) (Perlman and Ginn, 1990; Barker et al., 1991).

FOLLOW-UP

Follow-up cultures are indicated if there is a history of rheumatic fever in the patient or a household contact (Barker et al., 1991).

ACUTE BRONCHITIS

IMPORTANCE

Acute bronchitis is an inflammatory disorder of the tracheobronchial tree that results in acute cough without signs of pneumonia (Billas, 1990). An estimated 12 million physician visits per year are made for acute bronchitis, with annual costs upward of $300 million for physician visits and prescription costs (Billas, 1990).

SCREENING

There are no current recommendations on screening for acute bronchitis in asymptomatic patients.

DIAGNOSIS

The causative organism of acute bronchitis is usually viral, but a variety of bacterial organisms may cause or contribute to bronchitis (e.g., *Streptococcus pneumoniae, Mycoplasma pneumoniae, Chlamydia pneumoniae, B. catarrhalis, and Bordetella pertussis*) (Billas, 1990; Barker et al., 1991). Cough may be nonproductive initially but generally becomes mucopurulent. The duration of cough is two weeks or less. Sputum characteristics are not helpful in distinguishing etiology of cough (Barker et al., 1991). Pharyngitis, fatigue and headache often precede onset of cough. Examination of the chest is usually normal, but may reveal bronchi or rales without any evidence of consolidation

(Indicator 6). A detailed history must be obtained to rule in or out other possible causes for acute cough (Indicator 5). Acute cough is defined as lasting less than three weeks (Pratter et al., 1993). Bronchitis, sinusitis, and the common cold are probably the most common causes of acute cough. Cough secondary to irritants (e.g., tobacco smoke) and allergies (e.g., from allergic rhinitis) are the next most common causes of cough (Zervanos and Shute, 1994). Smokers with acute bronchitis should be encouraged to stop smoking, at least for the duration of the acute illness (Indicator 7) (Barker et al., 1991).

TREATMENT

Most authorities agree that treatment with antibiotics in patients who are otherwise healthy and free of systemic symptoms is not useful (Barker et al., 1991; Billas, 1990). Orr et al.,(1993) conducted a review of all randomized placebo-controlled trials of antibiotics for acute bronchitis published in the English language between 1980 and 1992. Four studies showed no significant benefit of using antibiotics, while two studies (one using erythromycin and the other using trimethoprim sulfa) did show benefit in decrease of subjective symptoms.

FOLLOW-UP

There are no clear indications for routine follow-up of acute bronchitis.

INFLUENZA

IMPORTANCE

Data from the 1993 NHIS indicated that there were approximately 133 million episodes of influenza-like illness annually in the United States, with an attack rate of 52.2 episodes per 100 persons per year (Benson and Marano, 1994). Most influenza symptoms are cause by influenza A virus, which is dispersed by sneezing, coughing, or talking. While generally a self-limited disease, pandemics of influenza have caused heavy death tolls (Wiselka, 1994). Influenza causes between

10,000 and 20,000 deaths in the United States annually, especially among
the elderly and those with chronic medical conditions (Fiebach and
Beckett, 1994). In addition, influenza can cause complications such as
pneumonitis, secondary pneumonia, Reye's syndrome, myositis and
myoglobinuria, myocarditis, and neurologic sequelae (Wiselka, 1994;
Barker et al., 1991).

SCREENING

There are no current recommendations on screening for influenza in
asymptomatic patients.

DIAGNOSIS

Uncomplicated influenza has an abrupt onset of systemic symptoms
including fever, chills, headache and myalgias. The fever generally
persists three to four days, but may persist up to seven days.
Respiratory symptoms (e.g., cough, hoarseness, nasal discharge,
pharyngitis) begin when systemic symptoms begin to resolve. Physical
findings include toxic appearance, cervical lymphadenopathy, hot skin,
watery eyes and, rarely, localized chest findings (e.g., rales).

TREATMENT

Treatment for uncomplicated influenza is generally symptomatic,
with rest, fluid intake, and aspirin or acetaminophen. Dyspnea,
hemoptysis, wheezing, purulent sputum, fever persisting more than seven
days, severe muscle pain, and dark urine, may indicate onset of
influenza complications (Barker et al., 1991). Amantadine has been
shown to decrease virus shedding and shorten duration of influenza
symptoms if treatment was started within 48 hours of symptom onset.
Common side-effects include headache, light headedness, dizziness and
insomnia. Amantadine should be considered for use in patients at high
risk who develop symptoms of a flu-like illness during an influenza
outbreak (Delker et al., 1980).[2] According to a 1979 National Institutes
of Health (NIH) consensus development conference, adults who should be

---

[2]Rimantadine is also an appropriate form of treatment.

considered for prophylaxis include those with chronic diseases, those whose activities are vital to community function and who have not been vaccinated, and persons in semi-closed institutional environments (NIH, 1979). However, because decisions about amantadine use are often subjective, amantadine use will not be employed as a quality indicator.

FOLLOW-UP

There are no clear indications for routine follow-up of influenza.

NASAL CONGESTION AND RHINORRHEA

IMPORTANCE

Nasal congestion was the principal reason for over eight million patient visits across all age groups in the United States in 1989 (NCHS, 1992). Nasal congestion may be due to a variety of causes, the principal of these being acute viral infection (i.e., common cold), allergic rhinitis and infectious sinusitis (acute or chronic) (Canadian Rhinitis Symposium, 1994). Other common causes include vasomotor rhinitis and rhinitis medicamentosa. Appropriate treatment rests in making distinctions among these causes. Other less common reasons for rhinitis include atrophic rhinitis and hormonal rhinitis and mechanical/obstructive rhinitis.

The Canadian Rhinitis Symposium convened in January of 1994 to develop a guide for assessing and treating rhinitis (Canadian Rhinitis Symposium, 1994). The guidebook is extensive, but essential elements for diagnosis and treatment are discussed below.

SCREENING

There are no current recommendations on screening for nasal congestion and rhinorrhea in asymptomatic patients.

DIAGNOSIS AND TREATMENT

The following descriptions may serve to differentiate between allergic rhinitis, infectious viral rhinitis (common cold), and sinusitis:

Allergic Rhinitis

Symptoms: Nasal congestion, sneezing, palatal itching, rhinorrhea with or without allergic conjunctivitis. Symptoms are seasonal or perennial and may be triggered by allergens such as pollens, mites, molds, and animal dander.

Physical exam: nasal mucosa is pale or hyperemic; edema with or without watery secretions are frequently present.

Treatment: Treatment of allergic rhinitis should include antihistamines, nasal cromolyn and/or nasal glucocorticoid sprays. Oral decongestants may be used for symptomatic relief. If prescribed, topical nasal decongestants are indicated for short term use only (Indicator 8).

Infectious Viral Rhinitis

Symptoms: Nasal congestion and rhinorrhea. Other symptoms of viral infectious rhinitis include mild malaise, sneezing, scratchy throat, and variable loss of taste and smell. Colds due to rhinoviruses typically last one week, and rarely as long as two weeks (Barker et al., 1991). Symptoms are generally of acute onset, unless chronic sinusitis is present (see below - chronic sinusitis). Symptoms of coexisting acute sinusitis may also be present (see Acute Sinusitis below).

Physical exam: Mucosa hyperemic and edematous with or without purulent secretions; physical exam should include nasal cavity and sinuses (for presence of sinusitis) and ears (for presence of otitis media) (Barker et al., 1991). Sinus tenderness and fever may be present with sinusitis

Treatment: Treatment of infectious viral rhinitis without sinusitis is symptomatic. Use of oral decongestants or short term nasal decongestants is appropriate but not necessary. For coexisting sinusitis, treatment should be with antibiotics in addition to decongestants (see acute sinusitis below)(Indicator 9).

Sinusitis

Symptoms/Physical Exam/Treatment: See discussions below on acute and chronic sinusitis.

FOLLOW-UP

There are no clear indications for routine follow-up of nasal congestion or rhinorrhea.

ACUTE SINUSITIS

IMPORTANCE

According to the 1991 National Ambulatory Medical Care Survey, sinusitis was the eighth most common diagnosis rendered by physicians for office visits in 1991. This translates into 1.7 percent of all visits among children and adults. Patients frequently mentioned symptoms which could be attributable to sinusitis--headache in 1.5 percent of visits and nasal congestion in 1.3 percent of visits. In adults 25 to 44 years of age, sinusitis accounted for 2.3 percent of visits and allergic rhinitis for 2.3 percent.

SCREENING

There are no current recommendations on screening for sinusitis in asymptomatic patients.

DIAGNOSIS

Acute sinusitis is defined as a sinus infection that lasts less than three weeks (Stafford, 1992). Acute sinusitis is a complication in about 0.5 percent of viral upper respiratory tract infections (Barker, 1991). Symptoms that may increase the likelihood of acute sinusitis being present include fever, malaise, cough, nasal congestion, toothache, purulent nasal discharge, little improvement with nasal decongestants, and headache or facial pain exacerbated by bending forward (Williams and Simel, 1993). Transillumination may improve the accuracy of diagnosis for maxillary sinusitis, but its usefulness is operator sensitive (Williams and Simel, 1993).

TREATMENT

Treatment is based on controlling infection and reducing tissue edema. Ten to fourteen days of antibiotics should be instituted for

241

treatment of acute sinusitis, although there is some recent evidence that three days may suffice (Williams et al., 1995; Balfour and Benfield, 1996; and Gehanno and Berche, 1996). Some have even recently questioned the utility of antibiotic therapy in acute sinusitis (van Buchem, 1997). For these reasons, our indicators do not specify a minimum time period for antibiotic treatment of acute sinusitis. In addition to antibiotics, oral or topical decongestants should be used. If a topical nasal decongestant is given, treatment should be limited to no more than four days (Barker et al., 1991; Stafford, 1992) (Indicator 8). Antihistamines, because of their drying action on the nasal mucosa, have no role in the treatment of most patients with acute sinusitis, except when patients also manifest symptoms of allergic rhinitis (thin, watery rhinorrhea, and sneezing) (Stafford, 1992).

FOLLOW-UP

If symptoms fail to improve after seven days, a ten to fourteen day course of therapy with another antibiotic should be prescribed (Stafford, 1992). If symptoms persist after two courses of antibiotics, referral to an otolaryngologist and/or more definitive diagnostic studies (e.g., x-ray, sinus CT, nasal endoscopy) are indicated (Indicator 10)(Stafford, 1992).

CHRONIC SINUSITIS

IMPORTANCE

The discussion for acute sinusitis also applies to chronic sinusitis.

SCREENING

There are no current recommendations on screening for acute sinusitis in asymptomatic patients.

DIAGNOSIS

Sinusitis that has continued for three months or more is considered chronic (Stafford, 1992). Chronic sinusitis appears to result from

episodes of prolonged, repeated, or inadequately treated acute
sinusitis. Chronic sinusitis generally presents with dull ache or
pressure across the midface, which patients characterize as a headache.
The headache may be worse in the morning and with head movement. In
addition, patients may also complain of nasal congestion and thick
pharyngeal secretions, blocked or popping ears, dental pain, chronic
cough, mild facial swelling, and eye pain (Godley, 1992).

Conditions that commonly predispose to chronic sinusitis include
previous acute sinusitis, allergic rhinitis, environmental irritants,
nasal polyposis, and viral infection (Godley, 1992).

Diagnosis rests on history, evaluation by nasal endoscopy, and CT
scanning (Bolger and Kennedy, 1992). In general, if the history is
strongly suggestive of chronic sinusitis, one should treat first with
antibiotics (see below). If medical therapy is unsuccessful or if the
disease recurs repeatedly, referral to an otolaryngologist for
endoscopic examination is indicated (Bolger and Kennedy, 1992).
Endoscopic examination is more specific for chronic sinusitis than is CT
scanning. If endoscopic findings are equivocal, a CT scan may
demonstrate underlying sinus disease. However, a CT is best performed
four to six weeks after optimal medical therapy is instituted to
optimize specificity (Bolger and Kennedy, 1992).

TREATMENT

Medical treatment should be attempted first. First-line therapy
for chronic disease is amoxicillin and clavulonic acid (Augmentin),
three times daily for 21 to 28 days (Bolger and Kennedy, 1992), or
trimethoprim-sulfamethoxazole, cefaclor, cefuroxime, and cefixime
(Godley, 1992) (Indicator 11). Other medications that may be used
include oral decongestants, nasal steroids, and antihistamines for
patients with an allergic component. If a topical nasal decongestant is
prescribed, treatment should be limited to no more than four days
(Indicator 8)(Barker et al., 1991; Stafford, 1992). If medical therapy
is unsuccessful or if the disease recurs without immunological cause,
referral to an otolaryngologist is indicated (Indicator 12)(Bolger and
Kennedy, 1992).

FOLLOW-UP

When medical therapy fails surgical treatment may be considered. Currently, endoscopic surgery is the method of choice (Bolger and Kennedy, 1992). Endoscopic examination and debridement of the operative cavity are required once or twice weekly for four to six weeks to promote healing and prevent stenosis of the sinus ostia. Complications of surgery include CSF rhinorrhea, diplopia, blindness and meningitis. However, the rates of complications are very low among experienced surgeons. In studies reporting success rates of surgery in consecutive patients, up to 93 percent of patients reported substantial symptomatic improvement in a two-year follow-up, and subsequent revision surgery is reported in seven to ten percent (Bolger and Kennedy, 1992). It should be noted that no randomized controlled trials or case-controlled studies for endoscopic surgery have been performed.

REFERENCES

Barker LR, JR Burton, and PD Zieve, Editors. 1991. *Principles of Ambulatory Medicine*, Third ed.Baltimore, MD: Williams and Wilkins.

Benson V and Marano MA. 1994. Current estimates from the National Health Interview Survey, 1993. National Center for Health Statistics. *Vital Health Statistics* 10(190).

Billas A. December 1990. Lower respiratory tract infections. *Primary Care* 17 (4): 811-24.

Bolger WE, and DW Kennedy. 30 September 1992. Changing concepts in chronic sinusitis. *Hospital Practice* 27 (9A): 20-2, 26-8.

Canadian Rhinitis Symposium. 1994. Assessing and treating rhinitis: A practical guide for Canadian physicians. Proceedings of the Canadian Rhinitis Symposium; Toronto, Ontario; January 14-15, 1994. *Canadian Medical Journal* 15 (Suppl. 4): 1-27.

Centers for Disease Control. 27 May 1994. Prevention and control of influenza: Part I, vaccines. *Morbidity and Mortality Weekly Report* 43 (RR-9): 1-13.

Delker LL, L Moser, H Robert et al. 1980. Amantadine: Does it have a role in prevention and treatment of influenza? *Annals of Internal Medicine* 92 (Part 1): 256-8.

Fiebach N, and W Beckett. 28 November 1994. Prevention of respiratory infections in adults: Influenza and pneumococcal vaccines. *Archives of Internal Medicine* 154: 2545-57.

Garibaldi RA. 28 June 1985. Epidemiology of community-acquired respiratory tract infections in adults: Incidence, etiology, and impact. *American Journal of Medicine* 78 (Suppl. 6B): 32-7.

Godley FA. May 1992. Chronic Sinusitis: An Update. *American Family Physician* 45 (5): 2190-9.

Komaroff A, TM Pass, MD Aronson et al.,January 1986. The prediction of streptococcal pharyngitis in adults. *Journal of General Internal Medicine* 1: 1-7.

Little PS, and I Williamson. 15 October 1994. Are antibiotics appropriate for sore throats? *British Medical Journal* 309: 1010-11.

National Center for Health Statistics. December 1994. *Current estimates from the National Health Interview Survey, 1993.* U.S. Department of Health and Human Services, Hyattsville, MD.

National Center for Health Statistics. April 1992. *National Ambulatory Medical Care Survey: 1989 summary*. U.S. Department of Health and Human Services, Hyattsville, MD.

National Center for Health Statistics. 1994. *National Ambulatory Medical Care Survey: 1991 summary*. U.S. Department of Health and Human Services, Hyattsville, MD.

National Center for Health Statistics. February 1993. *Prevalence of selected chronic conditions: United States, 1986-88*. U.S. Department of Health and Human Services, Hyattsville, MD.

National Institutes of Health Consensus Development Conference Summaries. *Amantadine: Does it have a role in the prevention and treatment of influenza?*, 51-6. Sponsored by the National Institute of Allergy and Infectious Diseases, October 15-16, 1979.

Orr PH, K Scherer, A Macdonald et al., 1993. Randomized placebo-controlled trials of antibiotics for acute bronchitis: A critical review of the literature. *Journal of Family Practice* 36 (5): 507-12.

Panzer RJ, ER Black, and PF Griner, Editors. 1991. *Diagnostic Strategies for Common Medical Problems*.Philadelphia, PA: American College of Physicians.

Perlman PE, and DR Ginn. January 1990. Respiratory infections in ambulatory adults: Choosing the best treatment. *Postgraduate Medicine* 87 (1): 175-84.

Pratter MR, T Bartter, S Akers et al., 15 November 1993. An algorithmic approach to chronic cough. *Annals of Internal Medicine* 119 (10): 977-83.

Shvartzman P. 15 October 1994. Careful prescribing is beneficial. *British Medical Journal* 309: 1011-12.

Stafford CT. November 1990. The clinician's view of sinusitis. *Otolaryngology-Head and Neck Surgery* 103 (Volume 5, Part 2): 870-5.

Williams JW, DR Holleman Jr., GP Samsa et al.,5 April 1995. Randomized controlled trial of 3 vs 10 days of trimethoprim/sulfamethoxazole for acute maxillary sinusitis. *Journal of the American Medical Association* 273 (13): 1015-21.

Williams JW, and DL Simel. 8 September 1993. Does this patient have sinusitis? Diagnosing acute sinusitis by history and physical examination. *Journal of the American Medical Association* 270 (10): 1242-6.

Wiselka M. 21 May 1994. Influenza: Diagnosis, management, and prophylaxis. *British Medical Journal* 308: 1341-5.

Wood RW, RK Tompkins, and BW Wolcott. November 1980. An efficient strategy for managing acute respiratory illness in adults. *Annals of Internal Medicine* 93 (5): 757-63.

Zervanos NJ, and KM Shute. March 1994. Acute, disruptive cough: Symptomatic therapy for a nagging problem. *Postgraduate Medicine* 95 (4): 153-68.

RECOMMENDED QUALITY INDICATORS FOR UPPER RESPIRATORY INFECTIONS

These indicators apply to men and women age 18 and older. These indicators were endorsed by a prior panel and reviewed but not rated by the current panel.

Pharyngitis

Indicator	Quality of Evidence	Literature	Benefits	Comments
Diagnosis				

1. For patient who present with a complaint of sore throat, a history/physical exam should document presence or absence of:
   a. fever;
   b. tonsillar exudate, and
   c. anterior cervical adenopathy.
	II	Komaroff, 1986	Alleviate sore throat. Prevent rheumatic heart disease. Prevent rheumatic fever.	If all three are present, the probability of streptococcal infections is greater than 40% and one would be inclined to treat empirically without culture.

Treatment				
2. Patients with sore throat and fever, tonsillar exudate and anterior cervical adenopathy should receive immediate treatment for presumed streptococcal infection.	II	Komaroff, 1986; Panzer, 1991	Decrease sore throat. Prevent rheumatic fever.	Since throat cultures and rapid antigen tests vary in their sensitivity and specificity, this combination of symptoms is sufficient to warrant antibiotic treatment without further laboratory testing.
3. Treatment of streptococcal throat infection should be with penicillin V, amoxicillin, or erythromycin for 10 days; or with a single injection of benzathine penicillin.	III	Barker et al., 1991	Decrease sore throat. Prevent rheumatic fever.	This is the current standard of care, although other antibiotics (e.g., ampicillin) are also effective.

4. If an antibiotic is NOT prescribed with the diagnosis of sore throat, a throat culture or rapid antigen test should be obtained if any of the following are present:
   a. fever;
   b. tonsillar exudate, and
   c. anterior cervical adenopathy.
	II	Komaroff, 1986	Prevent rheumatic fever.	Each finding increases the probability of streptococcal infection.

248

Bronchitis, Acute

Indicator	Quality of Evidence	Literature	Benefits	Comments
Diagnosis				
5. The history of patients presenting with cough of less than 3 weeks' duration should document presence or absence of fever and shortness of breath (dyspnea).	III	Barker et al., 1991	Decrease cough. Decrease shortness of breath. Prevent development of emphysema. Prevent development of sepsis.	These symptoms are consistent with possible pneumonia, which would require antibiotic treatment.
6. Patients presenting with acute cough should receive a physical examination of the chest for evidence of pneumonia.	III	Barker et al., 1991	Decrease cough. Decrease shortness of breath. Prevent development of emphysema. Prevent development of sepsis.	Signs of consolidation would lead one on a different diagnostic and treatment path.
Treatment				
7. If the history documents cigarette smoking in a patient with acute cough, encouragement to stop smoking should be documented.	III	Barker et al., 1991	Prevent future bronchitic episodes. Prevent smoking-related morbidity and mortality.	Smokers are predisposed to bronchitis. Symptomatic patients present a window of opportunity to counsel regarding smoking cessation.

Nasal Congestion

Indicator	Quality of Evidence	Literature	Benefits	Comments
Treatment				
8. If topical nasal decongestants are prescribed, duration of treatment should be for no longer than 4 days.	III	Stafford et al., 1992; Barker et al., 1991	Prevent rhinitis medicamentosa.	Long-term treatment with topical decongestants can cause rebound congestion (rhinitis medicamentosa).
9. Patients with nasal congestion and/or cough without a concurrent diagnosis of sinusitis, bronchitis, or pneumonia should not be prescribed antibiotics.	III	Stafford et al., 1992; Barker et al., 1991	May prevent emergence of antibiotic-resistant bacteria.	Expert panelists felt that antibiotics should not be prescribed without documentation of need, due to the increase in antibiotic-resistant bacteria.

249

Acute Sinusitis

Treatment

Indicator	Quality of Evidence	Literature	Benefits	Comments
10. If a patient with acute sinusitis does not improve after two courses of antibiotics, referral to an otolaryngologist or for a diagnostic test (CT, x-ray, ultrasound of the sinuses) is indicated.	III	Stafford et al., 1992	Decrease nasal congestion. Prevent development of chronic sinusitis.	Reevaluation of diagnosis and/or surgical treatment may be indicated.

Chronic Sinusitis

Treatment

Indicator	Quality of Evidence	Literature	Benefits	Comments
11. If a diagnosis of chronic sinusitis is made, the patient should be treated with at least 3 weeks of antibiotics.	III	Stafford et al., 1992	Decrease nasal congestion and other symptoms of chronic sinusitis.[1] Prevent recurrence of sinusitis.	It is generally agreed that a longer duration of treatment for chronic sinusitis is necessary than for acute sinusitis. However, the exact number of days has not been defined in RCTs. The literature cites 3 weeks as the standard of care.
12. If patient with chronic sinusitis has repeated symptoms after 2 separate 3 week trials of antibiotics, a referral to an otolaryngologist or for a diagnostic test (CT, x-ray, ultrasound of the sinuses) is indicated.	III	Bolger and Kennedy, 1992	Decrease nasal congestion and other symptoms of chronic sinusitis.[1] Prevent recurrence of sinusitis.	While medical treatment is still first-line therapy, surgical treatment may be indicated if two course of antibiotics fail to relieve symptoms.

Definitions and Examples

[1] Symptoms of chronic sinusitis include nasal congestions, fever, headache, facial pain, toothache, rhinorrhea, and purulent nasal discharge.

Quality of Evidence Codes

I	RCT
II-1	Nonrandomized controlled trials
II-2	Cohort or case analysis
II-3	Multiple time series
III	Opinions or descriptive studies

APPENDIX A: PANEL RATING SHEETS BY CONDITION

NOTE: This chapter has been revised from
Q1. Only new or revised indicators are being
rated.

DIAGNOSIS

3. Spirometry should be measured in patients
with moderate to severe asthma at least every
2 years.

```
1      3 2 2 1                  1       3 3 2
1 2 3 4 5 6 7 8 9   1 2 3 4 5 6 7 8 9   ( 1- 2)
   (5.0, 1.2, A)        (8.0, 1.0, A)
```

TREATMENT

7. Patients requiring chronic treatment with
systemic corticosteroids during any 12 month
period should have been prescribed inhaled
corticosteroids during the same 12 month
period.

```
          7 1 1                  1 6 2
1 2 3 4 5 6 7 8 9   1 2 3 4 5 6 7 8 9   ( 3- 4)
   (7.0, 0.3, A)        (8.0, 0.3, A)
```

10. All patients seen for an acute asthma
exacerbation should be evaluated with a
complete history including all of the
following:

a. time since onset of symptoms

```
1 4   2 1   1      1     2 1 2 1 1 1
1 2 3 4 5 6 7 8 9   1 2 3 4 5 6 7 8 9   ( 5- 6)
   (3.0, 1.4, I)        (6.0, 1.8, I)
```

b. all current medications

```
          3 2 4                  3 3 3
1 2 3 4 5 6 7 8 9   1 2 3 4 5 6 7 8 9   ( 7- 8)
   (8.0, 0.8, A)        (8.0, 0.7, A)
```

c. prior hospitalizations and emergency
department visits for asthma

```
          4 4 1                  4 3 2
1 2 3 4 5 6 7 8 9   1 2 3 4 5 6 7 8 9   ( 9- 10)
   (8.0, 0.6, A)        (8.0, 0.7, A)
```

d. prior episodes of respiratory
failure requiring intubation

```
            6 3                1 3 2 3
1 2 3 4 5 6 7 8 9   1 2 3 4 5 6 7 8 9   ( 11- 12)
   (8.0, 0.3, A)        (8.0, 0.9, A)
```

INDICATORS ADDED AFTER ROUND 1

25. Asthmatic patients newly prescribed
inhaled bronchodilaters should be
concurrently given either a spacer device or
instructions in proper use of an MDI.

```
          4 3 2                1 1 4 3
1 2 3 4 5 6 7 8 9   1 2 3 4 5 6 7 8 9   ( 13- 14)
   (8.0, 0.7, A)        (8.0, 0.7, A)
```

26. Patients with a new diagnosis of asthma
should have documentation of counseling for
self-management of asthma within one month of
diagnosis.

```
1 2         1 2 2 1   1   1   1 1 4 1
1 2 3 4 5 6 7 8 9   1 2 3 4 5 6 7 8 9   ( 15- 16)
   (7.0, 2.3, D)        (7.0, 1.6, D)
```

27. Patients who present with an
exacerbation of asthma should have
documentation of counseling for
self-management:

a. prior to discharge if hospitalized

```
2 2 1 1 1 1   1   2   1   1 2 2 1
1 2 3 4 5 6 7 8 9   1 2 3 4 5 6 7 8 9   ( 17- 18)
   (3.0, 1.9, I)        (6.0, 2.0, D)
```

b. at the time of presentation if not
hospitalized

```
2 2 1 1   1 1 1   2   1   1 2 2 1
1 2 3 4 5 6 7 8 9   1 2 3 4 5 6 7 8 9   ( 19- 20)
   (3.0, 2.1, D)        (6.0, 2.0, D)
```

Scales: 1 = low validity or feasibility; 9 = high validity or feasibility

DIAGNOSIS

1. Patients presenting with new-onset atrial fibrillation or atrial fibrillation of unknown duration should have documentation of the following in the medical record at the time of presentation:

    a. alcohol use

```
                  4 3 2              1 3 1 4
        1 2 3 4 5 6 7 8 9  1 2 3 4 5 6 7 8 9  ( 1- 2)
          (8.0, 0.7, A)      (8.0, 1.0, A)
                  4 3 2                1 3 1 4
```

    b. stimulant drug use

```
        1 2 3 4 5 6 7 8 9  1 2 3 4 5 6 7 8 9  ( 3- 4)
          (8.0, 0.7, A)      (8.0, 1.0, A)
```

2. Patients presenting with new-onset atrial fibrillation or atrial fibrillation of unknown duration should have thyroid function checked within the first two weeks of presentation.

```
                  2 4 3                2 2 5
        1 2 3 4 5 6 7 8 9  1 2 3 4 5 6 7 8 9  ( 5- 6)
          (8.0, 0.6, A)      (9.0, 0.7, A)
```

3. Patients presenting with new-onset atrial fibrillation or atrial fibrillation of unknown duration should have a chest radiograph performed within one week after presentation.

```
        2   1 1   1 4      1     1   1 1 3 2
        1 2 3 4 5 6 7 8 9  1 2 3 4 5 6 7 8 9  ( 7- 8)
          (6.0, 2.1, D)      (8.0, 1.8, I)
```

TREATMENT

4. Patients with atrial fibrillation of greater than 48 hours duration or of unknown duration who do not have contraindications to warfarin should receive warfarin if they are:

    a. under 65 with one or more other risk factors for stroke

```
                  1 2 6                1 4 4
        1 2 3 4 5 6 7 8 9  1 2 3 4 5 6 7 8 9  ( 9-10)
          (9.0, 0.4, A)      (8.0, 0.6, A)
                  1 4 4                1 3 5
```

    b. 65 years of age or older

```
        1 2 3 4 5 6 7 8 9  1 2 3 4 5 6 7 8 9  (11-12)
          (8.0, 0.6, A)      (9.0, 0.6, A)
```

5. Patients with chronic atrial fibrillation who have contraindications to warfarin or have declined warfarin therapy should receive aspirin if they are:

    a. under 65 with one or more other risk factors for stroke

```
                    3 6                2 3 4
        1 2 3 4 5 6 7 8 9  1 2 3 4 5 6 7 8 9  (13-14)
          (9.0, 0.3, A)      (8.0, 0.7, A)
                  2 4 3                1 3 5
```

    b. age 65 years or older

```
        1 2 3 4 5 6 7 8 9  1 2 3 4 5 6 7 8 9  (15-16)
          (8.0, 0.6, A)      (9.0, 0.6, A)
```

6a. Patients with atrial fibrillation who do not have contraindications to warfarin should be started on warfarin within two weeks of presenting with new onset ischemic or embolic stroke.

```
                  1 2 6                  5 4
        1 2 3 4 5 6 7 8 9  1 2 3 4 5 6 7 8 9  (17-18)
          (9.0, 0.4, A)      (8.0, 0.4, A)
```

6b. Patients with atrial fibrillation who do not have contraindications to warfarin should be started on warfarin within one week of presenting with new onset transient ischemic attack.

```
                    3 6                2 3 4
        1 2 3 4 5 6 7 8 9  1 2 3 4 5 6 7 8 9  (19-20)
          (9.0, 0.3, A)      (8.0, 0.7, A)
```

Scales: 1 = low validity or feasibility; 9 = high validity or feasibility

TREATMENT, CONT.

7. Patients with atrial fibrillation of
greater than 48 hours duration or of unknown
duration who are undergoing elective
electrical or chemical cardioversion should
receive anticoagulation for at least 3 weeks
prior to cardioversion unless they have had
a TEE within 24 hours of cardioversion that
indicates no clot.

```
                                    2 4 3                   2 3 4
                          1 2 3 4 5 6 7 8 9   1 2 3 4 5 6 7 8 9   ( 21- 22)
                            (8.0, 0.6, A)       (8.0, 0.7, A)
```

8. All patients with atrial fibrillation of
greater than 48 hours or of unknown duration
should receive anticoagulation for at least 4
weeks after cardioversion unless there are
contraindications to anticoagulation.

```
                                    2 5 2                   2 5 2
                          1 2 3 4 5 6 7 8 9   1 2 3 4 5 6 7 8 9   ( 23- 24)
                            (8.0, 0.4, A)       (8.0, 0.4, A)
```

FOLLOW-UP

9. Patients with atrial fibrillation started
on warfarin should have an INR checked within
1 week of the first dose.

```
                                    3 2 4                 1 1 3 4
                          1 2 3 4 5 6 7 8 9   1 2 3 4 5 6 7 8 9   ( 25- 26)
                            (8.0, 0.8, A)       (8.0, 0.8, A)
```

10. Patients on warfarin should have an INR
checked a minimum of every three months.

```
                              1       5 1 2               2 2 5
                          1 2 3 4 5 6 7 8 9   1 2 3 4 5 6 7 8 9   ( 27- 28)
                            (7.0, 1.0, A)       (9.0, 0.7, A)
```

Scales: 1 = low validity or feasibility; 9 = high validity or feasibility

DIAGNOSIS

1. Patients who receive thrombolytic therapy for treatment of acute stroke should receive a head CT or MRI after presenting with stroke and before initiation of thrombolytic treatment.

```
1   2 1     2 1 2 1   1       3 4
1 2 3 4 5 6 7 8 9   1 2 3 4 5 6 7 8 9   ( 1- 2)
   (7.0, 2.4, D)        (8.0, 1.7, A)
```

2. Patients who receive anticoagulant or antiplatelet therapy for treatment of acute stroke within 7 days of presentation should receive a head CT or MRI prior to the initiation of anticoagulant or antiplatelet treatment.

```
        1 1 3 1 3                 4 5
1 2 3 4 5 6 7 8 9   1 2 3 4 5 6 7 8 9   ( 3- 4)
   (7.0, 1.1, A)        (9.0, 0.4, A)
```

TREATMENT

3. Patients newly diagnosed with a stroke or TIA without a known cardiac source should be started on antiplatelet therapy within 1 week of the diagnosis unless a contraindication is documented.

```
            3 6               2 2 5
1 2 3 4 5 6 7 8 9   1 2 3 4 5 6 7 8 9   ( 5- 6)
   (9.0, 0.3, A)        (9.0, 0.7, A)
```

4. Patients with a documented history of stroke or TIA without a known cardiac source should be on daily antiplatelet treatment, unless a contraindication is documented.

```
          1 2   6           1 3   5
1 2 3 4 5 6 7 8 9   1 2 3 4 5 6 7 8 9   ( 7- 8)
   (9.0, 0.8, A)        (9.0, 1.0, A)
```

5. Patients presenting for care with carotid artery symptoms who are diagnosed with TIA or stroke should have a carotid artery imaging study within 6 months before or 1 month after the event, unless the medical record documents, in the same time period, that the patient is not a candidate for carotid surgery.

```
          2 5 2             2   4 3
1 2 3 4 5 6 7 8 9   1 2 3 4 5 6 7 8 9   ( 9- 10)
   (8.0, 0.4, A)        (8.0, 0.8, A)
```

6. Patients presenting for care with carotid artery symptoms, who are diagnosed with TIA and have carotid imaging evidence of >=70% stenosis on the side corresponding to the symptoms, should receive revascularization within 6 weeks of the diagnostic study unless there are contraindications.

```
        1 2 2 4             3 4 2
1 2 3 4 5 6 7 8 9   1 2 3 4 5 6 7 8 9   ( 11- 12)
   (8.0, 0.9, A)        (8.0, 0.6, A)
```

FOLLOW-UP

7. Patients who smoke and present with TIA or stroke but are not hospitalized should be counseled to stop smoking at the time they present with TIA or stroke.

```
          2 1 6             3   6
1 2 3 4 5 6 7 8 9   1 2 3 4 5 6 7 8 9   ( 13- 14)
   (9.0, 0.6, A)        (9.0, 0.7, A)
```

8. Patients who smoke and are admitted to the hospital with a TIA or stroke should be counseled to stop smoking before hospital discharge.

```
          2 1 6             2 1 6
1 2 3 4 5 6 7 8 9   1 2 3 4 5 6 7 8 9   ( 15- 16)
   (9.0, 0.6, A)        (9.0, 0.6, A)
```

Scales: 1 = low validity or feasibility; 9 = high validity or feasibility

INDICATORS ADDED AFTER ROUND 1

9.   Patients admitted with a newly diagnosed
stroke should have an assessment of the
following prior to discharge:

```
                                         1 2 2 4            3   6
    a. functional status       1 2 3 4 5 6 7 8 9  1 2 3 4 5 6 7 8 9  ( 17- 18)
                                  (8.0, 0.9, A)      (9.0, 0.7, A)
                                         1  2 1 1 4        1 1   1   6
    b. swallowing              1 2 3 4 5 6 7 8 9  1 2 3 4 5 6 7 8 9  ( 19- 20)
                                  (8.0, 1.4, I)      (9.0, 1.2, A)
```

10. Patients presenting with a new diagnosis
of stroke or TIA should have a neurological
examination at the time of presentation.

```
                                      1   1 3 4      1         2 6
                              1 2 3 4 5 6 7 8 9  1 2 3 4 5 6 7 8 9  ( 21- 22)
                                  (8.0, 0.9, A)      (9.0, 0.9, A)
```

Scales: 1 = low validity or feasibility; 9 = high validity or feasibility

DIAGNOSIS

1. A smoking history should be documented on the same day in patients who present with a new complaint of any of the following:

a. chronic cough (> 3 weeks duration)

```
          1 3 5                   2 1 6
1 2 3 4 5 6 7 8 9   1 2 3 4 5 6 7 8 9   ( 1- 2)
   (9.0, 0.6, A)       (9.0, 0.6, A)
```

b. shortness of breath

```
          1 3 5                   2 1 6
1 2 3 4 5 6 7 8 9   1 2 3 4 5 6 7 8 9   ( 3- 4)
   (9.0, 0.6, A)       (9.0, 0.6, A)
```

c. dyspnea on exertion

```
          1 4 4                   2 2 5
1 2 3 4 5 6 7 8 9   1 2 3 4 5 6 7 8 9   ( 5- 6)
   (8.0, 0.6, A)       (9.0, 0.7, A)
```

2. A lung exam should be documented on the same day in patients who present with a new complaint of any of the following:

a. chronic cough (> 3 weeks duration)

```
            4 5                 1 2 6
1 2 3 4 5 6 7 8 9   1 2 3 4 5 6 7 8 9   ( 7- 8)
   (9.0, 0.4, A)       (9.0, 0.4, A)
```

b. shortness of breath

```
            3 6                 1 2 6
1 2 3 4 5 6 7 8 9   1 2 3 4 5 6 7 8 9   ( 9- 10)
   (9.0, 0.3, A)       (9.0, 0.4, A)
```

c. dyspnea on exertion

```
            5 4                 1 2 6
1 2 3 4 5 6 7 8 9   1 2 3 4 5 6 7 8 9   ( 11- 12)
   (8.0, 0.4, A)       (9.0, 0.4, A)
```

3. COPD patients on bronchodilator therapy who have not had spirometry in the previous 12 months should have spirometry performed within 3 months after initiation of therapy.

```
          1 3 3 2               1   4 4
1 2 3 4 5 6 7 8 9   1 2 3 4 5 6 7 8 9   ( 13- 14)
   (7.0, 0.8, I)       (7.0, 0.7, A)
```

4. COPD patients on bronchodilator therapy should have one of the following tests within 6 months before or after initiation of therapy:

  - Hemoglobin
  - hematocrit
  - CBC
  - ABG
  - pulse oximetry.

```
3         1 3 2     2           2 2 2 1
1 2 3 4 5 6 7 8 9   1 2 3 4 5 6 7 8 9   ( 15- 16)
   (6.0, 2.0, D)       (7.0, 2.0, D)
```

5. COPD patients should have an ABG or pulse oximetry performed within 3 months of any of the following findings, unless hypoxemia ($PaO_2 < 55$) has been previously documented or the patient is already on chronic oxygen therapy:

a. laboratory detection of erythrocytosis (Hct >55)

```
          3 4 2                 1 4 4
1 2 3 4 5 6 7 8 9   1 2 3 4 5 6 7 8 9   ( 17- 18)
   (8.0, 0.6, A)       (8.0, 0.6, A)
```

b. notation of cyanosis or cor pulmonale in the medical record

```
          1 2 4 2               2 4 3
1 2 3 4 5 6 7 8 9   1 2 3 4 5 6 7 8 9   ( 19- 20)
   (8.0, 0.7, A)       (8.0, 0.6, A)
```

c. detection of FEV1 < 1 liter on spirometric evaluation.

```
          5 2 2                 2 3 4
1 2 3 4 5 6 7 8 9   1 2 3 4 5 6 7 8 9   ( 21- 22)
   (7.0, 0.7, A)       (8.0, 0.7, A)
```

Scales: 1 = low validity or feasibility; 9 = high validity or feasibility

TREATMENT

6. Newly diagnosed COPD patients who smoke should be counseled or referred for smoking cessation within 3 months before or after the new diagnosis of COPD.

```
            3 6                  2 1 6
1 2 3 4 5 6 7 8 9    1 2 3 4 5 6 7 8 9   ( 23- 24)
  (9.0, 0.3, A)        (9.0, 0.6, A)
```

7. All patients receiving regular bronchodilator treatment for COPD symptoms should be receiving ipratopium, unless intolerance is documented.

```
          1 3 3 2                3 4 2
1 2 3 4 5 6 7 8 9    1 2 3 4 5 6 7 8 9   ( 25- 26)
  (8.0, 0.8, A)        (8.0, 0.6, A)
```

8. Patients newly prescribed inhaled bronchodilaters should be concurrently given either a spacer device or instructions in proper use of an MDI.

```
          1 2 2 4            1   1 2 1 4
1 2 3 4 5 6 7 8 9    1 2 3 4 5 6 7 8 9   ( 27- 28)
  (8.0, 0.9, A)        (8.0, 1.3, A)
```

9. COPD patients should have a theophylline level checked within 1 week of either initiation or increase of theophylline dose.

```
          1 4 1 3              1 3 1 4
1 2 3 4 5 6 7 8 9    1 2 3 4 5 6 7 8 9   ( 29- 30)
  (7.0, 0.9, A)        (8.0, 1.0, A)
```

10. In patients receiving theophylline, both of the following should occur when serum theophylline level exceeds 20 ug/ml:

   a. The dose should be modified within 1 day of the measurement

```
          2 1 3 3          1   2 1 4 1
1 2 3 4 5 6 7 8 9    1 2 3 4 5 6 7 8 9   ( 31- 32)
  (8.0, 0.9, A)        (8.0, 1.2, I)
```

   b. Retesting of level should be performed within one week, unless theophylline was stopped.

```
          2 2 2 3              2 2 3 2
1 2 3 4 5 6 7 8 9    1 2 3 4 5 6 7 8 9   ( 33- 34)
  (8.0, 1.0, A)        (8.0, 0.9, A)
```

11. COPD patients should receive home oxygen if their baseline room air oxygen saturation is <88% at rest (not during an exacerbation).

```
            3 6                1 4 4
1 2 3 4 5 6 7 8 9    1 2 3 4 5 6 7 8 9   ( 35- 36)
  (9.0, 0.3, A)        (8.0, 0.6, A)
```

12. The following items should be documented in the medical record at the time of a COPD exacerbation:

   a. Outpatient COPD medications

```
          2 4 3            1 1 3 4
1 2 3 4 5 6 7 8 9    1 2 3 4 5 6 7 8 9   ( 37- 38)
  (8.0, 0.6, A)        (8.0, 0.8, A)
```

   b. Information on prior hospitalizations, urgent care, or ED visits for COPD (e.g., time of most recent visit or number per year)

```
          5 1 3            1 1 3   4
1 2 3 4 5 6 7 8 9    1 2 3 4 5 6 7 8 9   ( 39- 40)
  (7.0, 0.8, A)        (7.0, 1.2, A)
```

   c. Presence or absence of new cough

```
          2 1 2 4              2 2   5
1 2 3 4 5 6 7 8 9    1 2 3 4 5 6 7 8 9   ( 41- 42)
  (8.0, 1.0, A)        (9.0, 1.1, A)
```

   d. Vital signs, including respiratory rate, pulse, temperature, and blood pressure

```
            2 2 5              1 3 5
1 2 3 4 5 6 7 8 9    1 2 3 4 5 6 7 8 9   ( 43- 44)
  (9.0, 0.7, A)        (9.0, 0.6, A)
```

   e. A physical examination of the chest

```
            2 2 5                2 7
1 2 3 4 5 6 7 8 9    1 2 3 4 5 6 7 8 9   ( 45- 46)
  (9.0, 0.7, A)        (9.0, 0.2, A)
```

Scales: 1 = low validity or feasibility; 9 = high validity or feasibility

TREATMENT, CONT.

13. Patients admitted to the hospital for an exacerbation of COPD who have a history of coronary disease should have an EKG performed within 24 hours of admission.

```
            1 1 3 1 3                   6 3
1 2 3 4 5 6 7 8 9   1 2 3 4 5 6 7 8 9   ( 47- 48)
   (7.0, 1.1, A)        (8.0, 0.3, A)
```

14. A theophylline level should be obtained for patients on theophylline who meet any of the following conditions:

a. Present with an exacerbation of COPD

```
            1 2 5 1                   2 5 2
1 2 3 4 5 6 7 8 9   1 2 3 4 5 6 7 8 9   ( 49- 50)
   (8.0, 0.6, A)        (8.0, 0.4, A)
```

b. Are hospitalized with an exacerbation of COPD.

```
            1 1 4 3                   1 5 3
1 2 3 4 5 6 7 8 9   1 2 3 4 5 6 7 8 9   ( 51- 52)
   (8.0, 0.7, A)        (8.0, 0.4, A)
```

15. COPD patients who present with an exacerbation should receive inhaled bronchodilator therapy if their respiratory rate is >24.

```
1 1   2 1 1 2 1     1   1 1 1 2   2 1
1 2 3 4 5 6 7 8 9   1 2 3 4 5 6 7 8 9   ( 53- 54)
   (5.0, 1.9, D)        (6.0, 2.0, D)
```

16. Patients presenting with COPD exacerbation should have oxygen administered if the oxygen saturation is <88% or PO2 is <55 mm Hg.

```
            2 2 5               1 1 2 5
1 2 3 4 5 6 7 8 9   1 2 3 4 5 6 7 8 9   ( 55- 56)
   (9.0, 0.7, A)        (9.0, 0.8, A)
```

17. Patients presenting with COPD exacerbation should be admitted to the hospital if any of the following conditions are documented in the medical record on the date of presentation:

a. Acute Ischemia

```
            2 2 5           1   3 1 4
1 2 3 4 5 6 7 8 9   1 2 3 4 5 6 7 8 9   ( 57- 58)
   (9.0, 0.7, A)        (8.0, 1.1, A)
```

b. Pneumonia

```
1   1   3 3   1 1     1   3 1 3
1 2 3 4 5 6 7 8 9   1 2 3 4 5 6 7 8 9   ( 59- 60)
   (6.0, 1.4, I)        (7.0, 1.8, A)
```

c. Significant hypoxemia (saturation <88%, or PaO2 <55 mm Hg on room air in patients not on home oxygen).

```
2   2       4 1     1   1       4 2 1
1 2 3 4 5 6 7 8 9   1 2 3 4 5 6 7 8 9   ( 61- 62)
   (7.0, 2.3, D)        (7.0, 1.6, D)
```

18. Patients hospitalized with a COPD exacerbation should be admitted to a critical care bed while any of the following are present:

a. Severe dyspnea (breathing rate > 35 with accessory muscle use) despite initial therapeutic measures

```
1     1   1 4 1 1       2   1 1 2 1 2
1 2 3 4 5 6 7 8 9   1 2 3 4 5 6 7 8 9   ( 63- 64)
   (7.0, 1.4, I)        (7.0, 1.8, D)
```

b. Confusion or lethargy

```
            2 3 1 3               1 3 1 4
1 2 3 4 5 6 7 8 9   1 2 3 4 5 6 7 8 9   ( 65- 66)
   (7.0, 1.0, A)        (8.0, 1.0, A)
```

c. Severe hypoxemia (pO2 < 60 with FiO2 > 40%)

```
            1 5 3                   6 3
1 2 3 4 5 6 7 8 9   1 2 3 4 5 6 7 8 9   ( 67- 68)
   (8.0, 0.4, A)        (8.0, 0.3, A)
```

d. Severe respiratory acidosis (pH < 7.3)

```
            1 5 3                 1 3 5
1 2 3 4 5 6 7 8 9   1 2 3 4 5 6 7 8 9   ( 69- 70)
   (8.0, 0.4, A)        (9.0, 0.6, A)
```

Scales: 1 = low validity or feasibility; 9 = high validity or feasibility

TREATMENT, CONT.

19. COPD patients hospitalized for an
exacerbation should be discharged on home
oxygen if the last documented oxygen
saturation prior to discharge is <88%.

```
                    3 1 1 4              2 1 1 5
        1 2 3 4 5 6 7 8 9   1 2 3 4 5 6 7 8 9   ( 71- 72)
            (8.0, 1.2, I)       (9.0, 1.0, A)
```

20. Patients with a diagnosis of COPD who
present with a COPD exacerbation and whose
last documented oxygen saturation during the
exacerbation visit is < 88% or pO2 is <55
should either be hospitalized or discharged
on home oxygen treatment.

```
                  1   6 2                2 3 2 2
        1 2 3 4 5 6 7 8 9   1 2 3 4 5 6 7 8 9   ( 73- 74)
            (7.0, 0.4, A)       (7.0, 0.9, A)
```

INDICATORS ADDED AFTER ROUND 1

21. Asymptomatic smokers should receive
spirometry within one year of notation of 40
or more pack/years of cigarette use.

```
        2 2 1 2 1   1     1       1 1 4 2
        1 2 3 4 5 6 7 8 9   1 2 3 4 5 6 7 8 9   ( 75- 76)
            (3.0, 1.6, I)       (7.0, 1.2, I)
```

Scales: 1 = low validity or feasibility; 9 = high validity or feasibility

NOTE: This chapter has been revised from
Q1. Only new or revised indicators are being
rated.

SCREENING

2. Patients documented to be smokers should
have their smoking status indicated on more
than 50% of all office visits.

```
                                 4 2 3                  4   5
                    1 2 3 4 5 6 7 8 9  1 2 3 4 5 6 7 8 9  ( 1- 2)
                      (8.0, 0.8, A)      (9.0, 0.9, A)
```

TREATMENT

4. All smokers identified as attempting to
quit should be offered at least one
additional smoking cessation counseling visit
within 3 months.

```
                                 4 3 2              1 3 2 3
                    1 2 3 4 5 6 7 8 9  1 2 3 4 5 6 7 8 9  ( 3- 4)
                      (8.0, 0.7, A)      (8.0, 0.9, A)
```

5. All smokers attempting to quit who smoke
more than 10 cigarettes a day should be
offered nicotine replacement therapy except
in the presence of serious medical
precautions.

```
                               1 5 3              1 4 2 2
                    1 2 3 4 5 6 7 8 9  1 2 3 4 5 6 7 8 9  ( 5- 6)
                      (7.0, 0.4, A)      (7.0, 0.8, A)
```

FOLLOW-UP

6. All patients who receive a smoking
cessation intervention should have their
abstinence status documented within 4 weeks
of the completion of treatment.

```
                             1 1 4 1 2          2    3 2   2
                    1 2 3 4 5 6 7 8 9  1 2 3 4 5 6 7 8 9  ( 7- 8)
                      (7.0, 0.9, A)      (6.0, 1.6, D)
```

Scales: 1 = low validity or feasibility; 9 = high validity or feasibility

DIAGNOSIS

1. If a patient is diagnosed with pneumonia, on the day of diagnosis the provider should document:

  a. whether the cough is productive or nonproductive

```
1 1 2 1 2   1 1     1   1   1   2 2 2
1 2 3 4 5 6 7 8 9   1 2 3 4 5 6 7 8 9   ( 1-  2)
   (4.0, 1.8, D)       (7.0, 2.0, D)
```

  b. the presence or absence of a coexisting illness

```
            3 2 4                 3 2 4
1 2 3 4 5 6 7 8 9   1 2 3 4 5 6 7 8 9   ( 3-  4)
   (8.0, 0.8, A)       (8.0, 0.8, A)
```

  c. the presence or absence of recent upper respiratory symptoms

```
1 1 2 3 1     1     1   2   1   1 2 2
1 2 3 4 5 6 7 8 9   1 2 3 4 5 6 7 8 9   ( 5-  6)
   (4.0, 1.3, I)       (7.0, 2.4, D)
```

2. If a patient has a diagnosis of pneumonia, the following should be documented on the day of presentation:

  a. temperature

```
        2 2 5             1 3 5
1 2 3 4 5 6 7 8 9   1 2 3 4 5 6 7 8 9   ( 7-  8)
   (9.0, 0.7, A)       (9.0, 0.6, A)
```

  b. respiratory rate

```
        2 3 4             2 3 4
1 2 3 4 5 6 7 8 9   1 2 3 4 5 6 7 8 9   ( 9- 10)
   (8.0, 0.7, A)       (8.0, 0.7, A)
```

  c. heart rate

```
        3 2 4             1 3 5
1 2 3 4 5 6 7 8 9   1 2 3 4 5 6 7 8 9   ( 11- 12)
   (8.0, 0.8, A)       (9.0, 0.6, A)
```

  d. lung examination

```
        2 2 5             1 4 4
1 2 3 4 5 6 7 8 9   1 2 3 4 5 6 7 8 9   ( 13- 14)
   (9.0, 0.7, A)       (8.0, 0.6, A)
```

3. If a patient has a diagnosis of pneumonia the health care provider should offer a chest radiograph (CXR) on the day of presentation.

```
      2 2 1 4               2 2 5
1 2 3 4 5 6 7 8 9   1 2 3 4 5 6 7 8 9   ( 15- 16)
   (8.0, 1.1, A)       (9.0, 0.7, A)
```

4. If a patient has a diagnosis of pneumonia and suggestion of a pleural effusion on CXR, a lateral decubitus radiograph, ultrasound, or thorocentesis should be performed on the day of presentation.

```
      2 1 1 4 1           1   3 4 1
1 2 3 4 5 6 7 8 9   1 2 3 4 5 6 7 8 9   ( 17- 18)
   (8.0, 1.1, I)       (8.0, 0.8, A)
```

5. Patients over 65 years of age or with coexisting illness and a diagnosis of pneumonia, should receive the following blood tests on the day of presentation:

  a. white blood cell count

```
      2 4 3               1 3 5
1 2 3 4 5 6 7 8 9   1 2 3 4 5 6 7 8 9   ( 19- 20)
   (8.0, 0.6, A)       (9.0, 0.6, A)
```

  b. hemoglobin or hematocrit

```
1   1 2 2 1 2             1 1 4 3
1 2 3 4 5 6 7 8 9   1 2 3 4 5 6 7 8 9   ( 21- 22)
   (6.0, 1.4, I)       (8.0, 0.7, A)
```

  c. serum electrolytes

```
4 2 1 1 1           1   1     2 2 3
1 2 3 4 5 6 7 8 9   1 2 3 4 5 6 7 8 9   ( 23- 24)
   (4.0, 1.1, I)       (8.0, 1.9, D)
```

  d. BUN or creatinine

```
  1   4 1 3               1 3 5
1 2 3 4 5 6 7 8 9   1 2 3 4 5 6 7 8 9   ( 25- 26)
   (7.0, 1.0, A)       (9.0, 0.6, A)
```

6. Patients hospitalized for pneumonia should receive two sets of blood cultures on the day of hospitalization.

```
2   1 2     3 1             1 4 4
1 2 3 4 5 6 7 8 9   1 2 3 4 5 6 7 8 9   ( 27- 28)
   (5.0, 2.2, D)       (8.0, 0.6, A)
```

Scales: 1 = low validity or feasibility; 9 = high validity or feasibility

DIAGNOSIS, CONT.

7. Hospitalized persons with pneumonia should
have the following documented on the first
and second days of hospitalization:

```
                                        1 3 5              1 1 7
  a. temperature           1 2 3 4 5 6 7 8 9  1 2 3 4 5 6 7 8 9  ( 29- 30)
                             (9.0, 0.6, A)       (9.0, 0.3, A)
                                        2 3 4              2 1 6
  b. lung examination       1 2 3 4 5 6 7 8 9  1 2 3 4 5 6 7 8 9  ( 31- 32)
                             (8.0, 0.7, A)       (9.0, 0.6, A)
```

TREATMENT

8. Non-hospitalized persons <= 65 years of
age diagnosed with pneumonia without a known
bacteriologic etiology and without coexisting
illnesses should be offered an oral empiric
macrolide, unless allergic.

```
                                   1 3 2 3              3 4 2
                          1 2 3 4 5 6 7 8 9  1 2 3 4 5 6 7 8 9  ( 33- 34)
                             (8.0, 0.9, A)       (8.0, 0.6, A)
```

9. Non-hospitalized persons > 65 years of age
diagnosed with pneumonia without a known
bacteriologic etiology or with coexisting
illnesses should be offered one of the
following oral empiric antibiotic regimens:

  - a second generation cephalosporin
  - trimethoprim-sulfamethoxazole
  - a beta-lactam/beta-lactamase inhibitor
    combination

```
                                   1 4   4              2 4 3
                          1 2 3 4 5 6 7 8 9  1 2 3 4 5 6 7 8 9  ( 35- 36)
                             (7.0, 1.0, A)       (8.0, 0.6, A)
```

10. Hospitalized persons with non-severe
pneumonia without a known bacteriologic
etiology should be offered one of the
following empiric antibiotic regimens:

  - a second or third generation
    cephalosporin
  - a beta-lactam/beta-lactamase inhibitor
    combination.

```
                                   1 4 1 3              2 3 4
                          1 2 3 4 5 6 7 8 9  1 2 3 4 5 6 7 8 9  ( 37- 38)
                             (7.0, 0.9, A)       (8.0, 0.7, A)
```

11. Hospitalized persons with severe
pneumonia without a known bacteriologic
etiology should be offered one of the
following antibiotic regimens:

  - a macrolide and a third generation
    cephalosporin with anti-Pseudomonas
    activity
  - a macrolide and another anitpseudomonal
    agent such as imipenem/ciliastin,
    ciprofloxacin

```
                                   1 3 2 3              1 4 4
                          1 2 3 4 5 6 7 8 9  1 2 3 4 5 6 7 8 9  ( 39- 40)
                             (8.0, 0.9, A)       (8.0, 0.6, A)
```

12. Persons with CAP should be offered
antibiotics for 10-14 days, with the
exception of azithromycin, which may be given
for 5 days.

```
                          1 1 4 2     1    1 1    1   3 2 1
                          1 2 3 4 5 6 7 8 9  1 2 3 4 5 6 7 8 9  ( 41- 42)
                             (3.0, 1.1, I)       (7.0, 1.9, D)
```

FOLLOW-UP

13. Persons treated for pneumonia should
have follow-up contact with a provider
within 6 weeks after discharge or diagnosis.

```
                                   1 6   2              1 3 2 3
                          1 2 3 4 5 6 7 8 9  1 2 3 4 5 6 7 8 9  ( 43- 44)
                             (7.0, 0.6, A)       (8.0, 0.9, A)
```

Scales: 1 = low validity or feasibility; 9 = high validity or feasibility

INDICATORS ADDED AFTER ROUND 1

14. Patients with pneumonia with a new
effusion >= 10mm on lateral decubitus
radiograph or ultrasound, and an ipsilateral   2 1 2 4   1 4 4
infiltrate, should have a thorocentesis.   1 2 3 4 5 6 7 8 9 1 2 3 4 5 6 7 8 9 (45- 46)
                                                 (8.0, 1.0, A)   (8.0, 0.6, A)

WITH OR WITHOUT SYMPTOMS OF CAD

1."O" Patients 40-75 years old who have a
high risk stress test should be offered
coronary angiography within 6 weeks of
the stress test (unless they have
contraindications to revascularization).

```
                     2 1 3 3              1 2 2 4
            1 2 3 4 5 6 7 8 9  1 2 3 4 5 6 7 8 9  ( 1- 2)
              (8.0, 0.9, A)      (8.0, 0.9, A)
```

1."X" Patients > 75 years old who have a
high risk stress test should be offered
coronary angiography within 4 weeks of
the stress test (unless they have
contraindications to revascularization).

```
            1   1 1 2   2 1 1    1   1 1 1 3 2
            1 2 3 4 5 6 7 8 9  1 2 3 4 5 6 7 8 9  ( 3- 4)
              (5.0, 2.0, D)      (8.0, 1.4, I)
```

2."O" Patients 40-75 years old who have two
or more CAD risk factors and a newly
diagnosed low LVEF (<= 40%) should be offered
stress testing or coronary angiography within
3 months of the diagnosis of low LVEF (unless
an etiology of LV dysfunction other than CAD
is documented in the medical record or they
have contraindications to revascularization).

```
              2 1 1 1 4          1   1 2   3 2
            1 2 3 4 5 6 7 8 9  1 2 3 4 5 6 7 8 9  ( 5- 6)
              (6.0, 1.4, D)      (8.0, 1.6, I)
```

2."X" Patients > 75 years old who have two or
more CAD risk factors and a newly diagnosed
low LVEF (<= 40%) should be offered stress
testing or coronary angiography within 3
months of the diagnosis of low LVEF (unless
an etiology of LV dysfunction other than CAD
is documented in the medical record or they
have contraindications to revascularization).

```
            1 1 2 1 2   2      1   1   1 1   4 1
            1 2 3 4 5 6 7 8 9  1 2 3 4 5 6 7 8 9  ( 7- 8)
              (4.0, 1.7, D)      (8.0, 2.0, D)
```

3."O" Patients 40-75 years old who have an
ejection fraction <= 40% and a positive
stress test should be offered coronary
angiography within 4 weeks of the stress test
(unless they have contraindications to
revascularization).

```
                   2 2 4 1            1 4 2 2
            1 2 3 4 5 6 7 8 9  1 2 3 4 5 6 7 8 9  ( 9- 10)
              (8.0, 0.8, A)      (7.0, 0.8, A)
```

3."X" Patients > 75 years old who have an
ejection fraction <= 40% and a positive
stress test should be offered coronary
angiography within 4 weeks of the stress test
(unless they have contraindications to
revascularization).

```
            1   1 2 2   2 1    1 1   1 3 2 1
            1 2 3 4 5 6 7 8 9  1 2 3 4 5 6 7 8 9  ( 11- 12)
              (5.0, 1.7, D)      (7.0, 1.3, I)
```

Scales: 1 = low validity or feasibility; 9 = high validity or feasibility

Validity   Feasibility

STABLE ANGINA OR KNOWN CAD

4. Patients with newly diagnosed CAD should
have a 12-lead ECG at the time of diagnosis.

```
                              3   6              1 3 5
              1 2 3 4 5 6 7 8 9   1 2 3 4 5 6 7 8 9  ( 13- 14)
                (9.0, 0.7, A)       (9.0, 0.6, A)
```

5. Patients newly diagnosed with any
of the conditions listed below should
have a hemoglobin and/or hematocrit
measured at the time of diagnosis.

    a. angina

```
                          1   2 1 5             1 2 6
              1 2 3 4 5 6 7 8 9   1 2 3 4 5 6 7 8 9  ( 15- 16)
                (9.0, 1.0, A)       (9.0, 0.4, A)
```

    b. unstable angina

```
                              2 1 6             1 2 6
              1 2 3 4 5 6 7 8 9   1 2 3 4 5 6 7 8 9  ( 17- 18)
                (9.0, 0.6, A)       (9.0, 0.4, A)
```

    c. MI

```
                              1 2 6             1 2 6
              1 2 3 4 5 6 7 8 9   1 2 3 4 5 6 7 8 9  ( 19- 20)
                (9.0, 0.4, A)       (9.0, 0.4, A)
```

6."O" Patients < 75 years old newly diagnosed
with stable angina or CAD should be offered
stress testing or coronary angiography within
3 months of the diagnosis (unless they have
contraindications to revascularization).

```
              1   2 1   2 1 1 1    1   1   4 2 1
              1 2 3 4 5 6 7 8 9   1 2 3 4 5 6 7 8 9  ( 21- 22)
                (6.0, 2.1, D)       (7.0, 1.1, A)
```

6."X" Patients >= 75 years old newly
diagnosed with stable angina or CAD should be
offered stress testing or coronary
angiography within 3 months of the diagnosis
(unless they have contraindications to
revascularization).

```
              2   2 1 1   2 1    1   1   4 2 1
              1 2 3 4 5 6 7 8 9   1 2 3 4 5 6 7 8 9  ( 23- 24)
                (4.0, 2.1, D)       (7.0, 1.4, A)
```

Scales: 1 = low validity or feasibility; 9 = high validity or feasibility

UNSTABLE ANGINA

7. Patients being evaluated for "unstable
angina" or "rule out unstable angina"
should have an examination at the time of
evaluation documenting all of the following:

```
                              3 1 2 1   1 1        2        2 3 2
a. temperature            1 2 3 4 5 6 7 8 9   1 2 3 4 5 6 7 8 9   ( 25- 26)
                             (5.0, 1.7, D)       (8.0, 1.6, D)
                                  1 2 6                1 2 6
b. blood pressure         1 2 3 4 5 6 7 8 9   1 2 3 4 5 6 7 8 9   ( 27- 28)
                             (9.0, 0.4, A)       (9.0, 0.4, A)
                                  1 2 6                1 2 6
c. heart rate             1 2 3 4 5 6 7 8 9   1 2 3 4 5 6 7 8 9   ( 29- 30)
                             (9.0, 0.4, A)       (9.0, 0.4, A)
                                  1 2 6                1 2 6
d. heart exam             1 2 3 4 5 6 7 8 9   1 2 3 4 5 6 7 8 9   ( 31- 32)
                             (9.0, 0.4, A)       (9.0, 0.4, A)
                                  1 2 6                1 2 6
e. lung exam              1 2 3 4 5 6 7 8 9   1 2 3 4 5 6 7 8 9   ( 33- 34)
                             (9.0, 0.4, A)       (9.0, 0.4, A)
                                    3 6                  3 6
f. a 12-lead ECG          1 2 3 4 5 6 7 8 9   1 2 3 4 5 6 7 8 9   ( 35- 36)
                             (9.0, 0.3, A)       (9.0, 0.3, A)
```

8. Patients admitted with unstable angina
should be placed on cardiac monitoring
(i.e., telemetry).

```
                                  4 2 3                  5 4
                          1 2 3 4 5 6 7 8 9   1 2 3 4 5 6 7 8 9   ( 37- 38)
                             (8.0, 0.8, A)       (8.0, 0.4, A)
```

9. Patients admitted with unstable angina
should have cardiac enzymes measured every
6 to 8 hours for the first 24 hours of
admission.

```
                                1   2 2 4              1 3 5
                          1 2 3 4 5 6 7 8 9   1 2 3 4 5 6 7 8 9   ( 39- 40)
                             (8.0, 1.0, A)       (9.0, 0.6, A)
```

10. Patients admitted with unstable angina
should have a repeat ECG 12-36 hours after
admission.

```
                                  3 2 4                  4 5
                          1 2 3 4 5 6 7 8 9   1 2 3 4 5 6 7 8 9   ( 41- 42)
                             (8.0, 0.8, A)       (9.0, 0.4, A)
```

11. Patients admitted with unstable angina
who have any one of the conditions below
should have a measurement of LVEF by
echocardiogram, radionuclide scan, or
ventriculogram during their hospitalization
or within 10 days of discharge unless a prior
LVEF is documented in the past year:

```
                                1 2 2 4                2 2 5
a. a history of prior MI  1 2 3 4 5 6 7 8 9   1 2 3 4 5 6 7 8 9   ( 43- 44)
                             (8.0, 0.9, A)       (9.0, 0.7, A)
b. left bundle branch           2 1 1 5                2 3 4
block on their            1 2 3 4 5 6 7 8 9   1 2 3 4 5 6 7 8 9   ( 45- 46)
resting ECG                  (9.0, 1.0, A)       (8.0, 0.7, A)
                                2 1 3 1 2            1 3 1 4
c. cardiomegaly by        1 2 3 4 5 6 7 8 9   1 2 3 4 5 6 7 8 9   ( 47- 48)
examination                  (7.0, 1.1, I)       (8.0, 1.0, A)
                              1 2 2 1 3              2 2 5
d. cardiomegaly on        1 2 3 4 5 6 7 8 9   1 2 3 4 5 6 7 8 9   ( 49- 50)
chest X-ray                  (7.0, 1.2, I)       (9.0, 0.7, A)
                                  2 3 4                3 1 5
e. a diagnosis of heart   1 2 3 4 5 6 7 8 9   1 2 3 4 5 6 7 8 9   ( 51- 52)
failure                      (8.0, 0.7, A)       (9.0, 0.8, A)
```

Scales: 1 = low validity or feasibility; 9 = high validity or feasibility

UNSTABLE ANGINA, CONT.

12."O" Patients < 75 years old with a
discharge diagnosis of "unstable angina"
should be offered stress testing or coronary
angiography prior to or within 7 days of
hospital discharge (unless they have
contraindications to revascularization or
have had stress testing or coronary
angiography within 6 months prior to
discharge).

```
 1 2   1 1 1 1 2       1       3 3 2
1 2 3 4 5 6 7 8 9  1 2 3 4 5 6 7 8 9  ( 53- 54)
   (6.0, 2.2, D)       (8.0, 1.1, A)
```

12."X" Patients >= 75 years old with a
discharge diagnosis of "unstable angina"
should be offered stress testing or coronary
angiography prior to or within 7 days of
hospital discharge (unless they have
contraindications to revascularization or
have had stress testing or coronary
angiography within 6 months prior to
discharge).

```
 2 3 1   1 2           2       4 2 1
1 2 3 4 5 6 7 8 9  1 2 3 4 5 6 7 8 9  ( 55- 56)
   (3.0, 1.6, D)       (7.0, 1.3, D)
```

MYOCARDIAL INFARCTION

13. Patients hospitalized for the diagnosis
of an MI or "rule out MI" should have a
physical examination documenting all of the
following:

a. temperature

```
 1 1 2 1 2 1 1         1   2 3 3
1 2 3 4 5 6 7 8 9  1 2 3 4 5 6 7 8 9  ( 57- 58)
   (6.0, 1.6, I)       (8.0, 0.9, A)
```

b. blood pressure

```
         1 2 6               3 6
1 2 3 4 5 6 7 8 9  1 2 3 4 5 6 7 8 9  ( 59- 60)
   (9.0, 0.4, A)       (9.0, 0.3, A)
```

c. heart rate

```
           3 6               3 6
1 2 3 4 5 6 7 8 9  1 2 3 4 5 6 7 8 9  ( 61- 62)
   (9.0, 0.3, A)       (9.0, 0.3, A)
```

d. heart exam

```
           3 6               3 6
1 2 3 4 5 6 7 8 9  1 2 3 4 5 6 7 8 9  ( 63- 64)
   (9.0, 0.3, A)       (9.0, 0.3, A)
```

e. lung exam

```
         1 2 6               3 6
1 2 3 4 5 6 7 8 9  1 2 3 4 5 6 7 8 9  ( 65- 66)
   (9.0, 0.4, A)       (9.0, 0.3, A)
```

14. Patients hospitalized for the diagnosis
of an MI or "rule out MI" should have a
12-lead ECG within 20 minutes of
presentation.

```
     2   1 6           1   1 2 5
1 2 3 4 5 6 7 8 9  1 2 3 4 5 6 7 8 9  ( 67- 68)
   (9.0, 0.8, A)       (9.0, 0.9, A)
```

15. Patients hospitalized with an MI should
have an assessment of LVEF prior to discharge
if they have any risk factors for low LVEF
(unless it is noted during hospitalization
that prior to admission LVEF was <= 40%).

```
       1 2 1 5             1 3 5
1 2 3 4 5 6 7 8 9  1 2 3 4 5 6 7 8 9  ( 69- 70)
   (9.0, 0.9, A)       (9.0, 0.6, A)
```

Scales: 1 = low validity or feasibility; 9 = high validity or feasibility

MYOCARDIAL INFARCTION, CONT.

16. Patients hospitalized with an MI who
have a history of prior MI, but no risk
factors for low LVEF, should have an
assessment of LVEF during the hospitalization
or within 2 weeks of discharge (unless it
is noted during hospitalization that prior   2 1 2 4   1 4 4
to admission LVEF was <=40%).   1 2 3 4 5 6 7 8 9 1 2 3 4 5 6 7 8 9 (71- 72)
                                          (8.0, 1.0, A)   (8.0, 0.6, A)

17."O" Patients < 75 years old with an MI
should be offered symptom-limited stress
testing or coronary angiography within 8   1 3 3 2   1 5 3
weeks of the MI (unless they have   1 2 3 4 5 6 7 8 9 1 2 3 4 5 6 7 8 9 (73- 74)
contraindications to revascularization).   (8.0, 0.8, A)   (8.0, 0.4, A)

17."X" Patients >= 75 years old with an MI
should be offered symptom-limited stress
testing or coronary angiography within 8   1 2 2 1 1 1   1   2 3 2
weeks of the MI (unless they have   1 2 3 4 5 6 7 8 9 1 2 3 4 5 6 7 8 9 (75- 76)
contraindications to revascularization).   (5.0, 2.1, D)   (8.0, 1.1, A)

18."O" Patients < 75 years old hospitalized
with an MI who have any of the following
conditions after discharge but within 8 weeks
of the MI should be offered coronary
angiography within 2 weeks of the diagnosis
of the condition (unless they have   3 2 4   3 1 5
contraindications to revascularization):

   a. a high risk stress test   1 2 3 4 5 6 7 8 9 1 2 3 4 5 6 7 8 9 (77- 78)
                                          (8.0, 0.8, A)   (9.0, 0.8, A)
                                             1 3 3 2   4 2 3
   b. new heart failure   1 2 3 4 5 6 7 8 9 1 2 3 4 5 6 7 8 9 (79- 80)
                                          (8.0, 0.9, A)   (8.0, 0.8, A)
                                             2 2 4 1   3 3 3
   c. LVEF <= 40%   1 2 3 4 5 6 7 8 9 1 2 3 4 5 6 7 8 9 (81- 82)
                                          (8.0, 0.8, A)   (8.0, 0.7, A)
                                             2   2 5   3 1 5
   d. new severe mitral regurgitation   1 2 3 4 5 6 7 8 9 1 2 3 4 5 6 7 8 9 (83- 84)
                                          (9.0, 0.9, A)   (9.0, 0.8, A)
                                             2   2 5   2 2 5
   e. new ventricular septal defect   1 2 3 4 5 6 7 8 9 1 2 3 4 5 6 7 8 9 (85- 86)
                                          (9.0, 0.9, A)   (9.0, 0.7, A)

   f. sustained ventricular tachycardia or
   ventricular fibrillation which occurs >=48   2 1 2 4   2 2 5
   hr. after onset of the MI   1 2 3 4 5 6 7 8 9 1 2 3 4 5 6 7 8 9 (87- 88)
                                          (8.0, 1.0, A)   (9.0, 0.7, A)
                                             2 3 4   2 1 6
   g. angina at rest lasting >= 15 min. 1 2 3 4 5 6 7 8 9 1 2 3 4 5 6 7 8 9 (89- 90)
                                          (8.0, 0.7, A)   (9.0, 0.6, A)

Scales: 1 = low validity or feasibility; 9 = high validity or feasibility

Validity   Feasibility

MYOCARDIAL INFARCTION, CONT.

18."X" Patients >= 75 years old hospitalized
with an MI who have any of the following
conditions after discharge but within 8 weeks
of the MI should be offered coronary
angiography within 2 weeks of the diagnosis
of the condition (unless they have
contraindications to revascularization):

```
                               2 1 1 1 3   1     1       3 2 3
  a. a high risk stress test   1 2 3 4 5 6 7 8 9  1 2 3 4 5 6 7 8 9  ( 91- 92)
                                 (6.0, 1.7, D)       (8.0, 1.2, A)
                               1   2 1   1 4   1         3 3 2
  b. new heart failure         1 2 3 4 5 6 7 8 9  1 2 3 4 5 6 7 8 9  ( 93- 94)
                                 (6.0, 1.9, D)       (8.0, 1.3, A)
                               2     2 1 2 2   1         1 2 3 2
  c. LVEF <= 40%               1 2 3 4 5 6 7 8 9  1 2 3 4 5 6 7 8 9  ( 95- 96)
                                 (5.0, 1.8, D)       (8.0, 1.4, A)
                               1   2 1 1   2 2           1   3 2 3
  d. new severe mitral regurgitation  1 2 3 4 5 6 7 8 9  1 2 3 4 5 6 7 8 9  ( 97- 98)
                                 (6.0, 2.1, I)       (8.0, 1.0, A)
                                 2 1 1 1 2 2           1   2 3 3
  e. new ventricular septal defect  1 2 3 4 5 6 7 8 9  1 2 3 4 5 6 7 8 9  ( 99-100)
                                 (7.0, 1.7, I)       (8.0, 0.9, A)

  f. sustained ventricular tachycardia or
  ventricular fibrillation which occurs >=48   1 3 1   1 1 2    1       2 3 3
  hr. after onset of the MI    1 2 3 4 5 6 7 8 9  1 2 3 4 5 6 7 8 9  (101-102)
                                 (5.0, 2.0, I)       (8.0, 1.1, A)
                                 2     3 1 1 2   1         2 2 4
  g. angina at rest lasting >= 15 min.  1 2 3 4 5 6 7 8 9  1 2 3 4 5 6 7 8 9  (103-104)
                                 (6.0, 1.7, D)       (8.0, 1.2, A)
```

Scales: 1 = low validity or feasibility; 9 = high validity or feasibility

Validity   Feasibility

MYOCARDIAL INFARCTION, CONT.

19. "O" Patients < 75 years old who are
hospitalized with an MI complicated by any of
the following should be offered coronary
angiography prior to discharge (unless they
have contraindications to revascularization):

```
                                    1 3     5              3 1 5
a. a high risk stress test     1 2 3 4 5 6 7 8 9   1 2 3 4 5 6 7 8 9   (105-106)
                                  (9.0, 1.0, A)       (9.0, 0.8, A)
                                    1 4 1 3                  4 2 3
b. new heart failure           1 2 3 4 5 6 7 8 9   1 2 3 4 5 6 7 8 9   (107-108)
                                  (7.0, 0.9, A)       (8.0, 0.8, A)
                                    1 4 1 3              1 3 2 3
c. LVEF <= 40%                  1 2 3 4 5 6 7 8 9   1 2 3 4 5 6 7 8 9   (109-110)
                                  (7.0, 0.9, A)       (8.0, 0.9, A)
                                    2 1     6                1 1 2 5
d. new severe mitral regurgitation  1 2 3 4 5 6 7 8 9   1 2 3 4 5 6 7 8 9   (111-112)
                                  (9.0, 0.9, A)       (9.0, 0.8, A)
                                    2 1     6                1 1 1 6
e. new ventricular septal defect    1 2 3 4 5 6 7 8 9   1 2 3 4 5 6 7 8 9   (113-114)
                                  (9.0, 0.9, A)       (9.0, 0.7, A)
```

f. sustained ventricular tachycardia or
ventricular fibrillation >= 48 hr. after
onset of the MI

```
                                    1 1 1   6                3     6
                               1 2 3 4 5 6 7 8 9   1 2 3 4 5 6 7 8 9   (115-116)
                                  (9.0, 1.0, A)       (9.0, 0.7, A)
```

g. >5 min. of angina at rest occurring >=24
hr. after the onset of the MI

```
                                      2 3 4               1 2 2 4
                               1 2 3 4 5 6 7 8 9   1 2 3 4 5 6 7 8 9   (117-118)
                                  (8.0, 0.7, A)       (8.0, 0.9, A)
                                        1 2 6               1 2 6
h. shock                       1 2 3 4 5 6 7 8 9   1 2 3 4 5 6 7 8 9   (119-120)
                                  (9.0, 0.4, A)       (9.0, 0.4, A)
                                      2     7                2 1 6
i. pulmonary edema requiring intubation  1 2 3 4 5 6 7 8 9   1 2 3 4 5 6 7 8 9   (121-122)
                                  (9.0, 0.4, A)       (9.0, 0.6, A)
```

Scales: 1 = low validity or feasibility; 9 = high validity or feasibility

Validity   Feasibility

MYOCARDIAL INFARCTION, CONT.

19. "X" Patients >= 75 years old who are
hospitalized with an MI complicated by any of
the following should be offered coronary
angiography prior to discharge (unless they
have contraindications to revascularization):

a. a high risk stress test

```
          3   2   2   2      1         3 2 3
1 2 3 4 5 6 7 8 9   1 2 3 4 5 6 7 8 9   (123-124)
   (5.0, 2.0, D)       (8.0, 1.2, A)
```

b. new heart failure

```
          3 1 1   4         1         3 3 2
1 2 3 4 5 6 7 8 9   1 2 3 4 5 6 7 8 9   (125-126)
   (5.0, 1.7, D)       (8.0, 1.1, A)
```

c. LVEF <= 40%

```
      1 2 1 1 1 3           1       1 2 3 2
1 2 3 4 5 6 7 8 9   1 2 3 4 5 6 7 8 9   (127-128)
   (5.0, 1.7, D)       (8.0, 1.3, A)
```

d. new severe mitral regurgitation

```
      2 1 2   1   3                 1 1 1 3 3
1 2 3 4 5 6 7 8 9   1 2 3 4 5 6 7 8 9   (129-130)
   (5.0, 2.1, D)       (8.0, 1.0, A)
```

e. new ventricular septal defect

```
      2 1 2   1   3         1       1 1 2 4
1 2 3 4 5 6 7 8 9   1 2 3 4 5 6 7 8 9   (131-132)
   (5.0, 2.1, D)       (8.0, 1.3, A)
```

f. sustained ventricular tachycardia or
ventricular fibrillation >= 48 hr. after
onset of the MI

```
      3 1 1   1   3         1         3 1 4
1 2 3 4 5 6 7 8 9   1 2 3 4 5 6 7 8 9   (133-134)
   (5.0, 2.3, D)       (8.0, 1.2, A)
```

g. >5 min. of angina at rest occurring >=24
hr. after the onset of the MI

```
      1 2   1 1 2 2         1       1 2 3 2
1 2 3 4 5 6 7 8 9   1 2 3 4 5 6 7 8 9   (135-136)
   (6.0, 1.9, D)       (8.0, 1.2, A)
```

h. shock

```
      2   2 1 2   2         1         2 3 3
1 2 3 4 5 6 7 8 9   1 2 3 4 5 6 7 8 9   (137-138)
   (6.0, 1.8, D)       (8.0, 1.1, A)
```

i. pulmonary edema requiring intubation

```
      3   2   2   2         1         2 2 4
1 2 3 4 5 6 7 8 9   1 2 3 4 5 6 7 8 9   (139-140)
   (5.0, 2.0, D)       (8.0, 1.2, A)
```

Scales: 1 = low validity or feasibility; 9 = high validity or feasibility

Validity   Feasibility

SUDDEN DEATH

20."O" Patients < 75 years old admitted after
cardiac arrest should be offered a stress
test or coronary angiography before discharge
(unless they have contraindications to
revascularization or have had coronary
angiography).

```
        3     2 2   2         2          3 1 3
1 2 3 4 5 6 7 8 9   1 2 3 4 5 6 7 8 9   (141-142)
  (6.0, 1.9, D)       (7.0, 1.7, D)
```

20."X" Patients >= 75 years old admitted
after cardiac arrest should be offered a
stress test or coronary angiography before
discharge (unless they have contraindications
to revascularization or have had coronary
angiography).

```
2     2 1 1   1   2   1   1         3 2 2
1 2 3 4 5 6 7 8 9   1 2 3 4 5 6 7 8 9   (143-144)
  (4.0, 2.4, D)       (7.0, 1.8, D)
```

21."O" Patients < 75 years old admitted after
cardiac arrest and who have a positive stress
test during hospitalization should be offered
coronary angiography before discharge (unless
they have contraindications to
revascularization).

```
            1 2 1 5             1 2 1 5
1 2 3 4 5 6 7 8 9   1 2 3 4 5 6 7 8 9   (145-146)
  (9.0, 0.9, A)       (9.0, 0.9, A)
```

21."X" Patients >= 75 years old admitted
after cardiac arrest and who have a positive
stress test during hospitalization should be
offered coronary angiography before discharge
(unless they have contraindications to
revascularization).

```
1     2   2   1 1 2       1       1 2 2 3
1 2 3 4 5 6 7 8 9   1 2 3 4 5 6 7 8 9   (147-148)
  (5.0, 2.3, D)       (8.0, 1.3, A)
```

Scales: 1 = low validity or feasibility; 9 = high validity or feasibility

Validity   Feasibility

STABLE ANGINA OR KNOWN CAD

1. Patients newly diagnosed with CAD should
receive aspirin (at a dose of at least 81
mg/day continued indefinitely) within one
week of the diagnosis of CAD unless they have
a contraindication to aspirin.

```
                        2 7                 2   7
           1 2 3 4 5 6 7 8 9   1 2 3 4 5 6 7 8 9   ( 1- 2)
             (9.0, 0.2, A)       (9.0, 0.4, A)
```

2. Patients with a prior diagnosis of CAD
who are not on aspirin and do not have
contraindications to aspirin should receive
aspirin (at a dose of at least 81 mg/day
continued indefinitely) within one week of
any visit to a provider in which CAD
was addressed.

```
                       1 1 7                2   7
           1 2 3 4 5 6 7 8 9   1 2 3 4 5 6 7 8 9   ( 3- 4)
             (9.0, 0.3, A)       (9.0, 0.4, A)
```

3. Patients newly diagnosed with CAD who
smoke should have documentation of counseling
on smoking cessation at the time of the
diagnosis of CAD.

```
                        2 7             1 1 1 2 4
           1 2 3 4 5 6 7 8 9   1 2 3 4 5 6 7 8 9   ( 5- 6)
             (9.0, 0.2, A)       (8.0, 1.1, A)
```

UNSTABLE ANGINA

4. Patients with the diagnosis of unstable
angina should receive aspirin within 2 hours
of admission or presentation to the emergency
room.

```
                        3 6             1   1 2 5
           1 2 3 4 5 6 7 8 9   1 2 3 4 5 6 7 8 9   ( 7- 8)
             (9.0, 0.3, A)       (9.0, 0.9, A)
```

5. Patients admitted with the diagnosis of
unstable angina who have angina > 5 minutes
at rest associated with ischemic ST segment
changes and who do not have contraindications
to heparin should receive:

  a. heparin within 2 hours of the initial
  ECG that demonstrates ischemic changes

```
                       1 1 7                2 2 5
           1 2 3 4 5 6 7 8 9   1 2 3 4 5 6 7 8 9   ( 9- 10)
             (9.0, 0.3, A)       (9.0, 0.7, A)
```

  b. continuous heparin infusion or
  subcutaneous LMW heparin for at least
  24 hours (or until 26 hours after the ECG
  with ischemic changes)

```
                        2 7                 2 1 6
           1 2 3 4 5 6 7 8 9   1 2 3 4 5 6 7 8 9   ( 11- 12)
             (9.0, 0.4, A)       (9.0, 0.6, A)
```

6. Patients admitted with the diagnosis
of unstable angina who have angina > 5
minutes at rest associated with ischemic
ST segment changes should receive
beta-blockers within 4 hours (unless they
have contraindications to beta-blockers).

```
                        2 1 6               1 3 5
           1 2 3 4 5 6 7 8 9   1 2 3 4 5 6 7 8 9   ( 13- 14)
             (9.0, 0.6, A)       (9.0, 0.6, A)
```

Scales: 1 = low validity or feasibility; 9 = high validity or feasibility

Validity   Feasibility

MYOCARDIAL INFARCTION

7. Patients presenting with acute myocardial
infarction should receive at least 160 mg of
aspirin within 2 hours of presentation or
admission unless they have contraindications
to aspirin.

```
                              3 6                   1 3 5
          1 2 3 4 5 6 7 8 9   1 2 3 4 5 6 7 8 9   ( 15- 16)
            (9.0, 0.3, A)       (9.0, 0.6, A)
```

8."O" Patients < 75 years old presenting with
an acute myocardial infarction who are within
12 hours of the onset of MI symptoms and who
do not have contraindications to thrombolyis
or revascularization should receive a
thrombolytic agent within 1 hour of the time
their ECG initially shows either of the
following findings:

a. ST elevation > 0.1 mV in 2 or more
contiguous leads

```
                              1 3 5                 2 1 6
          1 2 3 4 5 6 7 8 9   1 2 3 4 5 6 7 8 9   ( 17- 18)
            (9.0, 0.6, A)       (9.0, 0.6, A)
                              2 3 4                 2 1 6
```

b. a LBBB not known to be old

```
          1 2 3 4 5 6 7 8 9   1 2 3 4 5 6 7 8 9   ( 19- 20)
            (8.0, 0.7, A)       (9.0, 0.6, A)
```

8."X" Patients >= 75 years old presenting
with an acute myocardial infarction who are
within 12 hours of the onset of MI symptoms
and who do not have contraindications to
thrombolyis or revascularization should
receive a thrombolytic agent within 1 hour of
the time their ECG initially shows either of
the following findings:

a. ST elevation > 0.1 mV in 2 or more
contiguous leads

```
                        1 3   4 1           1   3 1 4
          1 2 3 4 5 6 7 8 9   1 2 3 4 5 6 7 8 9   ( 21- 22)
            (7.0, 1.1, I)       (8.0, 1.1, A)
                        2 2 2 2 1             1 1 2 1 4
```

b. a LBBB not known to be old

```
          1 2 3 4 5 6 7 8 9   1 2 3 4 5 6 7 8 9   ( 23- 24)
            (6.0, 1.1, I)       (8.0, 1.2, A)
```

9. Patients admitted within 12 hours of the
onset of acute myocardial infarction who do
not have contraindications to heparin should
receive heparin (subcutaneously or IV) for at
least 24 hours unless they have received
streptokinase, APSAC, or urokinase.

```
                            1 2 5 1                 3 2 4
          1 2 3 4 5 6 7 8 9   1 2 3 4 5 6 7 8 9   ( 25- 26)
            (8.0, 0.6, A)       (8.0, 0.8, A)
```

10. Patients admitted with acute myocardial
infarction should receive a beta-blocker
within 12 hours of admission (unless they
have contraindications to beta-blockers).

```
                              3 6                   1 2 6
          1 2 3 4 5 6 7 8 9   1 2 3 4 5 6 7 8 9   ( 27- 28)
            (9.0, 0.3, A)       (9.0, 0.4, A)
```

Scales: 1 = low validity or feasibility; 9 = high validity or feasibility

Validity   Feasibility

MYOCARDIAL INFARCTION, CONT.

11. Patients admitted with acute myocardial
infarction and are known to have a LVEF <=
40% at admission should receive an ACE
inhibitor within the first 24 hours of
admission (unless they have contraindications
to ACE inhibitors).

```
2 2     1   3 1     1 1 1       1 1 4
1 2 3 4 5 6 7 8 9   1 2 3 4 5 6 7 8 9   ( 29- 30)
  (5.0, 2.6, D)       (8.0, 2.6, D)
```

12. Patients admitted with acute myocardial
infarction should NOT receive short-acting
nifedipine during the hospitalization.

```
          1 1   7             2 2 5
1 2 3 4 5 6 7 8 9   1 2 3 4 5 6 7 8 9   ( 31- 32)
  (9.0, 0.6, A)       (9.0, 0.7, A)
```

13. Patients admitted with acute myocardial
infarction should NOT receive any calcium
channel blocker if they have a reduced LVEF
(<=40%) or heart failure during the
hospitalization.

```
          1 1 1 6           2 2 5
1 2 3 4 5 6 7 8 9   1 2 3 4 5 6 7 8 9   ( 33- 34)
  (9.0, 0.7, A)       (9.0, 0.7, A)
```

14. Patients discharged after an acute
myocardial infarction who do not have
contraindications to aspirin should be
discharged on aspirin at a dose of at least
81 mg/day.

```
            2 7               4 5
1 2 3 4 5 6 7 8 9   1 2 3 4 5 6 7 8 9   ( 35- 36)
  (9.0, 0.2, A)       (9.0, 0.4, A)
```

15. Patients discharged after an acute
myocardial infarction should be discharged
on a beta-blocker (unless they have
contraindications to beta-blockers).

```
          1 2 6               3 6
1 2 3 4 5 6 7 8 9   1 2 3 4 5 6 7 8 9   ( 37- 38)
  (9.0, 0.4, A)       (9.0, 0.3, A)
```

16. Patients discharged after an acute
myocardial infarction who have an LVEF<= 40%
documented at any time during the
hospitalization should receive ACE inhibitors
at discharge (unless they have
contraindications to ACE inhibitors).

```
            2   7           1 1 7
1 2 3 4 5 6 7 8 9   1 2 3 4 5 6 7 8 9   ( 39- 40)
  (9.0, 0.4, A)       (9.0, 0.3, A)
```

REVASCULARIZATION

17. Patients with CAD who do not have
contraindications to revascularization should
be offered PTCA or CABS within 1 month of
coronary angiography if they have 3 vessel
CAD and an LVEF <= 40%.

```
          3 1 1 4           3 2 4
1 2 3 4 5 6 7 8 9   1 2 3 4 5 6 7 8 9   ( 41- 42)
  (8.0, 1.2, I)       (8.0, 0.8, A)
```

18. Patients with CAD who do not have
contraindications to revascularization
should be offered CABS within 1 month of
coronary angiography if they have left main
stenosis > 50%.

```
          2 1 1 5             2 2 5
1 2 3 4 5 6 7 8 9   1 2 3 4 5 6 7 8 9   ( 43- 44)
  (9.0, 1.0, A)       (9.0, 0.7, A)
```

Scales: 1 = low validity or feasibility; 9 = high validity or feasibility

DIAGNOSIS

1. Patients newly diagnosed with heart
failure who are beginning medical treatment
should receive an evaluation of their
ejection fraction within 1 month of the start
of treatment.

```
                      1 2 2 4                    3 2 4
          1 2 3 4 5 6 7 8 9    1 2 3 4 5 6 7 8 9   ( 1- 2)
            (8.0, 0.9, A)        (8.0, 0.8, A)
```

2. Patients newly diagnosed with heart
failure should have a history at the time of
the diagnosis documenting the presence or
absence of all of the following:

a. Prior myocardial infarction or cardiac
disease

```
                        1 3 5                    1 2 6
          1 2 3 4 5 6 7 8 9    1 2 3 4 5 6 7 8 9   ( 3- 4)
            (9.0, 0.6, A)        (9.0, 0.4, A)
```

b. Current symptoms of chest discomfort or
angina

```
                          4 5                    1 2 6
          1 2 3 4 5 6 7 8 9    1 2 3 4 5 6 7 8 9   ( 5- 6)
            (9.0, 0.4, A)        (9.0, 0.4, A)
```

c. History of hypertension

```
                      1     4 4                  1 2 6
          1 2 3 4 5 6 7 8 9    1 2 3 4 5 6 7 8 9   ( 7- 8)
            (8.0, 0.7, A)        (9.0, 0.4, A)
```

d. History of diabetes

```
                      1     4 4                  1 3 5
          1 2 3 4 5 6 7 8 9    1 2 3 4 5 6 7 8 9   ( 9- 10)
            (8.0, 0.7, A)        (9.0, 0.6, A)
```

e. Current medications

```
                          4 5                    1 3 5
          1 2 3 4 5 6 7 8 9    1 2 3 4 5 6 7 8 9   ( 11- 12)
            (9.0, 0.4, A)        (9.0, 0.6, A)
```

f. Alcohol use

```
                      1 5 3                      1   4 4
          1 2 3 4 5 6 7 8 9    1 2 3 4 5 6 7 8 9   ( 13- 14)
            (8.0, 0.4, A)        (8.0, 0.6, A)
```

g. Smoking status

```
                      1 3 5                        4 5
          1 2 3 4 5 6 7 8 9    1 2 3 4 5 6 7 8 9   ( 15- 16)
            (9.0, 0.6, A)        (9.0, 0.4, A)
```

3. Patients with a new diagnosis of heart
failure should have the following elements of
the physical examination documented at the
time of presentation:

a. Weight

```
                        3 6                        2 7
          1 2 3 4 5 6 7 8 9    1 2 3 4 5 6 7 8 9   ( 17- 18)
            (9.0, 0.3, A)        (9.0, 0.2, A)
```

b. Blood pressure

```
                          4 5                      3 6
          1 2 3 4 5 6 7 8 9    1 2 3 4 5 6 7 8 9   ( 19- 20)
            (9.0, 0.4, A)        (9.0, 0.3, A)
```

c. Lung exam

```
                          5 4                      3 6
          1 2 3 4 5 6 7 8 9    1 2 3 4 5 6 7 8 9   ( 21- 22)
            (8.0, 0.4, A)        (9.0, 0.3, A)
```

d. Cardiac exam

```
                          4 5                      3 6
          1 2 3 4 5 6 7 8 9    1 2 3 4 5 6 7 8 9   ( 23- 24)
            (9.0, 0.4, A)        (9.0, 0.3, A)
```

e. Abdominal exam

```
                      1 2 2 2 2                    5 4
          1 2 3 4 5 6 7 8 9    1 2 3 4 5 6 7 8 9   ( 25- 26)
            (7.0, 1.1, I)        (8.0, 0.4, A)
```

f. Lower extremity examination

```
                      3 3 3                        4 5
          1 2 3 4 5 6 7 8 9    1 2 3 4 5 6 7 8 9   ( 27- 28)
            (8.0, 0.7, A)        (9.0, 0.4, A)
```

g. Neck veins

```
                      1   1 2 5              1       4 4
          1 2 3 4 5 6 7 8 9    1 2 3 4 5 6 7 8 9   ( 29- 30)
            (9.0, 0.9, A)        (8.0, 0.8, A)
```

h. Heart rate

```
                          4 5                      3 6
          1 2 3 4 5 6 7 8 9    1 2 3 4 5 6 7 8 9   ( 31- 32)
            (9.0, 0.4, A)        (9.0, 0.3, A)
```

Scales: 1 = low validity or feasibility; 9 = high validity or feasibility

Validity   Feasibility

DIAGNOSIS, CONT.

4. Patients with a new diagnosis of heart
failure should be offered all of the
following studies within 1 month of the
diagnosis (unless performed within the prior
3 months):

a. Chest x-ray

```
                      1 4 1 3                 1 2 6
           1 2 3 4 5 6 7 8 9   1 2 3 4 5 6 7 8 9   ( 33- 34)
             (7.0, 0.9, A)        (9.0, 0.4, A)
```

b. EKG

```
                        3 2 4                   2 7
           1 2 3 4 5 6 7 8 9   1 2 3 4 5 6 7 8 9   ( 35- 36)
             (8.0, 0.8, A)        (9.0, 0.2, A)
```

c. Complete blood count

```
                      2 5   2                   2 2 5
           1 2 3 4 5 6 7 8 9   1 2 3 4 5 6 7 8 9   ( 37- 38)
             (7.0, 0.7, A)        (9.0, 0.7, A)
```

d. Serum sodium, potassium, and bicarbonate

```
                        4 2 3                 1 3 5
           1 2 3 4 5 6 7 8 9   1 2 3 4 5 6 7 8 9   ( 39- 40)
             (8.0, 0.8, A)        (9.0, 0.6, A)
```

e. Serum creatinine

```
                      1 4   4                   1 2 6
           1 2 3 4 5 6 7 8 9   1 2 3 4 5 6 7 8 9   ( 41- 42)
             (7.0, 1.0, A)        (9.0, 0.4, A)
```

f. Urinalysis

```
           1 1   3 3   1       1     1       3 4
           1 2 3 4 5 6 7 8 9   1 2 3 4 5 6 7 8 9   ( 43- 44)
             (4.0, 1.2, I)        (8.0, 1.7, A)
```

5. Patients with a diagnosis of heart
failure who are being treated with
medications for their heart failure should
have an evaluation of their ejection fraction
documented in the medical record.

```
             1     4 1 3       2   2 1   3     1
           1 2 3 4 5 6 7 8 9   1 2 3 4 5 6 7 8 9   ( 45- 46)
             (7.0, 1.0, A)        (5.0, 2.0, D)
```

6. Patients who are hospitalized for
symptoms of heart failure should have all of
the following elements of the physical
examination documented on the day of
hospitalization:

a. Weight

```
                      1 1 1 6                   1 2 6
           1 2 3 4 5 6 7 8 9   1 2 3 4 5 6 7 8 9   ( 47- 48)
             (9.0, 0.7, A)        (9.0, 0.4, A)
```

b. Blood pressure

```
                        2   7                   1 1 7
           1 2 3 4 5 6 7 8 9   1 2 3 4 5 6 7 8 9   ( 49- 50)
             (9.0, 0.4, A)        (9.0, 0.3, A)
```

c. Lung exam

```
                        3   6                   2 2 5
           1 2 3 4 5 6 7 8 9   1 2 3 4 5 6 7 8 9   ( 51- 52)
             (9.0, 0.7, A)        (9.0, 0.7, A)
```

d. Cardiac exam

```
                        3   6                   2 1 6
           1 2 3 4 5 6 7 8 9   1 2 3 4 5 6 7 8 9   ( 53- 54)
             (9.0, 0.7, A)        (9.0, 0.6, A)
```

e. Abdominal exam

```
                      1 1 3 3 1                 2 3 4
           1 2 3 4 5 6 7 8 9   1 2 3 4 5 6 7 8 9   ( 55- 56)
             (7.0, 0.9, A)        (8.0, 0.7, A)
```

f. Lower extremity examination

```
                        2 1 6                   1 1 7
           1 2 3 4 5 6 7 8 9   1 2 3 4 5 6 7 8 9   ( 57- 58)
             (9.0, 0.6, A)        (9.0, 0.3, A)
```

g. Neck veins

```
                      1   1 2 5             1   1 2 5
           1 2 3 4 5 6 7 8 9   1 2 3 4 5 6 7 8 9   ( 59- 60)
             (9.0, 0.9, A)        (9.0, 0.9, A)
```

h. Heart rate

```
                          4 5                   1 1 7
           1 2 3 4 5 6 7 8 9   1 2 3 4 5 6 7 8 9   ( 61- 62)
             (9.0, 0.4, A)        (9.0, 0.3, A)
```

Scales: 1 = low validity or feasibility; 9 = high validity or feasibility

DIAGNOSIS, CONT.

7. Patients who are hospitalized for heart
failure should have the following performed
within one day of hospitalization:

	2 3 4 2 2 5

a. Serum electrolytes
```
                    2 3 4              2 2 5
1 2 3 4 5 6 7 8 9   1 2 3 4 5 6 7 8 9   ( 63- 64)
   (8.0, 0.7, A)       (9.0, 0.7, A)
                    2 3 4              2 2 5
```
b. Serum creatinine
```
1 2 3 4 5 6 7 8 9   1 2 3 4 5 6 7 8 9   ( 65- 66)
   (8.0, 0.7, A)       (9.0, 0.7, A)
```

TREATMENT

8. Patients with a diagnosis of heart
failure who have an ejection fraction of less
than 40% and no contraindications to ACE
inhibitors should be receiving an ACE
inhibitor.
```
                      1   8              4 5
1 2 3 4 5 6 7 8 9   1 2 3 4 5 6 7 8 9   ( 67- 68)
   (9.0, 0.2, A)       (9.0, 0.4, A)
```

9. Patients with the diagnosis of heart
failure who are started on an ACE inhibitor
should have a potassium checked within 1 week
of starting the ACE inhibitor.
```
1   2   2   2 2     1       2 1 2 2 1
1 2 3 4 5 6 7 8 9   1 2 3 4 5 6 7 8 9   ( 69- 70)
   (5.0, 2.0, D)       (7.0, 1.7, I)
```

10. Patients with the diagnosis of heart
failure who are on an ACE inhibitor should
have the following checked every year:

a. Serum potassium
```
      1     1 3 2 2        1   1 3 4
1 2 3 4 5 6 7 8 9   1 2 3 4 5 6 7 8 9   ( 71- 72)
   (7.0, 1.2, A)       (8.0, 0.9, A)
```

b. Serum creatinine
```
      1     1 3 2 2        1   1 3 4
1 2 3 4 5 6 7 8 9   1 2 3 4 5 6 7 8 9   ( 73- 74)
   (7.0, 1.2, A)       (8.0, 0.9, A)
```

11. Patients with the diagnosis of heart
failure who are started on a diuretic should
have a potassium level checked within 1 week
of the start of treatment
```
1     1 1 2 1 1 2   1       1   2 4 1
1 2 3 4 5 6 7 8 9   1 2 3 4 5 6 7 8 9   ( 75- 76)
   (6.0, 1.9, I)       (8.0, 1.4, A)
```

12. Patients with the diagnosis of heart
failure in whom diuretic dose is increased
should have a potassium level checked within
1 week of the increase in dose
```
1 1 2   2 1 1 1     1       1 2 1 4
1 2 3 4 5 6 7 8 9   1 2 3 4 5 6 7 8 9   ( 77- 78)
   (5.0, 1.9, D)       (7.0, 1.6, I)
```

13. Patients with the diagnosis heart
failure and an ejection fraction of less than
40% who are not on ACE inhibitors should be
on hydralazine/nitrate, in the absence of
contraindications.
```
      2 1 2 2 2        1   5 1 2
1 2 3 4 5 6 7 8 9   1 2 3 4 5 6 7 8 9   ( 79- 80)
   (7.0, 1.2, I)       (7.0, 0.8, A)
```

14. Patients with a new diagnosis of heart
failure who are started on medical treatment
for heart failure should have dietary
counseling within 1 month of the start of
medical treatment
```
         4 3 2      1 2 1 3 2
1 2 3 4 5 6 7 8 9   1 2 3 4 5 6 7 8 9   ( 81- 82)
   (8.0, 0.7, A)       (8.0, 1.1, I)
```

Scales: 1 = low validity or feasibility; 9 = high validity or feasibility

Validity   Feasibility

FOLLOW-UP

15. Patients who have been hospitalized for
heart failure should have follow-up contact
within 4 weeks of discharge.

                              1 3 2 3   3 3 3
1 2 3 4 5 6 7 8 9   1 2 3 4 5 6 7 8 9   (83- 84)
(8.0, 0.9, A)   (8.0, 0.7, A)

16. Patients who have been hospitalized for
heart failure should have the following
physical examination elements performed
during the first post-discharge visit:

                               2 1 6   1 3 5

   a. Weight

1 2 3 4 5 6 7 8 9   1 2 3 4 5 6 7 8 9   (85- 86)
(9.0, 0.6, A)   (9.0, 0.6, A)
                               2 2 5   1 2 6

   b. Blood pressure

1 2 3 4 5 6 7 8 9   1 2 3 4 5 6 7 8 9   (87- 88)
(9.0, 0.7, A)   (9.0, 0.4, A)
                            1 1 3 4   2 3 4

   c. Lung exam

1 2 3 4 5 6 7 8 9   1 2 3 4 5 6 7 8 9   (89- 90)
(8.0, 0.8, A)   (8.0, 0.7, A)
                             2 3 4   1 4 4

   d. Cardiac exam

1 2 3 4 5 6 7 8 9   1 2 3 4 5 6 7 8 9   (91- 92)
(8.0, 0.7, A)   (8.0, 0.6, A)
                     1 1 2 3 2   1 1 4 3

   e. Abdominal exam

1 2 3 4 5 6 7 8 9   1 2 3 4 5 6 7 8 9   (93- 94)
(8.0, 1.2, A)   (8.0, 0.7, A)
                           1 1 2 5   1 3 5

   f. Lower extremity examination

1 2 3 4 5 6 7 8 9   1 2 3 4 5 6 7 8 9   (95- 96)
(9.0, 0.8, A)   (9.0, 0.6, A)
                     1 2 1 5   1   4 4

   g. Neck veins

1 2 3 4 5 6 7 8 9   1 2 3 4 5 6 7 8 9   (97- 98)
(9.0, 1.0, A)   (8.0, 0.8, A)
                           1 3 5   3 6

   h. Heart rate

1 2 3 4 5 6 7 8 9   1 2 3 4 5 6 7 8 9   (99-100)
(9.0, 0.6, A)   (9.0, 0.3, A)

17. Patients who have been hospitalized for
heart failure should have the following
laboratory tests performed within 4 weeks of
discharge:

                    1   4 1 1 1 1   1   1 1 4 2

   a. Creatinine

1 2 3 4 5 6 7 8 9   1 2 3 4 5 6 7 8 9   (101-102)
(4.0, 1.4, I)   (8.0, 1.3, A)
                    1   4 1 1 1 1   1   1 1 4 2

   b. Potassium

1 2 3 4 5 6 7 8 9   1 2 3 4 5 6 7 8 9   (103-104)
(4.0, 1.4, I)   (8.0, 1.3, A)

Scales: 1 = low validity or feasibility; 9 = high validity or feasibility

SCREENING

1."O" Men under age 75 with preexisting heart
disease who are not on pharmacological
therapy for hyperlipidemia should have total
cholesterol, HDL, and LDL levels documented
at least every 5 years.

```
              1 4 1 3              3 2 4
1 2 3 4 5 6 7 8 9  1 2 3 4 5 6 7 8 9  ( 1- 2)
   (7.0, 0.9, A)      (8.0, 0.8, A)
```

1."X" Women under age 75 with preexisting
heart disease who are not on pharmacological
therapy for hyperlipidemia should have total
cholesterol, HDL, and LDL levels documented
at least every 5 years.

```
              1 3 2 1 2              3 3 3
1 2 3 4 5 6 7 8 9  1 2 3 4 5 6 7 8 9  ( 3- 4)
   (7.0, 1.1, I)      (8.0, 0.7, A)
```

2."O" Men under age 75 with newly diagnosed
coronary disease should have had total
cholesterol, HDL, and LDL documented within 2
years before or within 4 months after the
diagnosis is first noted in the medical
record.

```
              3 3 3              2 3 4
1 2 3 4 5 6 7 8 9  1 2 3 4 5 6 7 8 9  ( 5- 6)
   (8.0, 0.7, A)      (8.0, 0.7, A)
```

2."X" Women under age 75 with newly diagnosed
coronary disease should have had total
cholesterol, HDL, and LDL documented within 2
years before or within 4 months after the
diagnosis is first noted in the medical
record.

```
              3 3 1 2              2 4 3
1 2 3 4 5 6 7 8 9  1 2 3 4 5 6 7 8 9  ( 7- 8)
   (7.0, 0.9, I)      (8.0, 0.6, A)
```

DIAGNOSIS

3."O" Men under age 75 with preexisting
coronary disease who have a total cholesterol
level exceeding 200 mg/dl should have a
measure of their LDL cholesterol documented
within 2 years before or 3 months after the
200 mg/dl level.

```
2 2 2 1         2 1  1       1 3 3
1 2 3 4 5 6 7 8 9  1 2 3 4 5 6 7 8 9  ( 9- 10)
   (3.0, 2.1, D)      (8.0, 1.8, D)
```

3."X" Women under age 75 with preexisting
coronary disease who have a total cholesterol
level exceeding 200 mg/dl should have a
measure of their LDL cholesterol documented
within 2 years before or 3 months after the
200 mg/dl level.

```
2 1 2 1  1      2 1  1       1 4 2
1 2 3 4 5 6 7 8 9  1 2 3 4 5 6 7 8 9  ( 11- 12)
   (3.0, 2.3, D)      (8.0, 1.7, D)
```

4. Patients without preexisting coronary
disease who are started on pharmacological
treatment for hyperlipidemia should have had
at least 2 measurements of their cholesterol
(total or LDL) documented in the year before
the start of pharmacological treatment.

```
              4 2 3              2 4 3
1 2 3 4 5 6 7 8 9  1 2 3 4 5 6 7 8 9  ( 13- 14)
   (8.0, 0.8, A)      (8.0, 0.6, A)
```

Scales: 1 = low validity or feasibility; 9 = high validity or feasibility

TREATMENT

5. "O" Men under age 75 with preexisting
coronary disease who have an untreated LDL
cholesterol level >130 mg/dl should begin
diet or drug therapy within 3 months of the   1   2 2 4   3 3 3
high LDL measurement.   1 2 3 4 5 6 7 8 9 1 2 3 4 5 6 7 8 9 (15- 16)
                                                (8.0, 1.0, A)   (8.0, 0.7, A)

5. "X" Women under age 75 with preexisting
coronary disease who have an untreated LDL
cholesterol level >130 mg/dl should begin
diet or drug therapy within 3 months of the   1   2 1 1 2 2   3 4 2
high LDL measurement.   1 2 3 4 5 6 7 8 9 1 2 3 4 5 6 7 8 9 (17- 18)
                                                (7.0, 1.7, I)   (8.0, 0.6, A)

6. "O" Men under age 75 with preexisting
coronary disease who have an LDL level >130
mg/dl after 6 months of dietary
cholesterol-lowering treatment should receive   4 3 2   3 4 2
pharmacological therapy for hyperlipidemia   1 2 3 4 5 6 7 8 9 1 2 3 4 5 6 7 8 9 (19- 20)
within 2 months of measurement.   (8.0, 0.7, A)   (8.0, 0.6, A)

6. "X" Women under age 75 with preexisting
coronary disease who have an LDL level >130
mg/dl after 6 months of dietary
cholesterol-lowering treatment should receive   1 1 2 1 3 1   3 5 1
pharmacological therapy for hyperlipidemia   1 2 3 4 5 6 7 8 9 1 2 3 4 5 6 7 8 9 (21- 22)
within 2 months of measurement.   (7.0, 1.3, I)   (8.0, 0.4, A)

FOLLOW-UP

7. Patients in whom pharmacological therapy
for hyperlipidemia has been initiated should
have their total cholesterol, HDL, and LDL   3 4 2   3 4 2
rechecked within 4 months.   1 2 3 4 5 6 7 8 9 1 2 3 4 5 6 7 8 9 (23- 24)
                                                (8.0, 0.6, A)   (8.0, 0.6, A)

8. Patients receiving pharmacological
therapy for hyperlipidemia who have had a
dosage or medication change should have total
cholesterol, HDL, and LDL rechecked within 4   1 3 3 2   1 2 4 2
months of the change.   1 2 3 4 5 6 7 8 9 1 2 3 4 5 6 7 8 9 (25- 26)
                                                (8.0, 0.8, A)   (8.0, 0.7, A)

Scales: 1 = low validity or feasibility; 9 = high validity or feasibility

DIAGNOSIS

2. All patients with average blood pressures
of >140 systolic and/or >90 diastolic as
determined on at least 3 separate visits
should have a diagnosis of hypertension   2 1 6   1 2 6
documented in the record.   1 2 3 4 5 6 7 8 9   1 2 3 4 5 6 7 8 9   (1- 2)
                                            (9.0, 0.6, A)   (9.0, 0.4, A)

INDICATORS ADDED AFTER ROUND 1

7. First-line treatment for Stage 1
hypertension is lifestyle modification. The
medical record should indicate counseling for
at least one of the following interventions
prior to initiating pharmacotherapy:

  - weight reduction if obese
  - increase physical activity if sedentary
  - low sodium diet   1 2 4 2   1   1 2 2 3
  - alcohol intake reduction if alcohol
    drinker   1 2 3 4 5 6 7 8 9   1 2 3 4 5 6 7 8 9   (3- 4)
                                            (8.0, 0.7, A)   (8.0, 1.2, A)

8. First-line treatment for Stage 2-3
hypertension is lifestyle modification. The
medical record should indicate counseling for
at least one of the following interventions
prior to initiating pharmacotherapy:

  - weight reduction if obese
  - increase physical activity if sedentary
  - low sodium diet   4 3 2   1   1 2 3 2
  - alcohol intake reduction if alcohol
    drinker   1 2 3 4 5 6 7 8 9   1 2 3 4 5 6 7 8 9   (5- 6)
                                            (8.0, 0.7, A)   (8.0, 1.2, A)

11. First-line pharmacotherarpy for diabetics   3 1   1 1 3   2   3 2 2
should include an ACE inhibitor, a calcium
channel blocker, or a thiazide diuretic. 1 2 3 4 5 6 7 8 9   1 2 3 4 5 6 7 8 9   (7- 8)
                                            (4.0, 2.0, I)   (7.0, 2.0, D)

Scales: 1 = low validity or feasibility; 9 = high validity or feasibility

INDICATORS ADDED AFTER ROUND 1

13. Patients who present with acute cough
should have the presence or absence of the
following items documentated at the time of
presentation:

                                              1 2 4 2   1 1 4 3
  a. cigarette smoking   1 2 3 4 5 6 7 8 9   1 2 3 4 5 6 7 8 9   (1- 2)
                                        (8.0, 0.7, A)   (8.0, 0.7, A)

  b. history of chronic cough or sputum   2   1 3 3   2 1 1 3 2
  production   1 2 3 4 5 6 7 8 9   1 2 3 4 5 6 7 8 9   (3- 4)
                                        (7.0, 1.3, D)   (8.0, 1.2, I)

  c. history of previous episodes of acute   2   1 2 2 1 1   1 1 1 1 3 2
  bronchitis in the prior year   1 2 3 4 5 6 7 8 9   1 2 3 4 5 6 7 8 9   (5- 6)
                                        (6.0, 1.6, D)   (8.0, 1.3, I)

9. Patients with nasal congestion and/or
cough, who do not have underlying lung
disease, should not be prescribed antibiotics
unless they have a concurrent diagnosis of   1   2 3 3   1 1   3 4
sinusitis or pneumonia.   1 2 3 4 5 6 7 8 9   1 2 3 4 5 6 7 8 9   (7- 8)
                                        (8.0, 0.9, A)   (8.0, 1.0, A)

Scales: 1 = low validity or feasibility; 9 = high validity or feasibility

APPENDIX B: CROSSWALK TABLE OF ORIGINAL AND FINAL INDICATORS

Chapter 1 - Asthma

	Indicator Proposed by Staff		Indicator Voted on by Panel	Comments/Disposition
Diagnosis				
1.	Patients with the diagnosis of moderate-to-severe asthma should have had some historical evaluation of asthma precipitants within six months (before or after) of diagnosis.	1.	Patients with the diagnosis of moderate-to-severe asthma should have had some historical evaluation of asthma precipitants within six months (before or after) of diagnosis.	INCLUDED BASED ON Q1 PANEL RATING
2.	Patients with the diagnosis of moderate-to-severe asthma should have baseline spirometry or peak flow performed within six months of diagnosis.	2.	Patients with the diagnosis of moderate-to-severe asthma should have baseline spirometry or peak flow performed within six months of diagnosis.	INCLUDED BASED ON Q1 PANEL RATING
3.	Spirometry should be measured in patients with chronic asthma at least every 2 years.	--	Spirometry should be measured in patients with chronic **moderate to severe** asthma at least every 2 years.	DROPPED due to low validity score
Treatment				
4.	Patients with the diagnosis of moderate-to-severe asthma should have been prescribed a beta2-agonist inhaler for symptomatic relief of exacerbations to use as needed.	3.	Patients with the diagnosis of moderate-to-severe asthma should have been prescribed a beta2-agonist inhaler for symptomatic relief of exacerbations to use as needed.	INCLUDED BASED ON Q1 PANEL RATING
5.	Patients who report using a beta2-agonist inhaler more than 3 times per day on a daily basis (not only during an exacerbation) should be prescribed a longer acting bronchodilator (theophylline) and/or an anti-inflammatory agent (inhaled corticosteroids, cromolyn).	4.	Patients who report using a $beta_2$-agonist inhaler more than 3 times per day on a daily basis (not only during an exacerbation) should be prescribed a longer acting bronchodilator (theophylline) and/or an anti-inflammatory agent (inhaled corticosteroids, cromolyn).	INCLUDED BASED ON Q1 PANEL RATING
6.	Patients with moderate-to-severe asthma should not receive beta-blocker medications (e.g., atenolol, propranolol).	5.	Patients with moderate-to-severe asthma should not receive beta-blocker medications (e.g., atenolol, propranolol).	INCLUDED BASED ON Q1 PANEL RATING
7.	Patients requiring chronic treatment with systemic corticosteroids during any 12 month period should have been prescribed inhaled corticosteroids during that same 12 month period.	6.	Patients requiring chronic treatment with systemic corticosteroids during any 12 month period should have been prescribed inhaled corticosteroids during that same 12 month period.	ACCEPTED

Indicator Proposed by Staff		Indicator Voted on by Panel		Comments/Disposition
8.	Patients on chronic theophylline (dose > 600 mg/day for at least 6 months) should have at least one serum theophylline level determination per year.	7.	Patients on chronic theophylline (dose > 600 mg/day for at least 6 months) should have at least one serum theophylline level determination per year.	INCLUDED BASED ON Q1 PANEL RATING
9.	Patients with the diagnosis of moderate-to-severe asthma should have a documented flu vaccination in the fall/winter of the previous year (September - January).	8.	Patients with the diagnosis of moderate-to-severe asthma should have a documented flu vaccination in the fall/winter of the previous year (September - January).	INCLUDED BASED ON Q1 PANEL RATING
Treatment of Exacerbations				
10.	All patients seen for an acute asthma exacerbation should be evaluated with a complete history including all of the following: a. time of onset, b. all current medications, c. prior hospitalizations and emergency department visits for asthma, d. prior episodes of respiratory insufficiency due to asthma.	9. -- a. b. c.	All patients seen for an acute asthma exacerbation should be evaluated with a complete history including all of the following: a. time ~~of~~ since onset **of symptoms**, b. all current medications, c. prior hospitalizations and emergency department visits for asthma, d. prior episodes of respiratory ~~insufficiency due to asthma~~ **failure requiring intubation.**	MODIFIED: Panelists felt that intubation is a more specific measure of severity. **"a" DROPPED due to low validity score.** Panelists felt this was not critical to determining treatment. **"b, c, d" ACCEPTED AS MODIFIED**
11.	Patients presenting to the physician's office with an asthma exacerbation or historical worsening of asthma symptoms should be evaluated with PEF or forced expiratory volume at 1 second (FEV_1).	10.	Patients presenting to the physician's office with an asthma exacerbation or historical worsening of asthma symptoms should be evaluated with PEF or forced expiratory volume at 1 second (FEV_1).	INCLUDED BASED ON Q1 PANEL RATING
12.	At the time of an exacerbation, patients on theophylline should have theophylline level measured.	11.	At the time of an exacerbation, patients on theophylline should have theophylline level measured.	INCLUDED BASED ON Q1 PANEL RATING
13.	A physical exam of the chest should be performed on patients presenting with an asthma exacerbation in the physician's office or emergency room.	12.	A physical exam of the chest should be performed on patients presenting with an asthma exacerbation in the physician's office or emergency room.	INCLUDED BASED ON Q1 PANEL RATING
14.	Patients presenting to the physician's office or ER with an FEV_1 or PEF < 70% of baseline should be treated with beta$_2$-agonists before discharge.	13.	Patients presenting to the physician's office or ER with an FEV_1 or PEF < 70% of baseline should be treated with beta$_2$-agonists before discharge.	INCLUDED BASED ON Q1 PANEL RATING
15.	Patients who receive treatment with beta$_2$-agonists in the physician's office or ER for FEV_1 < 70% of baseline should have an FEV_1 or PEF repeated prior to discharge.	14.	Patients who receive treatment with beta$_2$-agonists in the physician's office or ER for FEV_1 < 70% of baseline should have an FEV_1 or PEF repeated prior to discharge.	INCLUDED BASED ON Q1 PANEL RATING

Indicator Proposed by Staff		Indicator Voted on by Panel		Comments/Disposition
16.	Patients with an FEV1 or PEF < 70% of baseline after treatment for asthma exacerbation in the physician's office should be placed on an oral corticosteroid taper.	15.	Patients with an FEV$_1$ or PEF < 70% of baseline after treatment for asthma exacerbation in the physician's office should be placed on an oral corticosteroid taper.	INCLUDED BASED ON Q1 PANEL RATING
17.	Patients who have a PEF or FEV$_1$ < 40% of baseline after treatment with beta$_2$-agonists should not be discharged from the physician's office.	16.	Patients who have a PEF or FEV$_1$ < 40% of baseline after treatment with beta$_2$-agonists should not be discharged from the physician's office.	INCLUDED BASED ON Q1 PANEL RATING
Inpatient Diagnosis and Treatment				
18.	Patients admitted to the hospital for asthma exacerbation should have oxygen saturation measured.	17.	Patients admitted to the hospital for asthma exacerbation should have oxygen saturation measured.	INCLUDED BASED ON Q1 PANEL RATING
19.	Hospitalized patients should receive systemic steroids (either PO or IV).	18.	Hospitalized patients should receive systemic steroids (either PO or IV).	INCLUDED BASED ON Q1 PANEL RATING
20.	Hospitalized patients should receive treatment with beta$_2$-agonists.	19.	Hospitalized patients should receive treatment with beta$_2$-agonists.	INCLUDED BASED ON Q1 PANEL RATING
21.	Hospitalized patients with oxygen saturation < 90% should receive supplemental oxygen, unless pCO2 > 40 is previously documented.	20.	Hospitalized patients with oxygen saturation < 90% should receive supplemental oxygen, unless pCO$_2$ > 40 is previously documented.	INCLUDED BASED ON Q1 PANEL RATING
22.	Hospitalized patients with pCO$_2$ > 40 should receive at least one additional blood gas measurement to evaluate response to treatment, unless pCO$_2$ > 40 is previously documented.	21.	Hospitalized patients with pCO$_2$ > 40 should receive at least one additional blood gas measurement to evaluate response to treatment, unless pCO$_2$ > 40 is previously documented.	INCLUDED BASED ON Q1 PANEL RATING
23.	Hospitalized patients should not receive sedative drugs (e.g., anxiolytics), except if on a ventilator, physiologically dependent on sedatives, or in alcohol withdrawal.	22.	Hospitalized patients should not receive sedative drugs (e.g., anxiolytics), except if on a ventilator, physiologically dependent on sedatives, or in alcohol withdrawal.	INCLUDED BASED ON Q1 PANEL RATING
		23. (25)	**Asthmatic patients newly prescribed inhaled bronchodilaters should be concurrently given either a spacer device or instructions in proper use of an MDI.**	PROPOSED AND ACCEPTED BY Q2 PANEL. Indicator proposed in order to be consistent with Chapter 4 (COPD).
Follow-up				
24.	Patients with a hospitalization for asthma exacerbation should receive outpatient follow-up contact within 14 days.	24.	Patients with a hospitalization for asthma exacerbation should receive outpatient follow-up contact within 14 days.	INCLUDED BASED ON Q1 PANEL RATING

Indicator Proposed by Staff		Indicator Voted on by Panel	Comments/Disposition
	-- (26)	Patients with a new diagnosis of asthma should have documentation of counseling for self-management of asthma within one month of diagnosis.	**PROPOSED BY Q2 PANEL BUT DROPPED** due to disagreement on validity. Panelists felt that requiring documentation of counseling was troublesome.
	-- (27)	Patients who present with an exacerbation of asthma should have documentation of counseling for self-management: a. prior to discharge if hospitalized; or, b. at the time of presentation if not hospitalized.	**PROPOSED BY Q2 PANEL, BUT DROPPED** due to low validity score. Panelists felt that the indicator would not apply universally.

289

Chapter 2 - Atrial Fibrillation

	Indicator Proposed by Staff		Indicator Voted on by Panel	Comments/Disposition
Diagnosis				
1.	Patients presenting with new-onset atrial fibrillation or atrial fibrillation of unknown duration should have documentation of the following in the medical record at the time of presentation:	1.	Patients presenting with new-onset atrial fibrillation or atrial fibrillation of unknown duration should have documentation of the following in the medical record at the time of presentation:	ACCEPTED
	a. alcohol use; and	a.	a. alcohol use; and	
	b. stimulant drug use.	b.	b. stimulant drug use.	
2.	Patients presenting with new-onset atrial fibrillation or atrial fibrillation of unknown duration should have a thyroid stimulating hormone (TSH) level checked within the first week of presentation.	2.	Patients presenting with new-onset atrial fibrillation or atrial fibrillation of unknown duration should have a thyroid ~~stimulating hormone (TSH)~~ **function** level checked within the first **two** weeks of presentation.	MODIFIED: Panelists wanted to make the requirement more generic. ACCEPTED AS MODIFIED BY Q2
3.	Patients presenting with new-onset atrial fibrillation or atrial fibrillation of unknown duration should have a chest radiograph performed in the first 24 hours after presentation.	--	Patients presenting with new-onset atrial fibrillation or atrial fibrillation of unknown duration should have a chest radiograph ~~performed in the first 24 hours after presentation~~ **within one week of presentation.**	DROPPED due to low validity score. Panelists felt that chest x-rays do not change the course of treatment.
Treatment				
4.	Patients with atrial fibrillation of greater than 48 hours duration who do not have contraindications to warfarin should receive warfarin if they are:	3.	Patients with atrial fibrillation of greater than 48 hours duration **or of unknown duration** who do not have contraindications to warfarin should receive warfarin if they are:	MODIFIED: Panelists felt that the indicator should also apply if the duration is unknown. ACCEPTED AS MODIFIED BY Q2
	a. under 65 with one or more other risk factors for stroke or;	a.	a. **under 65 with one or more other risk factors for stroke; or**	
	b. 65 years of age or older.	b.	b. **65 years of age or older.**	
5.	Patients with chronic atrial fibrillation who have contraindications to warfarin or have declined warfarin therapy should receive aspirin if they are:	4.	Patients with chronic atrial fibrillation who have contraindications to warfarin or have declined warfarin therapy should receive aspirin if they are:	ACCEPTED
	a. under 65 with one or more other risk factors for stroke	a.	a. **under 65 with one or more other risk factors for stroke**	
	b. age 65 years or older.	b.	b. **age 65 years or older.**	

Indicator Proposed by Staff		Indicator Voted on by Panel		Comments/Disposition
6.	Patients with atrial fibrillation who do not have contraindications to warfarin should be started on warfarin within one month of presenting with either of the following: a. new onset ischemic or embolic stroke; or b. new onset transient ischemic attack.	5.	Patients with atrial fibrillation who do not have contraindications to warfarin should be started on warfarin ~~within one month of presenting with either of the following:~~ **within 2 weeks of presenting with new onset ischemic or embolic stroke.**	MODIFIED: Panelists split the indicator because they wanted different time frames for stroke and TIA. They felt that the one month time frame between symptoms and treatment was too long. ACCEPTED AS MODIFIED
		6. (6)	Patients with atrial fibrillation who do not have contraindications to warfarin should be started on warfarin ~~within one month of presenting with either of the following:~~ **within 1 week of presenting with new onset transient ischemic attack.**	MODIFIED: Panelists felt that warfarin should be started sooner with a diagnosis of TIA than with ischemic or embolic stroke. ACCEPTED AS MODIFIED
7.	Patients with atrial fibrillation of greater than 48 hours duration who are undergoing elective electrical or chemical cardioversion should receive anticoagulation for at least 3 weeks prior to cardioversion.	7.	Patients with atrial fibrillation of greater than 48 hours duration **or of unknown duration** who are undergoing elective electrical or chemical cardioversion should receive anticoagulation for at least 3 weeks prior to cardioversion **unless they have had a transesophageal echocardiogram within 24 hours of cardioversion that indicates no clot.**	MODIFIED: Panelists felt that the indicator should also apply if the duration is unknown. There is no need for anticoagulant therapy if patient has had a transesophageal echocardiogram with no clot. ACCEPTED AS MODIFIED
8.	All patients with atrial fibrillation should receive anticoagulation for at least 4 weeks after cardioversion unless there are contraindications to anticoagulation.	8.	All patients with atrial fibrillation **of greater than 48 hours or unknown duration** should receive anticoagulation for at least 4 weeks after cardioversion unless there are contraindications to anticoagulation.	MODIFIED: Panelists felt that the population should be the same as for indicator 7. ACCEPTED AS MODIFIED
Follow-up				
9.	Patients with atrial fibrillation started on warfarin should have an INR checked within 1 week of the first dose.	9.	Patients with atrial fibrillation started on warfarin should have an INR checked within 1 week of the first dose.	ACCEPTED
10.	Patients on warfarin should have an INR checked a minimum of every three months.	10.	Patients on warfarin should have an INR checked a minimum of every three months.	ACCEPTED

Chapter 3 - Cerebrovascular Disease

	Indicator Proposed by Staff		Indicator Voted on by Panel	Comments/Disposition
Diagnosis				
1.	Patients who receive thrombolytic therapy for treatment of acute stroke should receive a head CT or MRI after presenting with stroke and before initiation of thrombolytic treatment.	--	Patients who receive thrombolytic therapy for treatment of acute stroke should receive a head CT or MRI after presenting with stroke and before initiation of thrombolytic treatment.	**DROPPED due to disagreement on validity.** Panelists were concerned with lack of evidence to support this indicator.
2.	Patients who receive anticoagulant or antiplatelet therapy for treatment of acute stroke within 7 days of presentation should receive a head CT or MRI prior to the initiation of anticoagulant or antiplatelet treatment.	1.	Patients who receive anticoagulant or antiplatelet therapy for treatment of acute stroke within 7 days of presentation should receive a head CT or MRI prior to the initiation of anticoagulant or antiplatelet treatment.	ACCEPTED
Treatment				
3.	Patients newly diagnosed with a stroke or TIA who are not already on antiplatelet or antithrombotic treatment should be started on antiplatelet therapy or antithrombotic therapy within 1 month of the diagnosis unless a contraindication is documented.	2.	Patients newly diagnosed with a stroke or TIA ~~who are not already on antiplatelet or antithrombotic treatment~~ **without a known cardiac source** should be started on antiplatelet therapy ~~or antithrombotic therapy~~ within 1 ~~month~~ **week** of the diagnosis unless a contraindication is documented.	MODIFIED: Panelists felt that antithrombolitic therapy is not a substitute for antiplatelet therapy, which should be done in any case, unless contraindicated. ACCEPTED AS MODIFIED
4.	Patients with a documented history of stroke or TIA should be on daily antiplatelet or antithrombotic treatment, unless a contraindication to antithrombotic treatment is documented.	3.	Patients with a documented history of stroke or TIA **without a known cardiac source** should be on daily antiplatelet ~~or antithrombotic~~ treatment, unless a contraindication to ~~antithrombotic treatment~~ is documented.	MODIFIED: Panelists felt that antithrombolitic therapy is not a substitute for antiplatelet therapy, which should be done in any case, unless contraindicated. ACCEPTED AS MODIFIED
5.	Patients presenting for care with carotid artery symptoms who are diagnosed with TIA or stroke should have a carotid artery imaging study within 6 months before or 1 month after the event, unless the medical record documents, in the same time period, that the patient is not a candidate for carotid surgery.	4.	Patients presenting for care with carotid artery symptoms who are diagnosed with TIA or stroke should have a carotid artery imaging study within 6 months before or 1 month after the event, unless the medical record documents, in the same time period, that the patient is not a candidate for carotid surgery.	ACCEPTED

Indicator Proposed by Staff	Indicator Voted on by Panel	Comments/Disposition
6. Patients presenting for care with carotid artery symptoms, who are diagnosed with TIA and have carotid imaging evidence of >=70% stenosis on the side corresponding to the symptoms, should receive endarterectomy or referral for endarterectomy within 2 weeks of the diagnostic study.	5. Patients presenting for care with carotid artery symptoms, who are diagnosed with TIA and have carotid imaging evidence of >=70% stenosis on the side corresponding to the symptoms, should receive endarterectomy or referral for endarterectomy or revascularization within 2 6 weeks of the diagnostic study unless there are contraindications.	MODIFIED: Panelists wanted to make to measure treatment rather than referral. ACCEPTED AS MODIFIED
	6. (9) Patients admitted with a newly diagnosed stroke should have an assessment of the following prior to discharge: a. functional status; and b. swallowing.	PROPOSED AND ACCEPTED BY Q2 PANEL. Panelists felt that functional status and swallowing are easy tests for patients sick enough to be hospitalized.
	7. (10) Patients presenting with a new diagnosis of stroke or TIA should have a neurological examination at the time of presentation.	PROPOSED AND ACCEPTED BY Q2 PANEL. Panelists felt that a neurological exam is important for treatment decisions.
Follow-up		
7. Patients who smoke and present with TIA but are not hospitalized should be counseled to stop smoking at the time they present with TIA.	8. Patients who smoke and present with TIA or stroke but are not hospitalized should be counseled to stop smoking at the time they present with TIA or stroke.	MODIFIED: Panelists felt that the indicator applies equally well to stroke patients. ACCEPTED AS MODIFIED
8. Patients who smoke and are admitted to the hospital with a TIA should be counseled to stop smoking before hospital discharge.	9. Patients who smoke and are admitted to the hospital with a TIA or stroke should be counseled to stop smoking before hospital discharge.	MODIFIED: Panelists felt that the indicator applies equally well to stroke patients. ACCEPTED AS MODIFIED

Chapter 4 - Chronic Obstructive Pulmonary Disease (COPD)

Indicator Proposed by Staff		Indicator Voted on by Panel		Comments/Disposition
Diagnosis				
1. A smoking history should be documented on the same day in patients who present with a new complaint of any of the following: a. chronic cough (> 3 weeks duration); b. shortness of breath; or c. dyspnea on exertion.	1. a. b. c.	A smoking history should be documented on the same day in patients who present with a new complaint of any of the following: a. **chronic cough (> 3 weeks duration);** b. **shortness of breath; or** c. **dyspnea on exertion.**	ACCEPTED
2. A lung exam should be documented same day in patients who present with a new complaint of any of the following: a. chronic cough (> 3 weeks duration); b. shortness of breath; or c. dyspnea on exertion.	2. a. b. c.	A lung exam should be documented on the same day in patients who present with a new complaint of any of the following: a. **chronic cough (> 3 weeks duration);** b. **shortness of breath; or** c. **dyspnea on exertion.**	MODIFIED: Corrected typo. **ACCEPTED AS MODIFIED**
3. COPD patients on bronchodilator therapy should have spirometry performed with and without bronchodilation within 3 months of initiation of therapy, unless spirometry was performed in the previous 12 months.	3.	COPD patients on bronchodilator therapy **who have not had spirometry in the previous 12 months** should have spirometry performed with ~~and without bronchodilation within 3 months of~~ ~~initiation of therapy, unless spirometry was~~ **after initiation of therapy,** ~~performed in the previous 12 months.~~	MODIFIED: Panelists clarified wording and time frame. They felt that the "with and without bronchodilation" should not be required. **ACCEPTED AS MODIFIED**
4. COPD patients on bronchodilator therapy should have one of the following tests within 6 months before or after initiation of therapy: • Hemoglobin; • hematocrit; • CBC; • ABG; or • pulse oximetry.	--	COPD patients on bronchodilator therapy should have one of the following tests within 6 months before or after initiation of therapy: • Hemoglobin; • hematocrit; • CBC; • ABG; or • pulse oximetry.	DROPPED due to low validity score. Panelists felt that the indicator overlapped with indicator 5. Also, the eligible population is not clearly defined.

294

Indicator Proposed by Staff		Indicator Voted on by Panel	Comments/Disposition
5. COPD patients should have an ABG performed within 3 months of any of the following findings, unless hypoxemia (PaO_2 < 55) has been previously documented or the patient is already on chronic O_2 therapy: a. laboratory detection of erythrocytosis (Hct >55); b. notation of cyanosis or cor pulmonale in the medical record; and c. detection of FEV_1 < 1 liter on spirometric evaluation.	4. a. b. c.	COPD patients should have an ABG or pulse oximetry performed within 3 months of any of the following findings, unless hypoxemia (PaO_2 < 55) has been previously documented or the patient is already on chronic O_2 therapy: a. laboratory detection of erythrocytosis (Hct >55); b. notation of cyanosis or cor pulmonale in the medical record; and c. detection of FEV_1 < 1 liter on spirometric evaluation.	MODIFIED: Panelists felt that either test is adequate to document hypoxemia. ACCEPTED AS MODIFIED
	-- (21)	Asymptomatic smokers should receive spirometry within one year of notation of 40 or more pack/years of cigarette use.	PROPOSED BY Q2 PANEL BUT DROPPED due to low validity score. Panelists thought this indicator was not consistent with ACP guidelines.
Treatment			
6. Newly diagnosed COPD patients should be counseled or referred for smoking cessation within 3 months before or after of the new diagnosis of COPD.	5.	Newly diagnosed COPD patients **who smoke** should be counseled or referred for smoking cessation within 3 months before or after of the new diagnosis of COPD.	MODIFIED: Panelists clarified that this indicator applies only to smokers. ACCEPTED AS MODIFIED
7. All patients receiving pharmacologic treatment for COPD symptoms (including daily theophylline or non-PRN beta-agonists) should also be receiving ipratopium, unless intolerance is documented.	6.	All patients receiving **regular bronchodilator** pharmacologic treatment for COPD symptoms ~~(including daily theophylline or non-PRN beta-agonists)~~ should also be receiving ipratopium, unless intolerance is documented.	MODIFIED: Panelists clarified wording with focus on regular treatment. ACCEPTED AS MODIFIED
8. Patients newly prescribed inhaled bronchodilaters should be concurrently offered either a spacer device or instructions in proper use of a MDI.	7.	Patients newly prescribed inhaled bronchodilaters should be concurrently ~~offered~~ **given** either a spacer device or instructions in proper use of an MDI.	MODIFIED: Panelists strengthened the wording of the indicator, but still wanted to allow for patient refusal. ACCEPTED AS MODIFIED
9. COPD patients should have a theophylline level checked within 1 week of either initiation or increase of theophylline dose.	8.	COPD patients should have a theophylline level checked within 1 week of either initiation or increase of theophylline dose.	ACCEPTED

Indicator Proposed by Staff		Indicator Voted on by Panel	Comments/Disposition
10. In patients receiving theophylline, both of the following should occur when serum theophylline level exceeds 20 μg/ml: a. The dose should be modified within 1 day of the measurement; and b. Re-testing of level should be performed within one week, unless theophylline was stopped.	9. a. b.	In patients receiving theophylline, both of the following should occur when serum theophylline level exceeds 20 μg/ml: a. **The dose should be modified within 1 day of the measurement; and** b. **Re-testing of level should be performed within one week, unless theophylline was stopped.**	ACCEPTED
11. COPD patients should be offered home oxygen if their baseline room air oxygen saturation is < 88% at rest (not during an exacerbation).	10.	COPD patients should ~~be offered~~ receive home oxygen if their baseline room air oxygen saturation is < 88% at rest (not during an exacerbation).	MODIFIED: Panelists strengthened the wording of the indicator. **ACCEPTED AS MODIFIED**
Treatment: Management of Acute Exacerbation			
12. The following items should be documented in the medical record at the time of a COPD exacerbation a. Outpatient COPD medications; b. Information on prior hospitalizations, urgent care, or ED visits for COPD (e.g., time of most recent visit or number per year); c. Presence or absence of new cough: d. Vital signs, including respiratory rate, pulse, temperature, and blood pressure; and, e. A physical examination of the chest	11. a. b. c. d. e.	The following items should be documented in the medical record at the time of a COPD exacerbation a. Outpatient COPD medications; b. Information on prior hospitalizations, urgent care, or ED visits for COPD (e.g., time of most recent visit or number per year); c. Presence or absence of new cough: d. Vital signs, including respiratory rate, pulse, temperature, and blood pressure; and, e. A physical examination of the chest	ACCEPTED
13. Patients admitted to the hospital for an exacerbation of COPD who have a history of coronary disease should have an EKG performed within 24 hours of admission.	12.	Patients admitted to the hospital for an exacerbation of COPD who have a history of coronary disease should have an EKG performed within 24 hours of admission.	ACCEPTED

Indicator Proposed by Staff	Indicator Voted on by Panel	Comments/Disposition
14. A theophylline level should be obtained for patients on theophylline who meet any of the following conditions: a. Present with an exacerbation of COPD; and b. Are hospitalized with an exacerbation of COPD.	13. A theophylline level should be obtained for patients on theophylline who meet any of the following conditions: a. Present with an exacerbation of COPD; and b. Are hospitalized with an exacerbation of COPD.	ACCEPTED
15. COPD patients who present with an exacerbation should be offered inhaled bronchodilator therapy if their respiratory rate is >24.	-- COPD patients who present with an exacerbation should be offered receive inhaled bronchodilator therapy if their respiratory rate is >24.	DROPPED due to low validity score. Panelists felt that respiratory rate is not measured well in practice.
16. Patients presenting with COPD exacerbation should have oxygen administered if the oxygen saturation is <88% or PO2 is <55 mm Hg.	14. Patients presenting with COPD exacerbation should have oxygen administered if the oxygen saturation is <88% or PO2 is <55 mm Hg.	ACCEPTED
17. Patients presenting with COPD exacerbation should be offered admission to the hospital if any of the following conditions are documented in the medical record on the date of presentation: a. Acute Ischemia; b. Pneumonia; or c. Significant hypoxemia (saturation <88%, or PaO2 <55 mm Hg on room air in patients not on home oxygen).	15. Patients presenting with COPD exacerbation should be offered admission admitted to the hospital if any of the following conditions are documented in the medical record on the date of presentation: a. Acute Ischemia; -- b. Pneumonia; or -- c. Significant hypoxemia (saturation <88%, or PaO2 <55 mm Hg on room air in patients not on home oxygen).	MODIFIED: Panelists wanted to strengthen wording. "a" ACCEPTED AS MODIFIED "b" DROPPED due to low validity score. "c" DROPPED due to disagreement on validity. Panelists were concerned about lack of evidence for hospitalization. Also, the applicable population is small.

Indicator Proposed by Staff		Indicator Voted on by Panel	Comments/Disposition
18. Patients hospitalized with a COPD exacerbation should be admitted to a monitored setting (that includes access to pulse oximetry and telemetry) while any of the following are present:	16.	Patients hospitalized with a COPD exacerbation should be admitted to a ~~monitored setting (that includes access to pulse oximetry and telemetry)~~ critical care bed while any of the following are present:	MODIFIED: Panelists felt that "monitored setting" was ambiguous. The patient needs to have immediate access to mechanical ventilation. "c" was modified to clarify definition of hypoxemia.
a. Severe dyspnea (breathing rate > 35 with accessory muscle use) despite initial therapeutic measures;	a.	a. Severe dyspnea (breathing rate > 35 with accessory muscle use) despite initial therapeutic measures;	ACCEPTED AS MODIFIED
b. Confusion or lethargy;	b.	b. Confusion or lethargy;	
c. Persistent or worsening hypoxemia (pO2 < 60 with FiO2 > 40%); or	c.	c. ~~Persistent or worsening~~ Severe hypoxemia ~~despite supplemental~~ oxygen (pO2 < 60 with FiO2 > 40%); or	
d. Severe respiratory acidosis (pH < 7.3).	d.	d. Severe respiratory acidosis (pH < 7.3).	
19. COPD patients hospitalized for an exacerbation should be discharged on home oxygen if the last documented oxygen saturation prior to discharge is <88%.	17.	COPD patients hospitalized for an exacerbation should be discharged on home oxygen if the last documented oxygen saturation prior to discharge is <88%.	ACCEPTED
20. Patients with a diagnosis of COPD who present with a COPD exacerbation and whose last documented oxygen saturation during the exacerbation visit is < 88% should either be hospitalized or discharged on home oxygen treatment.	18.	Patients with a diagnosis of COPD who present with a COPD exacerbation and whose last documented oxygen saturation during the exacerbation visit is < 88% or pO$_2$ is <55 should either be hospitalized or discharged on home oxygen treatment.	MODIFIED: Panelists felt that 0$_2$ saturation and pO$_2$ can be substituted for each other in diagnosis. ACCEPTED AS MODIFIED

298

Chapter 5 - Cigarette Counseling

	Indicator Proposed by Staff		Indicator Voted on by Panel	Comments/Disposition
Screening				
1.	Smoking status should be documented at least once for all patients.	1.	Smoking status should be documented at least once for all patients.	**INCLUDED BASED ON Q1 PANEL RATING**
2.	Patients documented to be smokers should have their smoking status indicated on at least 50% of all non-emergency visits.	2.	Patients documented to be smokers should have their smoking status indicated on ~~at least 50% of all non-emergency~~ office visits.	MODIFIED: Wording changed to strengthen indicator. The definition of "office visits" includes face-to-face contact with a clinician, not including emergency or lab visits. **ACCEPTED AS MODIFIED**
Treatment				
3.	There should be documentation that advice to quit smoking was given to all smokers at least once during the course of a year.	3.	There should be documentation that advice to quit smoking was given to all smokers at least once during the course of a year.	**INCLUDED BASED ON Q1 PANEL RATING**
4.	All smokers identified as attempting to quit should be offered at least one additional smoking cessation counseling visit within 3 months.	4.	All smokers identified as attempting to quit should be offered at least one additional smoking cessation counseling visit within 3 months.	**ACCEPTED**
5.	All smokers attempting to quit who smoke more than 5 cigarettes a day should be offered nicotine replacement therapy except in the presence of serious medical precautions.	5.	All smokers attempting to quit who smoke more than ~~5~~ 10 cigarettes a day should be offered nicotine replacement therapy except in the presence of serious medical precautions.	MODIFIED: The evidence for nicotine replacement therapy is more compelling for heavier smokers. **ACCEPTED AS MODIFIED**
Follow-up				
6.	All patients who receive a smoking cessation intervention should have their abstinence status documented within 2 weeks of the completion of treatment.	6.	All patients who receive a smoking cessation intervention should have their abstinence status documented within ~~2~~ 4 weeks of the completion of treatment.	MODIFIED: Panelists felt two weeks was too short. **ACCEPTED AS MODIFIED**

Chapter 6 - Community Acquired Pneumonia

	Indicator Proposed by Staff		Indicator Voted on by Panel	Comments/Disposition
Diagnosis				
1.	If patient has symptoms of pneumonia, on the day of admission the provider should document:	1.	If a patient ~~has symptoms of~~ **is diagnosed with** pneumonia, on the day of ~~admission~~ **diagnosis** the provider should document:	MODIFIED: Panelists felt that because the documentation of symptoms varies it is more feasible to apply this indicator to diagnosed patients.
a.	whether the cough is productive or nonproductive;	a.	**whether the cough is productive or nonproductive;**	"a, c" DROPPED due to low validity score. Panelists did not think that these symptoms would change treatment.
b.	The presence or absence of a coexisting illness; and	b.	**The presence or absence of a coexisting illness; and**	"b" ACCEPTED AS MODIFIED
c.	the presence or absence of recent upper respiratory symptoms.	c.	**the presence or absence of recent upper respiratory symptoms.**	
2.	If patient has symptoms of pneumonia, the following should be documented on the day of presentation:	2.	If a patient ~~has symptoms~~ **a diagnosis** of pneumonia, the following should be documented on the day of presentation:	MODIFIED: Panelists felt that because the documentation of symptoms varies it is more feasible to apply this indicator to diagnosed patients.
a.	temperature;	a.	**temperature;**	
b.	respiratory rate;	b.	**respiratory rate;**	
c.	heart rate; and	c.	**heart rate; and**	ACCEPTED AS MODIFIED
d.	lung examination.	d.	**lung examination.**	
3.	If a patient has both symptoms and signs of pneumonia, the health care provider should offer a chest radiograph (CXR) on the day of presentation.	3.	If a patient has ~~both symptoms and signs~~ **a diagnosis** of pneumonia, the health care provider should offer a chest radiograph (CXR) on the day of presentation.	MODIFIED: Panelists felt that because the documentation of symptoms varies it is more feasible to apply this indicator to diagnosed patients. ACCEPTED AS MODIFIED
4.	If a patient has both symptoms and signs of pneumonia and suggestion of a pleural effusion on CXR a lateral decubitus radiograph or ultrasound should be offered on the day of presentation to assess the size of the effusion.	4.	If a patient has ~~both symptoms and signs~~ **a diagnosis** of pneumonia and suggestion of a pleural effusion on CXR, a lateral decubitus radiograph, ~~or~~ ultrasound , **or thorocentesis** should be ~~offered~~ **performed** on the day of presentation ~~to assess the size of the effusion.~~	MODIFIED: Panelists felt that because the documentation of symptoms varies it is more feasible to apply this indicator to diagnosed patients. Panelists also indicated that thorocentesis is acceptable. ACCEPTED AS MODIFIED
5.	If a patient over 60 years of age has both symptoms and signs of pneumonia with coexisting illness, the health care provider should offer the following blood tests on the day of presentation:	5.	~~If a~~ **Patients** over ~~60~~ **65** years of age **or with coexisting illness, and a diagnosis** ~~has both symptoms and signs~~ of pneumonia ~~with coexisting illness, the health care provider~~ should ~~offer~~ **receive** the following blood tests on the day of presentation:	MODIFIED: Panelists felt that because the documentation of symptoms varies it is more feasible to apply this indicator to diagnosed patients. They also preferred a higher age cut-off and indicated that either a hemoglobin or hematocrit would be acceptable.
a.	white blood cell count;	a.	**white blood cell count;**	"a, d" ACCEPTED AS MODIFIED
b.	hemoglobin and hematocrit;	b.	**hemoglobin and or hematocrit;**	"b" DROPPED due to low validity score
c.	serum electrolytes; and	c.	**serum electrolytes; and**	"c" DROPPED due to low validity score.
d.	BUN or creatinine.	d.	**BUN or creatinine.**	Panelists were concerned about the lack of evidence on electrolytes.

6.	If patient has both symptoms and signs of pneumonia, and is hospitalized, the health care provider should offer two sets of blood cultures on the day of hospitalization.	~~If~~ Patients ~~has both symptoms and signs of pneumonia, and is hospitalized,~~ for pneumonia, ~~the health care provider should offer~~ receive two sets of blood cultures on the day of hospitalization.	DROPPED due to low validity score Panelists felt that the cost was not justified for an unproved benefit.
7.	Hospitalized persons with pneumonia should have the following documented on the first and second days of hospitalization: a. temperature; and b. lung examination.	Hospitalized persons with pneumonia should have the following documented on the first and second days of hospitalization: a. temperature; and b. lung examination.	ACCEPTED
7. (14)		**Patients with pneumonia with a new effusion >=10mm on lateral decubitus radiograph or ultrasound, and an ipsilateral infiltrate, should have a thoracentesis on the day the effusion is noted.**	PROPOSED AND ACCEPTED BY Q2 PANEL Panelists wanted to ensure treatment of significant effusions.
Treatment			
8.	Non-hospitalized persons <= 60 years of age diagnosed with pneumonia without a known bacteriologic etiology and without coexisting illnesses should be offered an oral empiric macrolide, unless allergic.	Non-hospitalized persons <= ~~60~~ **65** years of age diagnosed with pneumonia without a known bacteriologic etiology and without coexisting illnesses should be offered an oral empiric macrolide, unless allergic.	MODIFIED: Panelists preferred a higher age cut-off. ACCEPTED AS MODIFIED
9.	Non-hospitalized persons > 60 years of age diagnosed with pneumonia without a known bacteriologic etiology and with coexisting illnesses should be offered one of the following oral empiric antibiotic regimens: • a second generation cephalosporin; • trimethoprim-sulfamethoxazole; or • a beta-lactam/beta-lactamase inhibitor combination.	Non-hospitalized persons > ~~60~~ **65** years of age diagnosed with pneumonia without a known bacteriologic etiology ~~and~~ **or** with coexisting illnesses should be offered one of the following oral empiric antibiotic regimens: • a second generation cephalosporin; • trimethoprim-sulfamethoxazole; or • a beta-lactam/beta-lactamase inhibitor combination.	MODIFIED: Panelists preferred a higher age cut-off. ACCEPTED AS MODIFIED

301

Indicator Proposed by Staff		Indicator Voted on by Panel	Comments/Disposition
10. Hospitalized persons with non-severe pneumonia without a known bacteriologic etiology should be offered one of the following empiric antibiotic regimens: • a second or third generation cephalosporin; or • a beta-lactam/beta-lactamase inhibitor combination.	10.	Hospitalized persons with non-severe pneumonia without a known bacteriologic etiology should be offered one of the following empiric antibiotic regimens: • a second or third generation cephalosporin; or • a beta-lactam/beta-lactamase inhibitor combination.	ACCEPTED
11. Hospitalized persons with severe pneumonia without a known bacteriologic etiology should be offered one of the following antibiotic regimens: • a macrolide and a third generation cephalosporin with anti-Pseudomonas activity; or • a macrolide and another anitpseudomonal agent such as imipenem/ciliastin, ciprofloxacin.	11.	Hospitalized persons with severe pneumonia without a known bacteriologic etiology should be offered one of the following antibiotic regimens: • a macrolide and a third generation cephalosporin with anti-Pseudomonas activity; or • a macrolide and another anitpseudomonal agent such as imipenem/ciliastin, ciprofloxacin.	ACCEPTED
12. Persons with CAP should be offered antibiotics for 10-14 days, with the exception of azithromycin, which may be given for 5 days.	--	Persons with CAP should be offered antibiotics for 10-14 days, with the exception of azithromycin, which may be given for 5 days.	DROPPED due to low validity score. Panelists were concerned with the lack of evidence.
Follow-up			
13. Persons who have been hospitalized for pneumonia should have an appointment with a provider within 6 weeks after discharge.	12.	Persons ~~who have been hospitalized~~ treated for pneumonia should have an ~~appointment~~ follow-up contact with a provider within 6 weeks after discharge **or diagnosis.**	MODIFIED: Intent is to make sure the patient is improving. ACCEPTED AS MODIFIED

302

Chapter 7 - Coronary Artery Disease: Diagnosis and Screening

Indicator Proposed by Staff		Indicator Voted on by Panel		Comments/Disposition
With or without symptoms of CAD				
1. Patients 40-75 years old who have a high risk stress test should be offered coronary angiography within 4 weeks of the stress test (unless they have contraindications to revascularization or have had coronary angiography within 2 years prior to the stress test).	1.	Patients 40-75 years old who have a high risk stress test should be offered coronary angiography within ~~4 weeks~~ **6 weeks** of the stress test (unless they have contraindications to revascularization or ~~have had coronary angiography within 2 years of the stress test~~).		MODIFIED: Panelists felt that a high risk stress test would warrant angiography even if one had been done 1 or 2 years before. **ACCEPTED AS MODIFIED**
	-- (1)	Patients > 75 years old who have a high risk stress test should be offered coronary angiography within ~~4 weeks~~ **6 weeks** of the stress test (unless they have contraindications to revascularization or ~~have had coronary angiography within 2 years of the stress test~~).		**Panel considered indicator for patients > 75 but DROPPED due to low validity score.** Panelists felt that the benefits were less clear for older patients.
2. Patients 40-75 years old who have two or more CAD risk factors and a newly diagnosed low LVEF (<= 0.45) should be offered stress testing or coronary angiography within 3 months of the diagnosis of low LVEF (unless an etiology of LV dysfunction other than CAD is documented in the medical record or they have contraindications to revascularization or they have had stress testing or coronary angiography within the 2 years prior to the diagnosis of low LVEF).	--	Patients 40-75 years old who have two or more CAD risk factors and a newly diagnosed low LVEF (<= 0.45 <=**40%**) should be offered stress testing or coronary angiography within 3 months of the diagnosis of low LVEF (unless an etiology of LV dysfunction other than CAD is documented in the medical record or they have contraindications to revascularization ~~or they have had stress testing or coronary angiography within the 2 years prior to the diagnosis of low LVEF~~).		**DROPPED due to low validity score.** Panelists felt that the benefits of treatment were unclear. They were also concerned about the lack of evidence.
	-- (2)	Patients > 75 years old who have two or more CAD risk factors and a newly diagnosed low LVEF (<= 0.45 <=**40%**) should be offered stress testing or coronary angiography within 3 months of the diagnosis of low LVEF (unless an etiology of LV dysfunction other than CAD is documented in the medical record or they have contraindications to revascularization ~~or they have had stress testing or coronary angiography within the 2 years prior to the diagnosis of low LVEF~~).		**Panel considered indicator for patients > 75 but DROPPED due to low validity score.**

303

Indicator Proposed by Staff		Indicator Voted on by Panel	Comments/Disposition
3. Patients 40-75 years old who have an ejection fraction <= 0.45 and a positive stress test should be offered coronary angiography within 4 weeks of the stress test (unless they have contraindications to revascularization or have had coronary angiography within 2 years of the stress test).	2.	Patients 40-75 years old who have an ejection fraction <= 0.45 <=40% and a positive stress test should be offered coronary angiography within 4 weeks of the stress test (unless they have contraindications to revascularization or have had coronary angiography within 2 years of the stress test).	MODIFIED: Panelists felt that a positive stress test and low EF test would warrant angiography even if one had been done 1 or 2 years before. LVEF <= 40% is clinically conservative and more appropriate for a quality indicator. ACCEPTED AS MODIFIED
	-- (3)	Patients >75 years who have an ejection fraction <= 0.45 <=40% and a positive stress test should be offered coronary angiography within 4 weeks of the stress test (unless they have contraindications to revascularization or have had coronary angiography within 2 years of the stress test).	Panel considered indicator for patients > 75 but DROPPED due to low validity.
Stable Angina or known CAD			
4. Patients < 75 years old with newly diagnosed CAD should have a 12-lead ECG within 3 months of diagnosis.	3.	Patients <75 years old with newly diagnosed CAD should have a 12-lead ECG within 3 months at the time of diagnosis	MODIFIED: Panelists felt the indicator applied regardless of age. ACCEPTED AS MODIFIED
5. Patients <75 years old with any of the conditions listed below should have a hemoglobin and/or hematocrit measured within 1 week of diagnosis: a. Angina; b. unstable angina, or c. MI.	4. a. b. c.	Patients <75 years old newly diagnosed with any of the conditions listed below should have a hemoglobin and/or hematocrit measured at the time of diagnosis: a. Angina; b. unstable angina, or c. MI.	MODIFIED: Panelists felt the indicator applied regardless of age. ACCEPTED AS MODIFIED
6. Patients 40-75 years old newly diagnosed with stable angina or CAD should be offered stress testing or coronary angiography within 3 months of the diagnosis (unless they have contraindications to revascularization).	--	Patients 40-75 < 75 years old newly diagnosed with stable angina or CAD should be offered stress testing or coronary angiography within 3 months of the diagnosis (unless they have contraindications to revascularization).	DROPPED due to disagreement on validity. Panelists felt that evidence of benefit was lacking.

304

Indicator Proposed by Staff		Indicator Voted on by Panel		Comments/Disposition
(6)	Patients >=75 years old newly diagnosed with stable angina or CAD should be offered stress testing or coronary angiography within 3 months of the diagnosis (unless they have contraindications to revascularization).	--	Patients >=75 years old newly diagnosed with stable angina or CAD should be offered stress testing or coronary angiography within 3 months of the diagnosis (unless they have contraindications to revascularization).	Panel considered indicator for patients >= 75 but DROPPED due to low validity score.
Unstable Angina				
7.	Patients < 75 years old being evaluated for "unstable angina" or "rule out unstable angina" should have an examination at the time of evaluation documenting all of the following: a. temperature; b. blood pressure; c. heart rate; d. heart exam; e. lung exam, and f. a 12-lead ECG.	5.	Patients ~~< 75 years old~~ being evaluated for "unstable angina" or "rule out unstable angina" should have an examination at the time of evaluation documenting all of the following: a. temperature; b. blood pressure; c. heart rate; d. heart exam; e. lung exam, and f. a 12-lead ECG.	MODIFIED: Panelists felt the indicator applied regardless of age. "a" DROPPED due to low validity score. Panelists felt there was no evidence for temperature as an indicator. "b-f" ACCEPTED AS MODIFIED
8.	Patients < 75 years old admitted with unstable angina should be placed on cardiac monitoring (i.e., telemetry).	6.	Patients ~~< 75 years old~~ admitted with unstable angina should be placed on cardiac monitoring (i.e., telemetry).	MODIFIED: Panelists felt that the indicator applied regardless of age. ACCEPTED AS MODIFIED
9.	Patients < 75 years old admitted with unstable angina should have cardiac enzymes measured every 6 to 8 hours for the first 24 hours of admission.	7.	Patients ~~< 75 years old~~ admitted with unstable angina should have cardiac enzymes measured every 6 to 8 hours for the first 24 hours of admission.	MODIFIED: Panelists felt that the indicator applied regardless of age. ACCEPTED AS MODIFIED
10.	Patients < 75 years old admitted with unstable angina should have a repeat ECG 12-36 hours after admission.	8.	Patients ~~< 75 years old~~ admitted with unstable angina should have a repeat ECG 12-36 hours after admission.	MODIFIED: Panelists felt that the indicator applied regardless of age. ACCEPTED AS MODIFIED

305

Indicator Proposed by Staff		Indicator Voted on by Panel	Comments/Disposition
11. Patients < 75 years old admitted with unstable angina who have any one of the conditions below should have a measurement of LVEF by echocardiogram, radionuclide scan, or ventriculogram during their hospitalization or within 10 days of discharge unless a prior LVEF is documented in the past year: a. a history of prior MI; b. left bundle branch block on their resting ECG; c. cardiomegaly by examination; d. cardiomegaly on chest X-ray, or e. a diagnosis of heart failure.	9.	Patients ~~< 75 years old~~ admitted with unstable angina who have any one of the conditions below should have a measurement of LVEF by echocardiogram, radionuclide scan, or ventriculogram during their hospitalization or within 10 days of discharge unless a prior LVEF is documented in the past year: a. a history of prior MI; b. left bundle branch block on their resting ECG; c. cardiomegaly by examination; d. cardiomegaly on chest X-ray, or e. a diagnosis of heart failure.	MODIFIED: Panelists felt that the indicator applied regardless of age. **ACCEPTED AS MODIFIED**
12. Patients 40-75 years old with a discharge diagnosis of "unstable angina" should be offered stress testing or coronary angiography prior to or within 7 days of hospital discharge (unless they have contraindications to revascularization or have had stress testing or coronary angiography within two years prior to discharge).	--	Patients ~~40-75~~ < 75 years old with a discharge diagnosis of "unstable angina" should be offered stress testing or coronary angiography prior to or within 7 days of hospital discharge (unless they have contraindications to revascularization or have had stress testing or coronary angiography ~~within two years~~ **6 months** prior to discharge).	**DROPPED due to disagreement on validity.** Panelists felt this test was not appropriate for all patients.
	(12)	Patients ~~40-75~~ >= 75 years old with a discharge diagnosis of "unstable angina" should be offered stress testing or coronary angiography prior to or within 7 days of hospital discharge (unless they have contraindications to revascularization or have had stress testing or coronary angiography ~~within two years~~ **6 months** prior to discharge).	Panel considered indicator for patients >= 75 but **DROPPED due to low validity score.**
Myocardial Infarction 13. Patients < 75 years old hospitalized for the diagnosis of an MI or "rule out MI" should have a physical examination documenting all of the following: a. temperature, b. blood pressure, c. heart rate, d. heart exam, and e. lung exam.	10. -- a. b. c. d.	Patients ~~< 75 years old~~ hospitalized for the diagnosis of an MI or "rule out MI" should have a physical examination documenting all of the following: a. temperature, b. blood pressure, c. heart rate, d. heart exam, and e. lung exam.	MODIFIED: Panelists felt that the indicator applied regardless of age. **"a"** DROPPED due to low validity score **"b-e" ACCEPTED AS MODIFIED**

Indicator Proposed by Staff		Indicator Voted on by Panel		Comments/Disposition
14.	Patients < 75 years old hospitalized for the diagnosis of an MI or "rule out MI" should have a 12-lead ECG within 20 minutes of presentation.	11.	Patients <75 years-old hospitalized for the diagnosis of an MI or "rule out MI" should have a 12-lead ECG within 20 minutes of presentation.	MODIFIED: Panelists felt that the indicator applied regardless of age. ACCEPTED AS MODIFIED
15.	Patients < 75 years old hospitalized with an MI should have an assessment of LVEF prior to discharge if they have any risk factors for low LVEF (unless it is noted during hospitalization that prior to admission LVEF was < 0.45).	12.	Patients <75 years-old hospitalized with an MI should have an assessment of LVEF prior to discharge if they have any risk factors for low LVEF (unless it is noted during hospitalization that prior to admission LVEF was <0.45 <=40%).	MODIFIED: Panel felt that the indicator applied regardless of age. LVEF <= 40% is clinically conservative and more appropriate for a quality indicator. ACCEPTED AS MODIFIED
16.	Patients < 75 years old hospitalized with an MI who have a history of prior MI, but no risk factors for low LVEF, should have an assessment of LVEF during the hospitalization or within 2 weeks of discharge (unless it is noted during hospitalization that prior to admission LVEF was < 0.45).	13.	Patients <75 years-old hospitalized with an MI who have a history of prior MI, but no risk factors for low LVEF, should have an assessment of LVEF during the hospitalization or within 2 weeks of discharge (unless it is noted during hospitalization that prior to admission LVEF was < 0.45 <=40%).	MODIFIED: Panelists felt that indicator applied regardless of age. LVEF <= 40% is clinically conservative and more appropriate for a quality indicator. ACCEPTED AS MODIFIED
17.	Patients with an MI should be offered symptom-limited stress testing or coronary angiography within 8 weeks after the MI (unless they have contraindications to revascularization or have had coronary angiography within two years of the MI).	14.	Patients < 75 years old with an MI should be offered symptom-limited stress testing or coronary angiography within 8 weeks after of the MI (unless they have contraindications to revascularization or have had coronary angiography within two years of the MI).	MODIFIED: Panelists felt that these tests may not always be appropriate for older patients. They also did not consider a prior angiography sufficient basis for an exception to the indicator. ACCEPTED AS MODIFIED
--		(17)	Patients >= 75 years old with an MI should be offered symptom-limited stress testing or coronary angiography within 8 weeks after of the MI (unless they have contraindications to revascularization or have had coronary angiography within two years of the MI).	Panel considered indicator for patients >=75 but DROPPED due to low validity score.

Indicator Proposed by Staff		Indicator Voted on by Panel	Comments/Disposition
18. Patients < 75 years old hospitalized with an MI who have any of the following conditions after discharge but within 8 weeks of the MI should be offered coronary angiography within 2 weeks of the diagnosis of the condition (unless they have contraindications to revascularization or have had coronary angiography within two years of the MI):	15.	Patients < 75 years old hospitalized with an MI who have any of the following conditions after discharge but within 8 weeks of the MI should be offered coronary angiography within 2 weeks of the diagnosis of the condition (unless they have contraindications to revascularization or ~~have had coronary angiography within two years of the MI~~):	MODIFIED: Panelists did not consider a prior angiography sufficient basis for an exception to the indicator. LVEF <= 40% is clinically conservative and more appropriate for a quality indicator.
a. a high risk stress test;	a.	a. a high risk stress test;	
b. new heart failure;	b.	b. new heart failure;	
c. LVEF <= 0.45;	c.	c. LVEF <= 0.45 <=40%;	"a- g" ACCEPTED AS MODIFIED
d. new severe mitral regurgitation;	d.	d. new severe mitral regurgitation;	
e. new ventricular septal defect;	e.	e. new ventricular septal defect;	
f. sustained ventricular tachycardia or ventricular fibrillation which occurs >=48 hr. after onset of the MI;	f.	f. sustained ventricular tachycardia or ventricular fibrillation which occurs >= 48 hr. after onset of the MI;	
g. angina at rest lasting>=15 min., or	g.	g. angina at rest lasting>= 15 min., ~~or~~	
h. shock.	--	h. ~~shock.~~	"h" DROPPED by staff prior to panel meeting.
	16. (18)	Patients >= 75 years old years old hospitalized with an MI who have any of the following conditions after discharge but within 8 weeks of the MI should be offered coronary angiography within 2 weeks of the diagnosis of the condition (unless they have contraindications to revascularization or ~~have had coronary angiography within two years of the MI~~):	Panel considered indicator for patients >= 75 but DROPPED "a, b, c, d, f, g" due to low validity scores.
	--	a. a high risk stress test;	
	--	b. new heart failure;	
	--	c. LVEF <= 0.45 <=40%;	
	--	d. new severe mitral regurgitation;	
	a.	e. new ventricular septal defect;	"e" ACCEPTED AS MODIFIED
	--	f. sustained ventricular tachycardia or ventricular fibrillation which occurs 48 hr. after onset of the MI;	
	--	g. angina at rest lasting15 min., ~~or~~	
	--	h. ~~shock.~~	"h" DROPPED BY STAFF PRIOR TO PANEL

308

Indicator Proposed by Staff		Indicator Voted on by Panel	Comments/Disposition
19. Patients < 75 years old who are hospitalized with an MI complicated by any of the following should be offered coronary angiography prior to discharge (unless they have contraindications to revascularization or have had coronary angiography within two years of the MI):	17.	Patients < 75 years old who are hospitalized with an MI complicated by any of the following should be offered coronary angiography prior to discharge (unless they have contraindications to revascularization or ~~have had coronary angiography within two years of the MI~~):	MODIFIED: Panelists did not consider a prior angiography sufficient basis for an exception to the indicator. LVEF <= 40% is clinically conservative and more appropriate for a quality indicator.
a. a high risk stress test;	a.	a. a high risk stress test;	ACCEPTED AS MODIFIED
b. new heart failure;	b.	b. new heart failure;	
c. LVEF <= 0.45;	c.	c. LVEF <= 0.45 <= 40%;	
d. new severe mitral regurgitation;	d.	d. new severe mitral regurgitation;	
e. new ventricular septal defect;	e.	e. new ventricular septal defect;	
f. sustained ventricular tachycardia or ventricular fibrillation 48 hr. after onset of the MI;	f.	f. sustained ventricular tachycardia or ventricular fibrillation 48 hr. after onset of the MI;	
g. > 5 min. of angina at rest occurring >=24 hr. after the onset of the MI;	g.	g. > 5 min. of angina at rest occurring >=24 hr. after the onset of the MI;	
h. shock, or	h.	h. shock, or	
i. pulmonary edema requiring intubation.	i.	i. pulmonary edema requiring intubation.	
	-- (19)	Patients >= 75 years old who are hospitalized with an MI complicated by any of the following should be offered coronary angiography prior to discharge (unless they have contraindications to revascularization or ~~have had coronary angiography within two years of the MI~~):	Panel considered indicator for patients >= 75 but DROPPED due to low validity score.
	a.	a. a high risk stress test;	
	b.	b. new heart failure;	
	c.	c. LVEF <= 0.45 <= 40%;	
	d.	d. new severe mitral regurgitation;	
	e.	e. new ventricular septal defect;	
	f.	f. sustained ventricular tachycardia or ventricular fibrillation >= 48 hr. after onset of the MI;	
	g.	g. > 5 min. of angina at rest occurring >=24 hr. after the onset of the MI;	
	h.	h. shock, or	
	i.	i. pulmonary edema requiring intubation.	

Indicator Proposed by Staff		Indicator Voted on by Panel	Comments/Disposition
Sudden Death			
20. Patients < 75 years old admitted after cardiac arrest should be offered a stress test or coronary angiography before discharge (unless they have contraindications to revascularization or have had coronary angiography within two years of the MI).	--	Patients < 75 years old admitted after cardiac arrest should be offered a stress test or coronary angiography before discharge (unless they have contraindications to revascularization or have had coronary angiography within two years of the MI).	**DROPPED due to low validity score.** Panelists felt these tests were not appropriate for all patients.
	-- (20)	Patients >= 75 years old admitted after cardiac arrest should be offered a stress test or coronary angiography before discharge (unless they have contraindications to revascularization or have had coronary angiography within two years of the MI).	**Panel considered indicator for patients >= 75 but DROPPED due to low validity score.** Panelists felt these tests were not appropriate for all patients.
21. Patients < 75 years old admitted after cardiac arrest and who have a positive stress test during hospitalization should be offered coronary angiography before discharge (unless they have contraindications to revascularization or have had coronary angiography within two years of the MI).	18.	Patients < 75 years old admitted after cardiac arrest and who have a positive stress test during hospitalization should be offered coronary angiography before discharge (unless they have contraindications to revascularization or have had coronary angiography within two years of the MI).	MODIFIED: Panelists did not consider a prior angiography sufficient basis for an exception to the indicator.

ACCEPTED AS MODIFIED |
| | -- (21) | Patients >= 75 years old admitted after cardiac arrest and who have a positive stress test during hospitalization should be offered coronary angiography before discharge (unless they have contraindications to revascularization or have had coronary angiography within two years of the MI). | **Panel considered indicator for patients >= 75 but DROPPED due to low validity score.** |

Chapter 8 - Coronary Artery Disease: Prevention and Treatment

	Indicator Proposed by Staff		Indicator Voted on by Panel	Comments/Disposition
	Stable Angina or known CAD			
1.	Patients newly diagnosed with CAD should be offered aspirin (at a dose of at least 81 mg/day continued indefinitely) within one week of the diagnosis of CAD unless they have a contraindication to aspirin.	1.	Patients newly diagnosed with CAD should be offered ~~offered~~ **receive** aspirin (at a dose of at least 81 mg/day continued indefinitely) within one week of the diagnosis of CAD unless they have a contraindication to aspirin.	MODIFIED: Panelists wanted to strengthen wording. **ACCEPTED AS MODIFIED**
2.	Patients with a prior diagnosis of CAD who are not on aspirin and do not have contraindications to aspirin should be offered aspirin (at a dose of at least 81 mg/day continued indefinitely) within one week of any visit to a provider in which CAD was addressed.	2.	Patients with a prior diagnosis of CAD who are not on aspirin and do not have contraindications to aspirin should ~~be offered~~ **receive** aspirin (at a dose of at least 81 mg/day continued indefinitely) within one week of any visit to a provider in which CAD was addressed.	MODIFIED: Panelists wanted to strengthen wording. **ACCEPTED AS MODIFIED**
3.	Patients newly diagnosed with CAD who smoke should have documentation of counseling on smoking cessation within 3 months of the diagnosis of CAD.	3.	Patients newly diagnosed with CAD who smoke should have documentation of counseling on smoking cessation ~~within 3 months~~ **at the time of the diagnosis of CAD.**	MODIFIED: Panelists felt that counseling is most effective when immediate. **ACCEPTED AS MODIFIED**
	Unstable Angina			
4.	Patients admitted with the diagnosis of unstable angina should receive aspirin within 24 hours of admission.	4.	Patients admitted ~~with the diagnosis~~ of unstable angina should receive aspirin within ~~24~~ **2** hours of admission **or presentation to the emergency room.**	MODIFIED: Panelists felt that aspirin should be given as soon as possible, and definitely within 2 hours. **ACCEPTED AS MODIFIED**
5.	Patients admitted with the diagnosis of definite unstable angina who do not have contraindications to heparin should receive: a. heparin within 2 hours of the initial ECG that demonstrates ischemic changes; and b. continuous heparin infusion for at least 24 hours (or until 26 hours after the ECG with ischemic changes).	5.	Patients admitted with the diagnosis of ~~definite~~ unstable angina **who have angina > 5 minutes at rest associated with ischemic ST segment changes** who do not have contraindications to heparin should receive:	MODIFIED: Indicator modified to clarify the definition of unstable angina. Subcutaneous heparin is also acceptable. **ACCEPTED AS MODIFIED**
		a.	**heparin within 2 hours of the initial ECG that demonstrates ischemic changes; and**	
		b.	**continuous heparin infusion or subcutaneous LMW heparin for at least 24 hours (or until 26 hours after the ECG with ischemic changes).**	

311

	Indicator Proposed by Staff		Indicator Voted on by Panel	Comments/Disposition
6.	Patients <75 years old admitted with the diagnosis of unstable angina who have angina > 5 minutes at rest associated with ischemic ST segment changes should receive beta-blockers within 4 hours (unless they have contraindications to beta-blockers).	6.	Patients <75 years old admitted with the diagnosis of unstable angina who have angina > 5 minutes at rest associated with ischemic ST segment changes should receive beta-blockers within 4 hours (unless they have contraindications to beta-blockers).	MODIFIED: Panelists felt that all patients with these symptoms should receive beta-blockers. ACCEPTED AS MODIFIED
Myocardial Infarction				
7.	Patients presenting with acute myocardial infarction should receive at least 160 mg of aspirin within 12 hours of presentation unless they have contraindications to aspirin.	7.	Patients presenting with acute myocardial infarction should receive at least 160 mg of aspirin within ~~12~~ 2 hours of presentation **or admission** unless they have contraindications to aspirin.	MODIFIED: The time frame was shortened to strengthen the indicator. ACCEPTED AS MODIFIED
8.	Patients <75 years old presenting with an acute myocardial infarction who are within 12 hours of the onset of MI symptoms and who do not have contraindications to thrombolysis or revascularization should receive a thrombolytic agent within 1 hour of the time their ECG initially shows either of the following findings:	8.	Patients <75 years old presenting with an acute myocardial infarction who are within 12 hours of the onset of MI symptoms and who do not have contraindications to thrombolysis or revascularization should receive a thrombolytic agent within 1 hour of the time their ECG initially shows either of the following findings:	ACCEPTED
a.	ST elevation > 0.1 mV in 2 or more contiguous leads, or	a.	ST elevation > 0.1 mV in 2 or more contiguous leads, or	
b.	a LBBB not known to be old.	b.	a LBBB not known to be old.	
		9. (8)	Patients >=75 years old presenting with an acute myocardial infarction who are within 12 hours of the onset of MI symptoms and who do not have contraindications to thrombolysis or revascularization should receive a thrombolytic agent within 1 hour of the time their ECG initially shows either of the following findings:	Panel considered indicator for patients >= 75 and ACCEPTED "a" but DROPPED "b" due to low validity score.
		a.	ST elevation > 0.1 mV in 2 or more contiguous leads, or	
		--	a LBBB not known to be old.	

312

	Indicator Proposed by Staff		Indicator Voted on by Panel	Comments/Disposition
9.	Patients admitted within 12 hours of the onset of acute myocardial infarction who do not have contraindications to heparin should receive heparin (subcutaneously or IV) for at least 24 hours unless they have received streptokinase, APSAC, or urokinase.	10.	Patients admitted within 12 hours of the onset of acute myocardial infarction who do not have contraindications to heparin should receive heparin (subcutaneously or IV) for at least 24 hours unless they have received streptokinase, APSAC, or urokinase.	ACCEPTED
10.	Patients admitted with acute myocardial infarction whose LVEF is either unknown at admission or >= 45%, should receive either a beta-blocker or an ACE inhibitor or both within 12 hours of admission (unless they have contraindications to both beta-blockers and ACE inhibitors).	11.	Patients admitted with acute myocardial infarction whose LVEF is either unknown at admission or >= 45%, should receive either a beta-blocker or an ACE inhibitor or both within 12 hours of admission (unless they have contraindications to both beta-blockers and ACE inhibitors).	MODIFIED: ACE inhibitors and beta-blockers are different treatments, and the timing of ACE treatment has less consensus. ACCEPTED AS MODIFIED
11.	Patients admitted with acute myocardial infarction and are known to have a LVEF <= 0.45 at admission should receive an ACE inhibitor within the first 24 hours of admission (unless they have contraindications to ACE inhibitors).	--	Patients admitted with acute myocardial infarction and are known to have a LVEF <= 0.45 **40%** at admission should receive an ACE inhibitor within the first 24 hours of admission (unless they have contraindications to ACE inhibitors).	DROPPED due to low validity score.
12.	Patients admitted with acute myocardial infarction should NOT receive short-acting nifedipine during the hospitalization.	12.	Patients admitted with acute myocardial infarction should NOT receive short-acting nifedipine during the hospitalization.	ACCEPTED
13.	Patients admitted with acute myocardial infarction should NOT receive any calcium channel blocker if they have a reduced LVEF (<0.45) or heart failure during the hospitalization.	13.	Patients admitted with acute myocardial infarction should NOT receive any calcium channel blocker if they have a reduced LVEF (<0.45) (<= 40%) or heart failure during the hospitalization.	MODIFIED: Panelists felt that LVEF <= 40% is clinically conservative and more appropriate for a quality indicator. ACCEPTED AS MODIFIED
14.	Patients discharged after an acute myocardial infarction who do not have contraindications to aspirin should be discharged on aspirin at a dose of at least 81 mg/day.	14.	Patients discharged after an acute myocardial infarction who do not have contraindications to aspirin should be discharged on aspirin at a dose of at least 81 mg/day.	ACCEPTED

313

Indicator Proposed by Staff		Indicator Voted on by Panel	Comments/Disposition
15.	Patients discharged after an acute myocardial infarction who have either an LVEF>=45% documented during hospitalization or an unknown LVEF, should be discharged on a beta-blocker or an ACE inhibitor or both (unless they have contraindications to both beta-blockers and ACE inhibitors).	15. Patients discharged after an acute myocardial infarction who have either an LVEF>=45% documented during hospitalization or an unknown LVEF, should be discharged on a beta-blocker or an ACE inhibitor or both (unless they have contraindications to both beta-blockers and ACE inhibitors).	MODIFIED: ACE inhibitors and beta-blockers are different treatments, and the timing of ACE treatment has less consensus. **ACCEPTED AS MODIFIED**
16.	Patients discharged after an acute myocardial infarction who have an LVEF<= 45% documented at any time during the hospitalization should receive ACE inhibitors at discharge (unless they have contraindications to ACE inhibitors).	16. Patients discharged after an acute myocardial infarction who have an LVEF<= 45% **40%** documented at any time during the hospitalization should receive ACE inhibitors at discharge (unless they have contraindications to ACE inhibitors).	MODIFIED: Panelists felt that LVEF <= 40% is clinically conservative and more appropriate for a quality indicator. **ACCEPTED AS MODIFIED**
Revascularization			
17.	Patients < 75 years old with CAD who do not have contraindications to revascularization should be offered PTCA or CABS within 1 month of coronary angiography if they have 3 vessel CAD and an LVEF < 0.45.	17. Patients < 75 years old with CAD who do not have contraindications to revascularization should be offered PTCA or CABS within 1 month of coronary angiography if they have 3 vessel CAD and an LVEF < 0.45 <= 40%.	MODIFIED: Panelists felt that LVEF <= 40% is clinically conservative and more appropriate for a quality indicator. They also wanted the indicator to apply regardless of age. **ACCEPTED AS MODIFIED**
18.	Patients < 75 years old with CAD who do not have contraindications to revascularization should be offered CABS within 1 month of coronary angiography if they have left main stenosis > 50%.	18. Patients < 75 years old with CAD who do not have contraindications to revascularization should be offered CABS within 1 month of coronary angiography if they have left main stenosis > 50%.	MODIFIED: Panelists wanted the indicator to apply to all patients. **ACCEPTED AS MODIFIED**

314

Chapter 9 - Heart Failure

Indicator Proposed by Staff		Indicator Voted on by Panel		Comments/Disposition
Diagnosis				
1.	Patients newly diagnosed with heart failure who are beginning medical treatment should receive an evaluation of their ejection fraction within 1 month of the start of treatment.	1.	Patients newly diagnosed with heart failure who are beginning medical treatment should receive an evaluation of their ejection fraction within 1 month of the start of treatment.	ACCEPTED
2.	Patients newly diagnosed with heart failure should have a history at the time of the diagnosis documenting the presence or absence of all of the following:	2.	Patients newly diagnosed with heart failure should have a history at the time of the diagnosis documenting the presence or absence of all of the following:	"a-f" ACCEPTED
	a. Prior myocardial infarction or cardiac disease;		a. Prior myocardial infarction or cardiac disease;	
	b. Current symptoms of chest discomfort or angina;		b. Current symptoms of chest discomfort or angina;	
	c. History of hypertension;		c. History of hypertension;	
	d. History of diabetes;		d. History of diabetes;	
	e. Current medications; and		e. Current medications; and	
	f. Alcohol use.		f. Alcohol use; and	
			g. Smoking status.	"g" PROPOSED AND ACCEPTED BY Q2 PANEL. Panelists added smoking because it is a treatable risk factor.
3.	Patient with a new diagnosis of heart failure should have the following elements of the physical examination documented at the time of presentation:	3.	Patients with a new diagnosis of heart failure should have the following elements of the physical examination documented at the time of presentation:	"a-f" ACCEPTED
	a. Weight;		a. Weight;	
	b. Blood Pressure		b. Blood Pressure;	
	c. Lung Exam;		c. Lung Exam;	
	d. Cardiac Exam		d. Cardiac Exam;	
	e. Abdominal exam; or		e. Abdominal exam; or	
	f. Lower extremity examination.		f. Lower extremity examination;	
			g. Neck veins; and	"g, h" PROPOSED AND ACCEPTED BY Q2 PANEL. Panelists considered checking neck veins and heart rate important parts of the cardiac exam.
			h. Heart rate.	

315

Indicator Proposed by Staff		Indicator Voted on by Panel		Comments/Disposition
4. Patients with a new diagnosis of heart failure should be offered all of the following studies within 1 month of the diagnosis (unless performed within the prior 3 months):		4. Patients with a new diagnosis of heart failure should be offered all of the following studies within 1 month of the diagnosis (unless performed within the prior 3 months):		
	a. Chest x-ray;		a. Chest x-ray;	"a–e" ACCEPTED
	b. EKG;		b. EKG;	
	c. Complete blood count;		c. Complete blood count;	
	d. Serum sodium, potassium, and bicarbonate;		d. Serum sodium, potassium, and bicarbonate;	
	e. Serum creatinine; and		e. Serum creatinine; and	
	f. Urinalysis.		f. Urinalysis.	"f" DROPPED due to low validity score. Panelists felt this test was not useful.
5. Patients with a diagnosis of heart failure who are being treated with medications for their heart failure should have one of the following documented in the medical record at least every two years:		5. Patients with a diagnosis of heart failure who are being treated with medications for their heart failure should have one of the following an evaluation of their ejection fraction documented in the medical record at least every two years:		MODIFIED: Panelists felt that ejection fraction measurement does not have to occur every two years, but that one should be noted in the chart. ACCEPTED AS MODIFIED
	a. a previously measured ejection fraction, or		a. a previously measured ejection fraction, or	
	b. a new evaluation of their ejection fraction.		b. a new evaluation of their ejection fraction.	
6. Patients who are hospitalized for symptoms of heart failure should have all of the following elements of the physical examination documented on the day of hospitalization:		6. Patients who are hospitalized for symptoms of heart failure should have all of the following elements of the physical examination documented on the day of hospitalization:		
	a. Weight;		a. Weight;	"a–f" ACCEPTED
	b. Blood pressure;		b. Blood pressure;	
	c. Lung exam;		c. Lung exam;	
	d. Cardiac exam;		d. Cardiac exam;	
	e. Abdominal exam; or		e. Abdominal exam; or	
	f. Lower extremity examination.		f. Lower extremity examination;	
			g. Neck veins; and	"g, h" PROPOSED AND ACCEPTED BY Q2 PANEL. Panelists considered checking neck veins and heart rate important parts of the cardiac exam.
			h. Heart rate.	

Indicator Proposed by Staff		Indicator Voted on by Panel	Comments/Disposition
7. Patients who are hospitalized for heart failure should have the following performed within one day of hospitalization: a. Serum electrolytes; and b. Serum creatinine.	7.	Patients who are hospitalized for heart failure should have the following performed within one day of hospitalization: a. Serum electrolytes; and b. Serum creatinine.	ACCEPTED
Treatment			
8. Patients with a diagnosis of heart failure who have an ejection fraction of less than 40% and no contraindications to ACE inhibitors should be receiving an ACE inhibitor.	8.	Patients with a diagnosis of heart failure who have an ejection fraction of less than 40% and no contraindications to ACE inhibitors should be receiving an ACE inhibitor.	ACCEPTED
9. Patients with the diagnosis of heart failure who are started on an ACE inhibitor should have a potassium checked within 1 week of after starting the ACE inhibitor.	--	Patients with the diagnosis of heart failure who are started on an ACE inhibitor should have a potassium checked within 1 week of after starting the ACE inhibitor.	**DROPPED due to low validity score.** Panelists felt that the time frame is not supported by evidence.
10. Patients with the diagnosis of heart failure who are on an ACE inhibitor should have the following checked every year: a. Serum potassium; and b. Serum creatinine.	9.	Patients with the diagnosis of heart failure who are on an ACE inhibitor should have the following checked every year: a. **Serum potassium; and** b. **Serum creatinine.**	ACCEPTED
11. Patients with the diagnosis of heart failure who are started on a diuretic should have a potassium level checked within 1 week of the start of treatment.	--	Patients with the diagnosis of heart failure who are started on a diuretic should have a potassium level checked within 1 week of the start of treatment.	**DROPPED due to low validity score.** Panelists felt that the time frame is not supported by evidence.
12. Patients with the diagnosis of heart failure in whom diuretic dose is increased should have a potassium level checked within 1 week of the increase in dose.	--	Patients with the diagnosis of heart failure in whom diuretic dose is increased should have a potassium level checked within 1 week of the increase in dose.	**DROPPED due to low validity score.** Panelists felt that time frame is not supported by evidence.
13. Patients with the diagnosis heart failure and an ejection fraction of less than 40% who are not on ACE inhibitors should be on hydralzine/isosorbide dinitrate, in the absence of contraindications.	10.	Patients with the diagnosis heart failure and an ejection fraction of less than 40% who are not on ACE inhibitors should be on hydralzine/isosorbide dinitrate, in the absence of contraindications.	MODIFIED: Panelists wanted the indicator to be more generic. **ACCEPTED AS MODIFIED**
14. Patients with a new diagnosis of heart failure who are started on medical treatment for heart failure should have dietary counseling within 1 month of the start of medical treatment.	11.	Patients with a new diagnosis of heart failure who are started on medical treatment for heart failure should have dietary counseling within 1 month of the start of medical treatment.	ACCEPTED

317

Indicator Proposed by Staff		Indicator Voted on by Panel	Comments/Disposition
Follow-up			
15. Patients who have been hospitalized for heart failure should have follow-up contact within 4 weeks of discharge.	12.	Patients who have been hospitalized for heart failure should have follow-up contact within 4 weeks of discharge.	ACCEPTED
16. Patients who have been hospitalized for heart failure should have the following physical examination elements performed during the first post-discharge visit: a. Weight; b. Blood pressure; c. Lung exam; d. Cardiac exam; e. Abdominal exam; and f. Lower extremity examination.	13. a. b. c. d. e. f. g. h.	Patients who have been hospitalized for heart failure should have the following physical examination elements performed during the first post-discharge visit: a. **Weight;** b. **Blood pressure;** c. **Lung exam;** d. **Cardiac exam;** e. **Abdominal exam; and** f. **Lower extremity examination;** g. Neck veins; and h. Heart rate.	**"a-f" ACCEPTED** **"g, h" PROPOSED AND ACCEPTED BY Q2 PANEL.** Panelists considered checking neck veins and heart rate important parts of the cardiac exam.
17. Patients who have been hospitalized for heart failure should have the following laboratory tests performed within 4 weeks of discharge: a. Creatinine; and b. Potassium.	--	Patients who have been hospitalized for heart failure should have the following laboratory tests performed within 4 weeks of discharge: a. **Creatinine; and** b. **Potassium.**	**DROPPED due to low validity score.** Panelists felt that tests are not an appropriate indicator of quality.

318

Chapter 10 - Hyperlipidemia

	Indicator Proposed by Staff		Indicator Voted on by Panel	Comments/Disposition
Screening				
1.	Men under age 70 with preexisting heart disease who are not on pharmacological therapy for hyperlipidemia should have cholesterol level documented at least every 5 years.	1.	Men under age ~~70~~ 75 with preexisting heart disease who are not on pharmacological therapy for hyperlipidemia should have total cholesterol, **HDL, and LDL** level documented at least every 5 years.	MODIFIED: Panelists felt that 75 years is a conservative age cut-off, and that HDL and LDL levels are essential. **ACCEPTED AS MODIFIED**
		2. (1)	Women under age ~~70~~ 75 with preexisting heart disease who are not on pharmacological therapy for hyperlipidemia should have total cholesterol, **HDL, and LDL** level documented at least every 5 years.	**PANEL ACCEPTED INDICATOR AS MODIFIED FOR WOMEN.**
2.	Men under age 70 with newly diagnosed coronary disease should have had total cholesterol documented within 2 years before or within 4 months after the diagnosis is first noted in the medical record.	3.	Men under age ~~70~~ 75 with newly diagnosed coronary disease should have had total cholesterol, **HDL, and LDL** documented within 2 years before or within 4 months after the diagnosis is first noted in the medical record.	MODIFIED: Panelists felt that 75 years is a conservative age cut-off, and that HDL and LDL levels are essential. **ACCEPTED AS MODIFIED**
		4. (2)	Women under age ~~70~~ 75 with newly diagnosed coronary disease should have had total cholesterol, **HDL, and LDL** documented within 2 years before or within 4 months after the diagnosis is first noted in the medical record.	**PANEL ACCEPTED INDICATOR AS MODIFIED FOR WOMEN.**
Diagnosis				
3.	Men under age 70 with preexisting coronary disease who have a total cholesterol level exceeding 200 mg/dl should have a measure of their LDL cholesterol documented within 2 years before or 3 months after the 200 mg/dl level.	-- (3)	Men under age ~~70~~ 75 with preexisting coronary disease who have a total cholesterol level exceeding 200 mg/dl should have a measure of their LDL cholesterol documented within 2 years before or 3 months after the 200 mg/dl level.	DROPPED due to low validity score.

319

Indicator Proposed by Staff		Indicator Voted on by Panel		Comments/Disposition
	-- (3)	Women under age ~~70~~ 75 with preexisting coronary disease who have a total cholesterol level exceeding 200 mg/dl should have a measure of their LDL cholesterol documented within 2 years before or 3 months after the 200 mg/dl level.		DROPPED due to low validity score.
4. Patients without preexisting coronary disease who are started on pharmacological treatment for hyperlipidemia should have had at least 2 measurements of their cholesterol (total or LDL) documented in the year before the start of pharmacological treatment.	5.	Patients without preexisting coronary disease who are started on pharmacological treatment for hyperlipidemia should have had at least 2 measurements of their cholesterol (total or LDL) documented in the year before the start of pharmacological treatment.		ACCEPTED
Treatment				
5. Men under age 70 with preexisting coronary disease who have an untreated LDL cholesterol level >130 mg/dl should begin diet or drug therapy within 3 months of the high LDL measurement.	6.	Men under age ~~70~~ 75 with preexisting coronary disease who have an untreated LDL cholesterol level >130 mg/dl should begin diet or drug therapy within 3 months of the high LDL measurement.		MODIFIED: Panelists felt that 75 years is a more conservative age cut-off. ACCEPTED AS MODIFIED
	7. (5)	Women under age ~~70~~ 75 with preexisting coronary disease who have an untreated LDL cholesterol level >130 mg/dl should begin diet or drug therapy within 3 months of the high LDL measurement.		PANEL ACCEPTED INDICATOR AS MODIFIED FOR WOMEN.
6. Men under age 70 with preexisting coronary disease who have an LDL level >130 mg/dl after 6 months of dietary cholesterol-lowering treatment should receive one of the following within 2 months: • pharmacological therapy for hyperlipidemia; or • a repeat LDL measurement.	8.	Men under age ~~70~~ 75 with preexisting coronary disease who have an LDL level >130 mg/dl after 6 months of dietary cholesterol-lowering treatment should receive **pharmacological therapy for hyperlipidemia** ~~one of the following within 2 months of measurement.~~		MODIFIED: Panelists did not feel that just getting a repeat LDL is adequate. ACCEPTED AS MODIFIED
	9. (6)	Women under age ~~70~~ 75 with preexisting coronary disease who have an LDL level >130 mg/dl after 6 months of dietary cholesterol-lowering treatment should receive **pharmacological therapy for hyperlipidemia** ~~one of the following within 2 months of measurement.~~		PANEL ACCEPTED INDICATOR AS MODIFIED FOR WOMEN.

320

Indicator Proposed by Staff		Indicator Voted on by Panel	Comments/Disposition
Follow-up			
7. Patients in whom pharmacological therapy for hyperlipidemia has been initiated should have their cholesterol rechecked within 4 months.	10.	Patients in whom pharmacological therapy for hyperlipidemia has been initiated should have their total cholesterol, **HDL, and LDL** rechecked within 4 months.	MODIFIED: Panelists felt that HDL and LDL levels are essential. **ACCEPTED AS MODIFIED**
8. Patients receiving pharmacological therapy for hyperlipidemia who have had a dosage or medication change should have cholesterol rechecked within 4 months of the change.	11.	Patients receiving pharmacological therapy for hyperlipidemia who have had a dosage or medication change should have total cholesterol, **HDL, and LDL** rechecked within 4 months of the change.	MODIFIED: Panelists felt that HDL and LDL levels are essential. **ACCEPTED AS MODIFIED**

Chapter 11 - Hypertension

	Indicator Proposed by Staff		Indicator Voted on by Panel	Comments/Disposition
Screening				
1.	Systolic and diastolic blood pressure should be measured on patients otherwise presenting for care at least once each year.	1.	Systolic and diastolic blood pressure should be measured on patients otherwise presenting for care at least once each year.	INCLUDED BASED ON Q1 PANEL RATING
Diagnosis				
2.	All patients with average blood pressures of >140 systolic and/or >90 diastolic, as determined on at least 3 separate visits, should have a diagnosis of hypertension documented in the record.	2.	All patients with average blood pressures of >140 systolic and/or >90 diastolic, as determined on at least 3 separate visits, should have a diagnosis of hypertension documented in the record.	ACCEPTED
3.	Patients with a new diagnosis of stage 1-3 hypertension should have at least 3 measurements on different days with a mean SBP>140 and/or a mean DBP>90.	3.	Patients with a new diagnosis of stage 1-3 hypertension should have at least 3 measurements on different days with a mean SBP>140 and/or a mean DBP>90.	INCLUDED BASED ON Q1 PANEL RATING
4.	Initial history and physical of patients with hypertension should document assessment of at least 2 items from each of the following groups by the third visit: • History: Family or personal history of premature CAD, CVA, diabetes, hyperlipidemia; • Medication and substance abuse: Personal history of tobacco abuse, alcohol abuse, or taking of medications that may cause hypertension; • Physical examination: Examination of the fundi, heart sounds, abdomen for bruits, peripheral arterial pulses, neurologic system.	4.	Initial history and physical of patients with hypertension should document assessment of at least 2 items from each of the following groups by the third visit: • History: Family or personal history of premature CAD, CVA, diabetes, hyperlipidemia; • Medication and substance abuse: Personal history of tobacco abuse, alcohol abuse, or taking of medications that may cause hypertension; • Physical examination: Examination of the fundi, heart sounds, abdomen for bruits, peripheral arterial pulses, neurologic system.	INCLUDED BASED ON Q1 PANEL RATING
5.	Stage 1 hypertensive patients taking drugs that may cause hypertension should have the drug discontinued (at least temporarily) before pharmacotherapy is initiated.	5.	Stage 1 hypertensive patients taking drugs that may cause hypertension should have the drug discontinued (at least temporarily) before pharmacotherapy is initiated.	INCLUDED BASED ON Q1 PANEL RATING

322

Indicator Proposed by Staff		Indicator Voted on by Panel	Comments/Disposition
6. Initial laboratory tests should include at least 5 of the following: • Urinalysis; • Serum, plasma, or blood glucose; • Serum potassium; • Serum creatinine; • Serum cholesterol; or • Serum triglyceride.	6.	Initial laboratory tests should include at least 5 of the following: • Urinalysis; • Serum, plasma, or blood glucose; • Serum potassium; • Serum creatinine; • Serum cholesterol; or • Serum triglyceride.	INCLUDED BASED ON Q1 PANEL RATING
Treatment			
7. First-line treatment for Stage 1-2 hypertension is lifestyle modification. The medical record should indicate counseling for at least 1 of the following interventions prior to initiating pharmacotherapy: • weight reduction if obese; • increased physical activity if sedentary; • low sodium diet, or • alcohol intake reduction if alcohol drinker.	7.	First-line treatment for Stage 1-2 hypertension is lifestyle modification. The medical record should indicate counseling for at least 1 of the following interventions prior to initiating pharmacotherapy: • weight reduction if obese; • increased physical activity if sedentary; • low sodium diet, or • alcohol intake reduction if alcohol drinker.	MODIFIED: Panelists felt that this indicator is not appropriate for treatment of stage 2 hypertension. ACCEPTED AS MODIFIED
8. First-line treatment for Stage 3 hypertension is lifestyle modification. The medical record should indicate counseling for at least 1 of the following interventions: • weight reduction if obese; • increased physical activity if sedentary; • low sodium diet, or • alcohol intake reduction if alcohol drinker.	8.	First-line treatment for Stage 2-3 hypertension is lifestyle modification. The medical record should indicate counseling for at least 1 of the following interventions **prior to initiating pharmacotherapy**: • weight reduction if obese; • increased physical activity if sedentary; • low sodium diet, or • alcohol intake reduction if alcohol drinker.	MODIFIED: Lifestyle changes should be recommended before or concurrent to drug treatment. ACCEPTED AS MODIFIED
9. Stage 1-2 hypertensives whose blood pressure remains Stage 1-2 after 6 months lifestyle modification should receive pharmacotherapy, if not already on it.	9.	Stage 1-2 hypertensives whose blood pressure remains Stage 1-2 after 6 months lifestyle modification should receive pharmacotherapy, if not already on it.	INCLUDED BASED ON Q1 PANEL RATING
10. Stage 3 hypertensives should receive pharmacotherapy.	10.	Stage 3 hypertensives should receive pharmacotherapy.	INCLUDED BASED ON Q1 PANEL RATING

Indicator Proposed by Staff		Indicator Voted on by Panel	Comments/Disposition
11. First-line pharmacotherapy for diabetics should include an ACE inhibitor, a calcium channel blocker, or a thiazide diuretic.	--	First-line pharmacotherapy for diabetics should include an ACE inhibitor, a calcium channel blocker or a thiazide diuretic.	DROPPED due to low validity score.
Follow-up			
12. Hypertensive patients should visit the provider at least once each year.	11.	Hypertensive patients should visit the provider at least once each year.	INCLUDED BASED ON Q1 PANEL RATING
13. Hypertensive patients with consistent average SBP>160 or DBP>90 over 6 months should have one of the following interventions recorded in the medical record: • Change in dose or regimen of antihypertensives; or • Repeated education regarding lifestyle modifications.	12.	Hypertensive patients with consistent average SBP>160 or DBP>90 over 6 months should have one of the following interventions recorded in the medical record: • Change in dose or regimen of antihypertensives; or • Repeated education regarding lifestyle modifications.	INCLUDED BASED ON Q1 PANEL RATING

Chapter 12 - Upper Respiratory Infection

Indicator Proposed by Staff		Indicator Voted on by Panel		Comments/Disposition
Pharyngitis				
Diagnosis				
1.	For patient who present with a complaint of sore throat, a history/physical exam should document presence or absence of:	1.	For patients who present with a complaint of sore throat, a history/physical exam should document presence or absence of:	INCLUDED BASED ON Q1 PANEL RATING
	a. fever;		a. **fever;**	
	b. tonsillar exudate, and		b. **tonsillar exudate, and**	
	c. anterior cervical adenopathy.		c. **anterior cervical adenopathy.**	
Treatment				
2.	Patients with sore throat and fever, tonsillar exudate and anterior cervical adenopathy should receive immediate treatment for presumed streptococcal infection.	2.	Patients with sore throat and fever, tonsillar exudate and anterior cervical adenopathy should receive immediate treatment for presumed streptococcal infection.	INCLUDED BASED ON Q1 PANEL RATING
3.	Treatment of streptococcal throat infection should be with penicillin V, amoxicillin, or erythromycin for 10 days; or with a single injection of benzathine penicillin.	3.	Treatment of streptococcal throat infection should be with penicillin V, amoxicillin, or erythromycin for 10 days; or with a single injection of benzathine penicillin.	INCLUDED BASED ON Q1 PANEL RATING
4.	If an antibiotic is NOT prescribed with the diagnosis of sore throat, a throat culture or rapid antigen test should be obtained if any of the following are present:	4.	If an antibiotic is NOT prescribed with the diagnosis of sore throat, a throat culture or rapid antigen test should be obtained if any of the following are present:	INCLUDED BASED ON Q1 PANEL RATING
	a. fever;		a. **fever;**	
	b. tonsillar exudate, and		b. **tonsillar exudate, and**	
	c. anterior cervical adenopathy.		c. **anterior cervical adenopathy.**	
Acute Bronchitis				
Diagnosis				
5.	The history of patients presenting with cough of less than 3 weeks duration should document presence or absence of fever and shortness of breath (dyspnea).	5.	The history of patients presenting with cough of less than 3 weeks duration should document presence or absence of fever and shortness of breath (dyspnea).	INCLUDED BASED ON Q1 PANEL RATING
6.	Patients presenting with acute cough should receive a physical examination of the chest for evidence of pneumonia.	6.	Patients presenting with acute cough should receive a physical examination of the chest for evidence of pneumonia.	INCLUDED BASED ON Q1 PANEL RATING

Indicator Proposed by Staff		Indicator Voted on by Panel	Comments/Disposition
	7. (13)	Patients who present with acute cough should have the presence or absence of the following items documented at the time of presentation: a. cigarette smoking; -- b. history of chronic cough or sputum production; -- c. history of previous episodes of acute bronchitis in the prior year.	"a" PROPOSED AND ACCEPTED BY Q2 PANEL "b" PROPOSED BUT DROPPED BY Q2 PANEL due to disagreement on validity. "c" DROPPED due to low validity score. Panelists felt this level of documentation was not a reasonable requirement for all coughs.
Treatment 7. If the history documents cigarette smoking in a patient with acute cough, encouragement to stop smoking should be documented.	8.	If the history documents cigarette smoking in a patient with acute cough, encouragement to stop smoking should be documented.	INCLUDED BASED ON Q1 PANEL RATING
Nasal Congestion *Treatment* 8. If topical nasal decongestants are prescribed, duration of treatment should be for no longer than 4 days.	9.	If topical nasal decongestants are prescribed, duration of treatment should be for no longer than 4 days.	INCLUDED BASED ON Q1 PANEL RATING
9. Patients with nasal congestion and/or cough without a concurrent diagnosis of sinusitis, bronchitis, or pneumonia should not be prescribed antibiotics.	10.	Patients with nasal congestion and/or cough, who do not have underlying lung disease, ~~without a concurrent diagnosis of sinusitis, bronchitis, or pneumonia~~ should not be prescribed antibiotics unless they have concurrent diagnosis of sinusitis or pneumonia.	MODIFIED: Bronchitis was dropped because of the over-prescription of antibiotics in this population. ACCEPTED AS MODIFIED
10. If a patient with acute sinusitis does not improve after two courses of antibiotics, referral to an otolaryngologist or for a diagnostic test (CT, x-ray, ultrasound of the sinuses) is indicated.	11.	If a patient with acute sinusitis does not improve after two courses of antibiotics, referral to an otolaryngologist or for a diagnostic test (CT, x-ray, ultrasound of the sinuses) is indicated.	INCLUDED BASED ON Q1 PANEL RATING
Chronic Sinusitis *Treatment* 11. If a diagnosis of chronic sinusitis is made, the patient should be treated with at least 3 weeks of antibiotics.	12.	If a diagnosis of chronic sinusitis is made, the patient should be treated with at least 3 weeks of antibiotics.	INCLUDED BASED ON Q1 PANEL RATING

Indicator Proposed by Staff		Indicator Voted on by Panel	Comments/Disposition
12. If patient with chronic sinusitis has repeated symptoms after 2 separate 3 week trials of antibiotics, a referral to an otolaryngologist or for a diagnostic test (CT, x-ray, ultrasound of the sinuses) is indicated.	13.	If patient with chronic sinusitis has repeated symptoms after 2 separate 3 week trials of antibiotics, a referral to an otolaryngologist or for a diagnostic test (CT, x-ray, ultrasound of the sinuses) is indicated.	INCLUDED BASED ON Q1 PANEL RATING

327